Library of Congress Cataloging-in-Publication Data

Aging and Health: Linking Research and Public Policy.

Proceedings of the First International Symposium—Research and Public Policy on Aging and Health, held in Saskatoon, Sask. on February 8-10, 1988.
Includes bibliographies and index.
1. Aged—Health and hygiene—Congresses. 2. Gerontology—Research—Congresses. 3. Medical policy—Congresses. I. Lewis, Steven J. II. International Symposium—Research and Public Policy on Aging and Health (1st : Saskatoon, Sask.)
RA564.8.A3887   1989   362.1′9897   89-2626
ISBN 0-87371-160-2

LEWIS PUBLISHERS. INC.
121 South Main Strteet, Chelsea, Michigan 48118

Printed in the United States of America   2 3 4 5 6 7 8 9 0

Aging & Heal

Linking Research and Public F

Steven J. Lewis

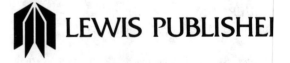 LEWIS PUBLISHEI

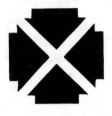

STEVEN J. LEWIS
Connections '88 Conference Coordinator
Executive Director
Saskatchewan Health Research Board
Saskatoon, Saskatchewan

PATRICIA BARAN
Editorial Assistant
Saskatchewan Health Research Board
Saskatoon, Saskatchewan

Preface

In the spring of 1987 the Saskatchewan Health Research Board, a small granting agency in a thinly populated Canadian prairie province, decided to put on a little seminar on aging and health in order to stimulate greater interest in the field among Saskatchewan investigators. Our little seminar grew into CONNECTIONS '88: First International Symposium—Research and Public Policy on Aging and Health, and was attended by a diverse audience of over 500 practitioners, administrators, academics, students, consumers, young people, and old people on February 8–10, 1988.

We considered it insufficiently challenging to hold the conference in a major city in a hospitable climate. We settled on Saskatoon, the home of the Saskatchewan Health Research Board and a city of 180,000 in the center of Canada's Great Plains whose considerable charms have as yet failed to establish its reputation as an international center of tourism. We chose February in the hope that the expectation of bracing weather would weed out the triflers who might attend the conference for reasons not entirely connected with the subject matter. (The weather was, all things considered, perfect: −32°C [about −25°F] for all three days, shrouding the city in an eerily beautiful ice fog rising off the South Saskatchewan River.)

This book is organized into five parts: Health Needs, Programs, and Policies; Money, Politics, and Public and Private Choices; Performing Effective Gerontological Research; Applying Gerontological Research Effectively; and Cementing Research and Policy Connections. It conveys the range and depth of ideas and findings that characterize gerontology in the late 1980s. We have included the papers of all the keynote speakers and invited presenters, and a good sampling of others.

Some themes and thrusts command attention.

Current Trends—What *are* current epidemiological, social, attitudinal, and program trends in aging and health? What are "the facts"? The papers collectively present a vast array of empirical data.

Aging in the Future—What is aging going to be like in the next century? Are we going to live healthier and longer lives, dropping dead after mercifully brief illnesses, having lived to the limits of effective cell replication? James Fries's morbidity compression theme is a point of departure for many of the papers.

Health Care Systems—What do we expect the health system for the elderly to accomplish, and can we afford it? Who decides, and on what basis? Robert Evans illuminates the assumptions behind many of the cliches of the times, combining analytical insights with some startling empirical footwork. And the chapters of the "political" panel—Barrett, Miller, and Mustard—remind us that public policy is not a science.

Ethics—Both private and public ethical decisions and policies permeate many presentations and discussions, with Andrew Malcolm's thoughtful remarks a frequently cited jumping-off point. An ancient and still unsolved philosophical conundrum challenges us to derive what we *should do* (the "ought") from what we *know* (the "is"). In health and health care, there are many "oughts" with a given set of resources and conditions. More or less uncritical fascination with medical technology has given way to thoughtful ethical scrutiny, which among other things attests to the growing maturity and reach of gerontology.

All chapters deal with gerontological research and policy and in one way or another revolve around these concepts. The topics range from making or not making tough choices (Malcolm and others) to applying research to practice (Archibald, Gaudet, Kessler); from consumer views (Oussoren, Rose, and, most elegantly, Fulton) to the workings of think tanks (Dobell); from conditions in Canada (numerous) to conditions in Australia (Crichton), Continental Europe (Amann), Holland (van Maanen), the United Kingdom (Johnson), China (Liu et al.), and the United States (numerous). Some address disorders of the mind (Parhad & Rohs; Schilder, Stewart & Richardson; Seggie & Tainsh), others breakdowns of the body and their human and financial tolls (Mitchell, Krutzen, & Sibley; Sibley & Blocka; Martin et al.). There are discussions of how research penetrates policymaking (Pringle, Roger, Grant, Adams, Marshall, Havens, and others), and how research can be made less mysterious and mystifying (Chappell, Gutman, McFarlane, and, I hope, everyone else by example).

As far as possible I have tried to edit the chapters to a high degree of conciseness while at the same time retaining a sense of their authors' "voices" and their interrelatedness. You will notice the many references to some of the seminal chapters (e.g., Fries, Evans, Verbrugge). Some chapters are presented in standard scientific form; others are edited transcripts of the oral presentations. Gerontology is a combination of social and biological science, scholarship, interaction, dissertation, commentary, and synthesis. So, too, is this book.

Our goal in organizing the conference was to present gerontology in its diversity, and to persuade people that translating research into sound public policy is an urgent necessity. Gerontology researchers cannot stay above the fray; public policy is all around us, and the stakes are high. We will have definitively succeeded when conferences like CONNECTIONS '88 have to be held in Toronto or London to draw a crowd, and when volumes like this are no longer unique by virtue of bringing together the perspectives of diverse communities—when, that is, all of us come to think of the linkage between gerontological research and policy as important, as essential, and as natural as ice fog in Saskatoon in February.

Steven J. Lewis

Acknowledgments

This volume is the product of many talented, able, and committed people, most prominent of whom are, of course, the authors. Their willingness to consider thoughtfully the vital relationship between research and public policy created not only a memorable and exciting conference, but also, we hope, a valuable and lasting contribution to gerontological research and policy development.

None of this could have come about had the Saskatchewan Health Research Board been unable to enlist the support of dozens of people. Those familiar with conference planning and organization will know the formidable tasks facing the committees. Our thanks to the committee chairmen—Phil Gaudet, Dave Gibson, Debra Gillis, Wayne Hindmarsh, Shan Landry, and Ed Marleau—and their colleagues for fifteen months of superb work.

No conference on the scale of CONNECTIONS '88 can be conceived without generous financial support. We received a sustaining grant from the National Health Research and Development Program of Health and Welfare Canada, whose enthusiastic endorsement of our idea and plans literally made it possible for us to proceed on the scale envisioned and ultimately realized. We received additional and generous public sector funding from the Medical Research Council of Canada, the Social Sciences and Humanities Research Council of Canada, the City of Saskatoon, the University of Saskatchewan, and Sherbrooke Community Centre in Saskatoon.

The private sector also contributed significantly to the conference. We thank the Canadian Imperial Bank of Commerce; Astra Pharma Inc.; Boehringer Ingelheim (Canada) Ltd.; Ciba-Geigy Canada Ltd.; Hoffmann-Laroche Limited; Merck Frosst Canada Inc.; Nordic Laboratories Inc.; Parke-Davis Canada Inc.; Rhône-Poulenc Pharma Inc.; Sandoz Canada Inc.; Squibb Canada Inc.; and Upjohn Company of Canada.

As Conference Coordinator I was most fortunate to have the unstinting and enthusiastic support and guidance of Una Ridley, Vice-Chairman of the Saskatchewan Health Research Board and CONNECTIONS '88 Chairman. As editor of this volume I am indebted to the good sense and advice of my editorial board colleagues Debra Gillis, Kurt Hall, Wayne Hindmarsh, Norma Stewart, Evelyn Swanson, and Elizabeth Troyer, and to Pat Baran and Barb Nisbet for preparing the manuscript. Their talent, precision, and good humor literally brought order out of chaos, and their contributions deserve a good deal more praise than a brief acknowledgment can convey.

This book owes a good deal to Lewis Publishers, especially Brian Lewis, whose early interest in producing a first-class version of the proceedings of the conference reinforced our perception that we were indeed onto an important and timely topic, and to our in-house editor, Janet Tarolli, whose editorial skill and advice have contributed significantly to the quality of the book.

Contributors

Mr. N. Duane Adams
Regional Director, Indian Health Services Branch, Health and Welfare Canada, 1855 Smith Street, Regina, SK, Canada S4P 2N5

Dr. Anton Amann
Professor, Institute of Sociology, University of Vienna, Alser Strasse 33, A - 1080, Vienna, Austria

Ms. Suellen Archibald
Director, Resident Care Services, Sherbrooke Community Centre, 301 Acadia Drive, Saskatoon, SK, Canada S7H 2E7

Mrs. Linda Bakken
Special Programs Consultant, Long Term Care Program Division, Manitoba Health Services Commission, P.O. Box 925, 599 Empress Street, Winnipeg, MB, Canada R3C 2T6

Hon. David Barrett
Member of Parliament, Parliament Buildings, Ottawa, ON, Canada K1A 0K9

Dr. Ronald Bayne
Chairman, Gerontology Research Council of Ontario, 88 Maplewood Avenue, Hamilton, ON, Canada L8M 1W9

Dr. Larry W. Chambers
Professor, Department of Clinical Epidemiology and Biostatistics, Faculty of Health Sciences, McMaster University, 1200 Main Street West, Hamilton, ON, Canada L8N 3Z5

Dr. Neena L. Chappell
National Health Scholar, Director, Centre on Aging, University of Manitoba, 338 Isbister Building, Winnipeg, MB, Canada R3T 2N2

DR. ANNE CRICHTON
Professor Emerita, Department of Health Care and Epidemiology,
Faculty of Medicine, University of British Columbia, Mather Building,
5804 Fairview Avenue, Vancouver, BC, Canada V6T 1W5

DR. CARL D'ARCY
Director, Applied Research Unit, Department of Psychiatry, Box 92,
University Hospital, Saskatoon, SK, Canada S7N 0X0

DR. A. ROD DOBELL
President, The Institute for Research on Public Policy, 3771 Haro
Road, Victoria, BC, Canada V8P 5C3

DR. ROBERT G. EVANS
Professor, Department of Economics, University of British Columbia,
Vancouver, BC, Canada V6T 1W5

MS. BRENDA FRASER
University School of Rural Planning and Development, University of
Guelph, Guelph, ON, Canada N1G 2W1

DR. JAMES F. FRIES
Associate Professor of Medicine, Division of Immunology, Department
of Medicine, Stanford University School of Medicine, Stanford
University Medical Center, Stanford, CA, USA 94305

MRS. PATRICIA FULTON
1632 West 40th Avenue, Vancouver, BC, Canada V6M 1V9

MR. PHIL GAUDET
President and Chief Executive Officer, The Good Samaritan Society,
Box 8190, Station F, Edmonton, AB, Canada T6H 5A2 (formerly
Executive Director of Saskatoon Home Care)

MS. LAN T. GIEN
Associate Professor, School of Nursing, Memorial University of
Newfoundland, St. John's, NF, Canada A1B 3V6

DR. PETER GLYNN
Assistant Deputy Minister, Health and Welfare Canada, Jeanne Mance
Building, Tunney's Pasture, Ottawa, ON, Canada K1A 1B4

DR. PETER R. GRANT
Associate Professor, Department of Psychology, University of
Saskatchewan, Saskatoon, SK, Canada S7N 0W0

DR. GLORIA M. GUTMAN
Director, Gerontology Research Centre, Simon Fraser University,
Burnaby, BC, Canada V5A 1S6

MS. BETTY HAVENS
Provincial Gerontologist, Manitoba Council on Aging, 175 Hargrave
Street, 7th Floor, Winnipeg, MB, Canada R3C 0V8

DR. DAVID R. J. JARRETT
162 Broomwood Road, London, England SW11 6JY (Formerly Acting
Section Head, Clinical Gerontology Services, Department of Medicine,
University Hospital, Saskatoon, SK, Canada)

PROFESSOR MALCOLM L. JOHNSON
Department of Health and Social Welfare, The Open University,
Walton Hall, Milton Keynes, England, MK7 6AA

MS. LINDA KESSLER
Nursing Unit Manager, Geriatric Assessment, University Hospital,
Saskatoon, SK, Canada S7N 0X0

MRS. PAT I. KRUTZEN
Research Nurse and Patient Assessor, Rheumatic Disease Unit,
University Hospital, Saskatoon, SK, Canada S7N 0X0

DR. CYNTHIA L. LEIBSON
Health Services Evaluation, Mayo 8 EB, Mayo Clinic, 200 1st Street
S.W., Rochester, MN, USA 55905

DR. WILLIAM T. LIU
Director, Pacific/Asian American Mental Health Research Center,
University of Illinois at Chicago, 7th Floor, 1033 W. Van Buren Street,
Chicago, IL, USA 60607

Mr. Andrew Malcolm
National News Desk, The New York Times, 229 West 43rd Street, New York, NY, USA 10036

Dr. Victor W. Marshall
Professor, Department of Behavioural Science, Faculty of Medicine, University of Toronto, Toronto, ON, Canada M5S 1A8

Dr. Alan D. Martin
Director, Sport and Exercise Sciences Research Institute, Max Bell Centre, University of Manitoba, Winnipeg, MB, Canada R3T 2N2

Dr. Bruce A. McFarlane
Professor of Sociology, Department of Sociology and Anthropology, Room B750 Loeb Building, Carleton University, Ottawa, ON, Canada K1S 5B6

Hon. Frank S. Miller
c/o Mr. Hugh K. N. MacKenzie, President, Enterprise Canada, 133 Richmond Street West, Suite 406, Toronto, ON, Canada M5H 2L3

Dr. J. Fraser Mustard
President, The Canadian Institute for Advanced Research, #701 - 179 John Street, Toronto, ON, Canada M5T 1X4

Dr. Sheila M. Neysmith
Associate Professor, Faculty of Social Work, University of Toronto, 246 Bloor Street West, Toronto, ON, Canada M5S 1A1

Mr. John Oussoren
Coordinator, Seniors' Education Centre, University Extension, University of Regina, Regina, SK, Canada S4S 0A2

Dr. Irma M. Parhad
Associate Professor, Departments of Pathology and Clinical Neurosciences, Room 2040 Health Sciences Centre, University of Calgary, 3330 Hospital Drive N.W., Calgary, AB, Canada T2N 4N1

Dr. Dorothy Pringle
Dean of Nursing, University of Toronto, 50 St. George Street, Toronto, ON, Canada M5S 1A1

Mr. W. F. (Rick) Roger
Vice-President, Finance and Management Services, Greater Victoria Hospital Society, 2101 Richmond Avenue, Victoria, BC, Canada V8R 4R7

Mrs. Donna L. Rose
Provincial Senior Citizens Advisory Council, P.O. Box 221, Bassano, AB, Canada T0J 0B0

Ms. Erna J. Schilder
Associate Professor, School of Nursing, 248 Bison Building, University of Manitoba, Winnipeg, MB, Canada R3T 2N2

Dr. Cope W. Schwenger
Professor, Department of Health Administration, Faculty of Medicine, University of Toronto, Toronto, ON, Canada M5S 1A8

Dr. Alexander Segall
National Health Scholar, Associate Professor, Department of Sociology, University of Manitoba, Winnipeg, MB, Canada R3T 2N2

Dr. Jo Seggie
Professor, Biomedical Sciences and Psychiatry, Department of Neurosciences, Faculty of Health Sciences, McMaster University, 1200 Main Street West, Hamilton, ON, Canada L8N 3Z5

Dr. John T. Sibley
Associate Professor of Medicine, Department of Medicine, University Hospital, Saskatoon, SK, Canada S7N 0X0

Dr. Norma J. Stewart
Associate Professor and Director, Nursing Research Unit, College of Nursing, University of Saskatchewan, Saskatoon, SK, Canada S7N 0W0

Dr. Thomas N. Taylor
Health Economist, Health Care Economics and Policy Analysis, The Upjohn Company, 7000 Portage Road, Kalamazoo, MI, USA 49001 (Formerly Assistant Professor, Department of Economics, Kalamazoo College, Kalamazoo, MI)

Dr. Hanneke M. Th. van Maanen
Associate Professor of Gerontology and Health Sciences, Faculty of
Nursing, University of Toronto, 50 St. George Street, Toronto, ON,
Canada M5S 1A1

Dr. Lois M. Verbrugge
Professor, Institute of Gerontology, The University of Michigan, 300
North Ingalls, Ann Arbor, MI, USA 48109–2007

Contents

PART IV: APPLYING GERONTOLOGICAL RESEARCH EFFECTIVELY

PART V: CEMENTING RESEARCH AND POLICY CONNECTIONS

PART I

Health Needs, Programs, and Policies

1. Reduction of the National Morbidity

JAMES F. FRIES

INTRODUCTION

The thesis of the compression of morbidity presents a paradigm for the aging process and suggests new approaches toward preventive gerontology. An allegory is that of Oliver Wendell Holmes, Sr.'s "one-hoss shay," which functioned perfectly over a long period of years until all parts simultaneously wore out and the shay collapsed into a pile of sawdust, nuts, and bolts. If a human organism can lead a long and vigorous life terminated by a sharp decline mandated by senescence, then a social and individual ideal for many might be reached.

The compression of morbidity represents a paradigm of aging in which if morbidity advances outstrip life expectancy gains, the health burden of the individual, and eventually the society, may be reduced (Fries, 1980, 1983a, 1984a, 1984c, 1987; Fries & Crapo, 1981; Gruenberg, 1977; Holmes, 1908; Schneider & Brody, 1983). A dynamic concept, the paradigm emphasizes that when one projects age-specific changes in mortality into the future and anticipates the social consequences, one must also carefully consider the accompanying (and often linked) changes in age-specific morbidity.

This chapter considers some conceptual misunderstandings, notes general improvement in the quality of models, discusses the continued slow compression of mortality, summarizes evidence for major reduction in incidence of chronic disease, presents a definition and classification of morbidity, reviews experimental evidence (including randomized controlled trials) for the ability to reduce and compress morbidity, discusses the trade-offs involved, notes the multidisciplinary nature of the evidence, and summarizes the mandate for a policy of prevention if we are to reduce morbidity.

Reprinted (abridged) with permission from *Gerontologica Perspecta* Vol. 1, 1987.
Aging and Health: Linking Research and Public Policy, © 1989 Lewis Publishers, Inc., Chelsea, Michigan 48118. Printed in U.S.A.

CONCEPTUAL ISSUES

In discussions of the compression of morbidity, there have been three areas which distract from an evolving consensus about critical health policy issues with an increasingly aged population.

First, there is the question of the correct use of tense (past, present, and future). When the compression of morbidity paradigm was introduced in 1980 (Fries, 1980), the phenomenon was viewed as a future possibility, with the future suggested as the early part of the 21st century. Subsequent elaboration (Fries & Crapo, 1981) emphasized the increasing national morbidity resulting from the exchange of acute disease deaths for more chronic ones—the major pattern throughout the century. With increasing evidence of the magnitude of the decline of chronic disease (principally atherosclerosis and, more recently, lung cancer) it became increasingly possible that reduction of morbidity might already be beginning to occur (Fries, 1983a). Hence, it became relevant to search for emerging evidence of the phenomenon of morbidity "compression." There is little disagreement that morbidity increased through the 1960s and, at least in most areas, through most or all of the 1970s. Attempts to "refute" phenomena of the 1980s or beyond with data from the 1960s and 1970s are superficial and misleading (Schneider & Guralnik, 1987; Crimmins, 1987).

Second, there has been an unfortunate emphasis on quantitative rather than substantive issues, and this has obscured broad areas of agreement (Manton, 1982; Myers & Manton, 1984a, 1984b). Yet the various predictions, as exemplified by life expectancy over age 100, differ by less than a year over the next 40-year period (Faber, 1982). With average life expectancy until recently increasing at a rate of three to four months each year, these differences are not conceptually important. It might help if projections of the future were limited by law to two significant digits (Faber, 1982).

Third, there is an all too frequent avoidance of the central issue. Morbidity, rather than mortality, represents the major national health problem, whether viewed in human or economic terms. Is it possible to wage a war against morbidity? What weapons might be utilized? How might forces be deployed? What are the targets? How do we measure progress?

The compression of morbidity thesis has consistently emphasized the *possibility* and not the *inevitability* of its occurrence. It is clearly possible to deploy resources so that future morbidity will be increased, as, for example, with large programs of artificial organs and life support systems. The science of prevention and postponement is presently a slight one, and will not grow optimally with only lip service to its importance (Schneider & Guralnik, 1987). Resources must be allocated for research, development, and implementation, both making use of what we already know and steadily increasing that knowledge.

IMPROVED MODELS: A CONSTRUCTIVE CHANGE

The Surgeon General, following the tone of the earlier LaLonde report for Canada, has set forth a strategy for attacking both morbidity and mortality, utilizing predominantly preventive approaches, and has summarized the data (*Healthy People*, 1979). Bartlett and Windsor have described the potential conflicts between preventive and curative approaches (1985). Taeuber (and others) have emphasized that the coming increases in numbers of elderly and in the need for care are almost entirely a product of increasing birth cohorts, with relatively little of the burden contributed by increasing life expectancy (Taeuber, 1983).

Goldman (1984) has presented a theoretical context in which "a full and healthy life, within the present parameters, with survival to see our children, and possibly our grandchildren mature, followed by a rapid, painless decline, is a worthy, reasonable, achievable, and morally justifiable goal." Economos (1982) has discussed models of aging in humans and experimental animals, noting an exponential decrease in vitality at advanced ages. Dilman (1984) has described and analyzed three models, somewhat interrelated, which describe the aging process, and has emphasized the role, potential and actual, of the compression of morbidity. Poterba and Summers (1985) have noticed a balance between declining morbidity and increasing longevity. Olshansky (1985, 1986, 1987) has described the present changes as the "fourth stage of the epidemiologic transition"—the age of delayed degenerative diseases.

Kohn (1982), examining the causes of death in very old people at autopsy, notes that senescence is not recorded as a cause of death, although it appears responsible for perhaps some 30% of presently autopsied deaths. He notes that senescence is a "universal, progressive, and ultimately fatal disease" and proposes that it be viewed as a disease and accepted as a valid cause of death. Steel and Barry (1985), in reviewing recent advances in geriatrics, describe the potential importance of prevention of aging problems and of the compression of morbidity. Russell (1986), on the other hand, discusses the possibility that there are cost offsets associated with prevention which need to be taken into account.

Trends in morbidity, over the years through 1980 (for which data are available) have been examined by several authors (Crimmins, 1987; Palmore, 1978, 1986, 1987; Verbrugge, 1984a, 1984b; Schneider & Guralnik, 1987). Verbrugge (1984a, 1984b) notes a probable increase in national morbidity over this period related to a decrease of acute conditions in ages over 45. Restricted activity and bed disability, she finds, have been relatively constant, and suggest that the stage has been set for a compression of morbidity in the future. Palmore (1978, 1986, 1987) has indicated the need for increasingly sophisticated analyses, including identification of age, period, and cohort effects. His adjusted analyses suggest the possibility of a decrease of morbidity over age 65 even in periods prior to 1980. Chirikos (1986), on the other hand, suggests that the rise in work-disability prevalence over this period is probably real.

Katz et al. (1983) have emphasized the term "active life expectancy," have proposed methods for its measurement and expression, and have urged collection of data directly assessing morbidity. Schneider and Guralnik, in recent writings (1987), recognize the need to assess the dynamic interplay between changes in morbidity and changes in mortality. Manton and Soldo, in their recent writings (Manton & Soldo, 1985; Soldo & Manton, 1985), present a much more dynamic model than previously. Manton now agrees with this author that "we have argued for an interpretation of mortality-morbidity dynamics which anticipates further progress in controlling the rate of chronic disease progression and thereby reduces the severity of the chronic degenerative diseases manifest at any age. This understanding implies increases in the number of productive, nondisabled years of life, but also any number of difficult trade-offs between social and individual benefits" (Soldo & Manton, 1985).

These several perspectives now converge in recognition of the interactions between age-specific mortality and age-specific morbidity, the importance of assessing their relative rates of change, and the necessity for development of better methods of obtaining the relevant data. The difficulties in conclusively assessing presently available data have been accurately, and often eloquently, described (Kovar, 1987).

THE COMPRESSION OF MORTALITY

Rectangularization

Since 1960, life expectancy from birth has increased approximately four years, while life expectancy from age 100 has increased only approximately three months (see Table 1). If the maximal average life expectancy were rising, we should expect changes in life expectancy to occur more equally across all ages as the entire curve shifted to the right. Instead, we see monotonically decreasing amounts of change. While there are many more centenarians because of increasing birth cohorts in the 1880s and because of markedly decreased rates of premature death, the average life expectancy for the individual reaching age 100 remains relatively fixed. Life expectancy from age 100 is a useful reference point, since virtually all premature deaths should have occurred before that point. Were the life span to be increasing without rectangularization, and the standard deviation of the age of death increasing, these figures would look quite different. All authors now appear to agree that the standard deviation of age of death is decreasing, however slowly (Myers & Manton, 1984b).

Table 1. Life Expectancy (Male/Female)

	Birth	60	70	80	90	100
			Years Expected from Age			
1960	66.6/73.2	15.9/19.6	10.3/12.5	6.1/7.0	3.4/3.7	2.1/2.1
1970	67.1/74.8	16.1/20.9	10.5/13.6	6.3/7.8	3.6/4.2	2.2/2.4
1980	69.9/77.5	17.3/22.2	11.2/14.8	6.8/8.7	3.8/4.6	2.3/2.6
			Changes in Life Expectancy			
			Males			
1960-1970	3.3	2.4	.9	.7	.4	.2
1970-1980	2.8	1.2	.7	.5	.2	.1
			Females			
1960-1970	4.3	2.6	2.3	1.7	.9	.3
1970-1980	2.7	1.3	1.2	.9	.4	.2

Source: Faber, J. F. (1982). *Life tables for the United States 1900-2050.* Actuarial Study No. 87, U.S. Dept. of Health and Human Services, SSA Pub. No. 11-11534.

Average Life Span (Maximum Average Life Expectancy)

The most recent data available on current life expectancy are summarized in Table 2. The lower bound for life span can be estimated from such data. Assuming that few individuals have a genetic life span below 65, the expected age at death for the most favored population groups who have reached age 65 provides an approximation of the lower bound. This age is currently 83.9 years for white females and rising. Since it is likely that the individuals currently dying before age 65 have a lower average maximal life expectancy than those dying after, this approximation should be somewhat optimistic. On the other hand, available data are always several years behind the current date.

Demeny (1984), making forecasts for the World Bank, has estimated that by year 2100 there will be no country with a life expectancy over 82.5 years. On the other hand, Faber (1982), using computer-based competing risk models without a term for senescence, projects that the average age at death for those females reaching their 65th birthday will be nearly 86 years by the year 2000. With life expectancy from birth currently increasing at a rate of three months each year, these differences in estimates represent only a differ-

Table 2. Life Expectancy, United States, 1982

	All	Male	Female	White Female
From birth	74.6	70.9	78.2	78.8
From age 65	16.8	14.5	18.8	18.9
From age 70	13.7	11.6	15.2	15.3

Source: Vital Statistics of the United States, 1985.

ence of a few years in the time of reaching senescent barriers; the various projections of mortality are not very different from each other. Of interest, the male-female gap has been recently declining in the United States and now stands at 7.3 years. In Japan it is less than six years.

Standard Deviation of Life Span (Maximal Average Life Expectancy)

Schneider and Guralnik (1987), and others, correctly point out that our original estimates of four years for the standard deviation of age of death are too narrow and lead to logical contradictions. With the assumption that about 2% of the population might live to age 100 or above, that the distribution is an untransformed normal distribution (not Gompertzian), and that the mean is 85 to 86 years, a better estimate would approximate seven years. This standard deviation is currently approximately nine years and is slowly decreasing (Fries, 1984c; Myers & Manton, 1984b).

THE DECLINING INCIDENCE OF CHRONIC DISEASE

Mortality from chronic disease, dominated by cardiovascular mortality, has been declining strikingly, at a rate of approximately 3% per year, for more than 10 years (Stern, 1979). Morbidity, however, is more importantly linked to the age-specific *incidence* of chronic disease—to the age at which disease becomes manifest rather than the age at death at which it ends. If age-specific incidence were relatively constant, declines in mortality might mean increases in morbidity. If incidence is declining, there may be less morbidity. It is therefore important to inspect data on age-specific incidence. Discussion here will be limited to incidence of cardiovascular disease and lung cancer, since these are numerically the most important, and because the best data are to be found in these areas. These data indicate that the principal reduction has been in incidence rather than in survival after the first clinical event.

Pell and Fayerweather (1985) found a steady decline in age-specific incidence rates of myocardial infarction among male employees of the Du Pont Company. Over a 20-year period, an average decline of 28.2% was observed. As would be expected from the compression of morbidity model, the declines were most striking at younger ages. Males aged an average of 30 years showed incidence rates declining by 50%; those at age 40, 39.4%; those at age 50, 25.9%; and those at age 60, 22.3%.

National hospital discharge survey data (Report of the Surgeon General, 1983) show steadily declining hospitalization rates of acute myocardial infarction. The Kaiser-Permanente study in Northern California (Friedman, 1979) confirmed these decreasing rates. The Minnesota Heart Survey (Gillum et al., 1983) reported a decline in hospitalization rates for acute myocardial infarction between 1970 and 1980. Analysis of the involved factors suggested that lifestyle (reduction in smoking and serum cholesterol) and hypertension control were the most important contributors to the observed decline in ischemic heart disease mortality rates (Goldman & Cook, 1984). Analysis of short-term hospital stays in United States hospitals (National Center for Health Statistics, 1965, 1968, 1974, 1978) over time suggests that the age-specific rates of hospitalization for cardiovascular disease increased more rapidly over a 13-year period (average increase of four years) than did life expectancy (two years) over the same period (Fries, 1983a).

The compression of morbidity model predicts, paradoxically, that even as mortality from coronary heart disease declines, 5- and 10-year survival after heart attack will decrease. Data from the Worcester heart attack study provide preliminary evidence that this phenomenon may be occurring in some locations (Goldberg et al., 1986). The theoretical models underlying prediction of coronary events and coronary death based originally on the Framingham data have recently been confirmed by the Multiple Risk Factor Intervention Trial Research Group (1986b).

Lung Cancer

The situation with regard to solid tumor incidence rates is relatively straightforward (Bailar & Smith, 1986). Since mortality rates for these tumors have remained essentially constant, incidence rates must almost exactly parallel mortality rates. Models predicting risk of developing lung cancer are related to exposure factors (such as pack-years of cigarette exposure) in which a reduction of exposure should logically result in later incidence. Recently, Horm and Kessler (1986) have documented falling rates of lung cancer for the first time in the United States. A decrease of 4% from 1982 to 1983 has the result of "7,000 fewer cases in 1983 alone. . . . Both incidence and mortality have been decreasing for men under 45 since at least 1973, and for men between 45 and 54 years of age since 1978" (Horm & Kessler, 1986). Lung cancer incidence, morbidity, and mortality, following this model, are continuing to increase in women, and are expected to do so for the next five to seven years. Stomach cancer, once among the most major of malignancies, has demonstrated marked declines in incidence, morbidity, and mortality, although the reasons for the decline are much less clear (Bailar & Smith, 1986).

A DEFINITION AND CLASSIFICATION OF MORBIDITY

Health, as defined by the World Health Organization, is "not merely the absence of disease, but total physical, social, and psychological well being"

(Constitution of the World Health Organization, 1948). Morbidity, then, in the broadest sense, may be defined as the absence of health.

Kovar (1987) and others have described the many difficulties in measurement of morbidity. In contrast to mortality data, which is adequately available, most of the required measurements of morbidity have not been made, and when made, are subject to a variety of biases, including ascertainment, normative expectation, changing definitions, and others. There is lack of a conceptual framework from which to view morbidity.

Major clinical advances in the measurement of morbidity (often termed patient outcome or health status) have recently been made, and tools for more accurate assessment are now available (Fries, 1983b). When questioned, patients categorize their desires for health under the headings of minimizing death, minimizing disability, minimizing symptoms, minimizing iatrogenic problems, and minimizing the adverse economic effects of illness. These four dimensions of morbidity (disability, discomfort, doctor- and drug-caused problems, and dollar costs) are often involved in health care decisions in complex ways. New instruments such as the Health Assessment Questionnaire (HAQ) provide a broader view of the various impacts and allow quantitation of their magnitude. It may be hoped that such measurements will become a standard part of longitudinal studies of the development of morbidity.

For purposes of examining the trade-offs associated with postponement or cure of particular conditions in the context of increasing morbidity with age, a classification of morbidity (Table 3) is helpful. It is clear from inspection of such an admittedly arbitrary classification that preventive approaches to most of the problems are currently available.

Many authors have attempted to quantitate the effects of these approaches on mortality; morbidity data will be discussed in the following section. Tarlov (1984, Table 4) has provided estimates of potentially postponable death and accompanying economic impact for major disease categories. Siegel and Davidson (1984) note the Public Health Service estimate that lifestyle alone accounts for 54, 37, 50, and 49% of mortality from heart disease, cancer, cardiovascular disease, and arteriosclerosis, respectively. Stamler (1985) has reviewed the approaches to coronary heart disease, anticipating the ability to continue a 3% per year reduction over the next several years. Hertzman has projected health care costs in Canada in the year 2026 ranging from essentially stable costs with preventive scenarios to approximately a tripling of costs with official projections, using standard data (Schwenger & Cross, 1980). Salkever (1986) estimates present morbidity costs at over $100 billion a year in current U.S. dollars.[1]

Fuchs (1984) observes that the health status of the elderly at any given age has improved in recent decades, that "health care spending among the elderly is not so much a function of time since birth as it is a function of time to death," and that "adjustment for age-sex differences in survival status elimi-

Table 3.   A Classification of Morbidity (Selected Risk Factors in Parentheses)

Morbidity with Often-fatal Diseases

Atherosclerosis[a] (diet, inactivity, smoking, hypertension, obesity)—myocardial infarction, angina pectoris, intermittent claudication, congestive heart failure, peripheral occlusive disease, nonfatal stroke, multiple infarct dementia, impaired renal function

Cancer[a] (smoking, diet, alcohol)—cachexia, pain, structural interference with organ functions, iatrogenic toxicity

Emphysema[a] (smoking)—oxygen hunger, activity limitation, infection

Cirrhosis[a] (alcohol)—ascites, gastrointestinal bleeding, jaundice, dementia

Diabetes[a] (obesity, inactivity)—retinopathy, neuropathy, renal failure, hypoglycemia, atherosclerosis

Trauma[a] (seat belt nonuse, substance abuse)—quadriplegia, hemiplegia, amputation, brain damage, fractures

Morbidity Associated with Seldom-fatal Diseases

Osteoarthritis[a] (obesity, injury, inactivity)—musculoskeletal disability, pain

Back pain and intervertebral disk[a] (injury, poor conditioning)

Hernias[a] (obesity, poor conditioning)

Hemorrhoids[a] (obesity, inactivity)

Varicose veins[a] (obesity, inactivity)

Dental decay and gum disease[a] (inadequate prophylaxis)

Gallbladder disease[a] (obesity, diet)

Kidney stone (diet, hydration)

Ulcers[a] (stress, drugs, alcohol)

Upper respiratory infection

Bladder infection[a] (hydration, hygiene)

Depression (inactivity)

Anxiety (inactivity, stimulants)

Morbidity Associated with Senescence

Cataracts and corneal opacification[b]

Hearing loss[b]

Osteoporosis[a] (inactivity, diet)

Falls and fractures[a,b]

Memory loss[a]

Senile dementia

Incontinence

Constipation[a] (inactivity, diet)

Iatrogenic problems[a] (polypharmacy)

Dependence[a]

Agonal Terminal Morbidity

Pain, dependence, cost[a]

[a]Preventable with present knowledge.
[b]Effective treatment often possible.

nates most of the age-related increase in expenditures." He concludes that current predictions for health expenses over age 65 may be inflated by over 50%. Fries (1984b) has categorized chronic illness into two broad types: those with Gompertzian age-related incidence, for which preventive initiatives are likely to be most useful, and those with mid-life incidence characteristics (such as multiple sclerosis, rheumatoid arthritis, ulcerative colitis, Hodgkin's disease, acute leukemia) for which medical approaches to treatment and cure hold the most promise. Bayer et al. (1983) have reviewed the

Table 4.   Estimates of Potentially Postponable Deaths, Preventable Years of Life Lost, Preventable Economic Cost, by Selected Diagnostic Categories

Diagnostic Category and % Deaths Postponable	No. of Deaths Potentially Postponable[a]	Years of Life Lost Potentially Preventable[a]	Economic Costs $ Billions Potentially Preventable[a]
All (66%)	1,260,000	23,000,000	$302
Injuries (90%)	144,000 (3)	5,490,000 (2)	75 (1)
Circulatory dis. (67%)	665,000 (1)	8,385,000 (1)	57 (2)
Neoplasms (67%)	283,000 (2)	4,850,000 (3)	34 (3)
Respiratory dis. (76%)	98,000 (4)	1,359,000 (4)	25 (4)
Digestive dis. (55%)	41,000 (5)	779,000 (5)	23 (5)
Musculoskeletal (30%)	1,700	32,700	6
Infectious dis. (50%)	38,000	708,000	5

Source: Tarlov, A. (1984). *Henry J. Kaiser Family Foundation Annual Report.* Menlo Park, California.
[a]Rankings are shown in parentheses.

moral and economic issues surrounding care of the terminally ill patient; expenses during the last year of life are 18% of lifetime medical costs.

EXPERIMENTAL EVIDENCE OF THE ABILITY TO DECREASE MORBIDITY

An increasing clinical literature addresses questions of morbidity as well as mortality, and in some instances allows a comparison of the effects of experimental interventions both upon mortality and upon morbidity. The multiple risk factor intervention trial (MRFIT) is an instructive example (Multiple Risk Factor Intervention Trial Research Group, 1982). This large, randomized controlled trial of the effects of reduction of smoking, reduction of hypertension, and reduction of cholesterol was perhaps the most expensive scientific experiment ever performed, with a cost of over $115 million. Initial results on mortality were disappointing, since statistically significant differences between treatment and control subjects were not observed.

Morbidity data from this study, recently released (Multiple Risk Factor Intervention Trial Research Group, 1986a), show a far more encouraging picture. Whereas the interventions reduced coronary death by only 7%, eight measures of morbidity were decreased by an average of 23% (Table 5). Statistical significance was achieved with three of the morbidity measures (angina pectoris, congestive heart failure, and peripheral occlusive disease). A compression of morbidity thus appears to have been achieved, in a randomized controlled trial, by these lifestyle interventions, with a much greater effect upon the occurrence of morbid events than upon mortal ones.

These results are consistent with the classic Veterans' Administration cooperative study on antihypertensive agents (1970), in which treatment was

Table 5.   Multiple Risk Factor Intervention Trial Results After Seven Years

Endpoint	Intervention Group (%)	Control Group (%)	Percent Reduction	P-Value
Mortality				
Coronary death	1.79	1.93	7%	N.S.
Morbidity				
Myocardial infarction	4.57	5.02	9%	N.S.
Angina pectoris	10.05	12.69	21%	0.05
Intermittent claudication	3.92	4.46	12%	N.S.
Congestive heart failure	0.03	0.26	88%	0.05
Peripheral occlusive disease	2.27	2.72	16%	0.05
Stroke (nonfatal)	0.56	0.47	20%	N.S.
Left venticular hypertrophy	1.63	1.94	16%	N.S.
Impaired renal function	0.12	0.17	27%	N.S.
All morbidities			23%	

Source: Multiple Risk Factor Intervention Trial Research Group (1986a). Coronary heart disease death, nonfatal acute myocardial infarction, and other clinical outcomes in the multiple risk factor intervention trial. *Am J Cardiol, 58,* 1-13.
Note: N.S. = not significant.

found effective in preventing congestive heart failure and stroke (morbidity), but no statistically significant reduction in coronary heart disease deaths occurred. The Lipid Research Clinic coronary prevention trial (1984), another massive study, also failed to reduce total deaths, which were essentially identical between the two groups. Reduction in incidence of nonfatal coronary heart disease, however, was observed.

Oster and colleagues, in a series of cost-benefit analyses (Oster et al., 1984; Oster & Epstein, 1986), have computed the economic benefits of various lifestyle interventions. Economic costs of health care, being related to required health services, probably represent a satisfactory surrogate for morbidity. Large benefits ($20,000 for light smokers, $56,000 for heavy smokers) accrued to those who stopped smoking, and smaller amounts to those using nicotine chewing gum or who lowered serum cholesterol.

Rosenberg et al. (1985) studied the risk of nonfatal myocardial infarction, a measure of morbidity, after quitting smoking in men under 55 years of age. Current smokers had a relative risk of 2.9 compared with those who never smoked, ex-smokers declined to a relative risk of 2.0 after cessation of 12 to 23 months and to about 1.0 for abstainers of longer periods. A major effect of cessation of cigarette smoking upon morbidity was clearly identified. Paffenbarger et al. (1986) have studied the effect of physical activity upon mortality and longevity in a large longitudinal study. Death rates declined steadily with increasing amounts of exercise, ultimately contributing one to two more years of life. In contrast to these positive but relatively slight effects, Bairey (1986), Bortz (1982, 1987), Bruce (1984), Larson (1986), and others have noted dramatic changes in cardiovascular reserve and other measures of morbidity. Maximum oxygen uptake declines markedly more slowly in aerobically trained individuals with age.

Branch (1985), using crude binary lifestyle definitions and crude measures of outcome, noted that slowed down physical activities in women and cigarette smoking in men were associated with subsequent physical limitations. Spirduso (1980) has shown marked effects of physical training upon psychomotor speed; psychomotor speed is likely to be related to a number of adaptive behaviors.

Osteoporosis is a major cause of fractures and disability in the elderly, particularly women. Brody (1985) estimates that 650,000 fractures projected by the mid-21st century might be reduced by 50% if osteoporosis were treated by currently available techniques. A recent consensus panel has emphasized the need for adequate calcium intake and adequate weight-bearing exercise to retain bone strength. Lane et al. (1986) have documented increased bone density (CT scan of first lumbar vertebra) of 40% in regular runners as compared with community controls after careful pairwise matching, a very significant result. Osteoarthritis and associated musculoskeletal disability are increasingly the subject of risk factor analyses (Lane et al., 1986; Panush et al., 1986). Problems are more prevalent in the obese, the sedentary, those with prior injuries to joints, and those with other coincident diseases. No relationship of long-term running activity, postulated as possibly harmful, to subsequent development of osteoarthritis has been found, and in individuals without previous injury, some protective effect may be present (Lane et al., 1986; Panush et al., 1986).

The association of adverse lifestyles with increased morbidity is substantial. For example, from our own data, 2592 consecutive "healthy" insurees show a doubling of hospitalization rates together with a 20% decrease in self-reported health status for each pack of cigarettes smoked daily. Each hour per week in aerobic exercise was associated with a 10% improvement in reported health status and a significant reduction in work time lost. Health risk reductions of 19% after six months in 1900 subjects in a health promotion program were associated with significant decreases in doctor visits, work time lost, and hospitalization, and increases in reported health. Direct cost reductions averaged $160 per subject per year.

Lane et al. (1987) studied the development of musculoskeletal disability by year of age in a cross-sectional study comparing nearly 500 runners and a similar number of carefully matched community controls (Table 6). Reported disability by the Health Assessment Questionnaire, using measures of activities of daily living similar to those of Katz, showed virtually no decline with age in the active group. The rate of development of disability was nearly 10 times greater in the control population. Seidell et al. (1986), confirming earlier studies, note a strong association between increases in body weight and greater morbidity, with multiple complex interactions involving social and psychological factors.

Table 6. Rate of Development of Musculoskeletal Disability per Year of Age (50-72 Years)

Reported Disability (ADL)	Unit Decline/Year		
	All	Males	Females
All ages			
Runners	0.003	0.005	−0.001
Community controls	0.028	0.016	0.043
Comparison with age 30			
Runners	0.050	0.055	0.016
Community controls	0.100	0.075	0.140

Source: Lane, N. E., Bloch, D. A., Wood, P. D., et al. (1987). Aging, long-distance running, and the development of musculoskeletal disability: A controlled study. *Am J Med*, *82*, 772-780.
Note: ADL = Activities of daily living.

Williams and Lund (1986) have examined the impact of seat belt use laws in the recent United States experience, noting an inadequate compliance (approximately 50%) with the laws, and indicate that passive restraint systems may also be needed. The positive effects of seat belts include reduction in both mortality and injury, with injury being approximately 10 times as prevalent as death. Space does not permit detailed discussion of the risk factors associated with the other morbid conditions listed in Table 3, but discussions may be found in standard medical textbooks (Cecil & Loeb, 1987).

Space similarly does not permit detailed discussion of the major interactions of social and psychological factors, but these are clearly important. Berkman and Syme (1979) report important interactions between social networks and mortality. Relative risk of death of 2.3 for men and 2.8 for women for those most isolated versus those with most social ties were documented. Nesselroade, Schaie, and Baltes (1972) and Plemons, Willis, and Baltes (1978) note the modifiability of cognitive status in elders and provide a theoretical framework for its understanding. Loftus and Loftus (1980), Langer, Rodin, and Beck (1979), and others have described techniques for improving memory and cognitive function in later life. Valliant (1979) has studied the effect of coping behaviors on physical morbidity, finding strong effects. Rodin and Langer (1977) have described health benefits in both morbidity and mortality after environmental changes for the institutionalized aged which allow greater personal control of the environment for the individual.

The elderly show great variability in health care utilization, reflecting at least in part great variation in morbidity. Roos and Shapiro (1981), using the Manitoba data sets, found only a few elderly to be high users of care. Gurewitsch (1984), carefully studying a Swiss senior home, noted greatly reduced care requirements for those who were physically fit, had many interests, were independent and helpful, and lived in supportive environments. Such individuals required only 54 days of substantial care, as compared with 911 for the individuals without these characteristics.

It is clear from these and many other studies (Fries & Crapo, 1981; Fries, 1983a) that substantial reductions in morbidity of a great many types are currently theoretically possible. When direct comparisons are possible, the effects of interventions on morbidity appear stronger than the effects upon mortality.

TRADE-OFFS BETWEEN DEATH-STYLES

The purpose of the classification of Table 3 is to allow better estimation of benefits and offsets from postponement of morbidity. Note that only postponement of morbidity in the first category, associated with often-fatal disease, is likely to result in incurring some future morbidity as a partial offset. Morbidity reduction in nonfatal illness, in senescent morbidity, or in terminal morbidity incurs no such trade-off and represents a net gain. Note also that the risk factors for the morbidity associated with nonfatal illness and senescence are closely similar to those for morbidity associated with fatal disease.

A REQUIREMENT FOR MULTIDISCIPLINARY SCIENCE

This chapter reviews relevant literature from a number of fields, each of which contributes to our understanding. Only a few citations from each are included, but it is hoped that these may serve as entry points into the various literatures for readers interested in exploring other perspectives or who are not persuaded by these brief excursions. Morbidity may be considered from clinical, demographic, social, biologic, genetic, psychologic, or humanistic perspectives, but not adequately by any of these in isolation.

Much confusion has resulted from narrowness of study. Mathematical models that do not know that we grow old and then we die will ultimately prove invalid. Trees do not grow to heaven. Attempts to prove that the life span is increasing by demographic arguments which ignore the science of genetics will similarly fail. Life span, as other species characteristics (Rockstein, 1958), is subject to change resulting from selective pressure on mortality. No mechanism has been suggested by which this might be occurring. We might hope that arguments that fly in the face of current scientific consensus might be burdened with the need to suggest some plausible mechanism.

Two final caveats are important; either could greatly effect future projections. First, a breakthrough in altering the life span could occur. Like Schneider (Schneider & Reed, 1985), I believe such occurrence to be unlikely, at least over the near term. Certainly the Schneider discussion refutes evidence for major effects on mortality from known factors such as exercise (Bortz, 1987). Second, on the negative side, new scourges could appear which would roll back progress or even extinguish the race. AIDS, a preventable illness, is a new and major problem causing both morbidity and mortality. The possibility of nuclear holocaust hangs over us as a heavy threat. Such possibilities are not easily integrated into any models, although they could prove the dominant considerations.

A POLICY OF PREVENTION?

The central mandate of the compression of morbidity is that we begin to execute, as policy, that which we already know how to do. If we wish less morbidity, we must seek out and identify its antecedents. We must reduce morbidity in each of the several categories. We need research, development, and implementation, both serially and concurrently. Any other policy will prove more costly in human or any other terms.

NOTE

1. Dollar figures in this chapter are U.S. dollars.

REFERENCES

Bailar, J. C., & Smith, E. M. (1986). Progress against cancer? *New England Journal of Medicine, 314,* 1226–1232.

Bairey, C. N. (1986). Exercise and coronary artery disease. *Western Journal of Medicine, 144,* 205–211.

Bartlett, E. E., & Windsor, R. A. (1985). Health education and medicare: Competition or cooperation? *Health Education Quarterly, 12,* 219–229.

Bayer, R., Callahan, D., Fletcher, J., et al. (1983). The care of the terminally ill: Mortality and economics. *New England Journal of Medicine, 309*(4), 1490–1494.

Berkman, L. F., & Syme, S. L. (1979). Social networks, host resistance, and mortality: A nine-year follow-up study of Alameda County Residents. *American Journal of Epidemiology, 109,* 186–204.

Bortz, W. M. (1982). Disuse and aging. *JAMA: Journal of the American Medical Association, 248,*(10), 1203–1208.

Bortz, W. M. (1987). Disuse and extended morbidity. *Gerontologica Perspecta, 1,* 52–53.

Branch, L. G. (1985). Health practices and incident disability among the elderly. *American Journal of Public Health, 75,* 1436-1439.

Brody, J. A. (1985). Prospects for an aging population. *Nature, 315,* 463–466.

Bruce, R. A. (1984). Exercise, functional aerobic capacity, and aging—another viewpoint. *Sports & Exercise, 16*(1), 8–13.

Cecil & Loeb. (1987). *Textbook of medicine* (17th ed.), (Wyngaarden & Smith, Eds.). Philadelphia: W. B. Saunders.

Chirikos, T. N. (1986). Accounting for the historical rise in work-disability prevalence. *Milbank Quarterly, 64,* 271–301.

Constitution of the World Health Organization, 1948. (1964). In *Basic documents* (15th ed.). Geneva: WHO.

Crimmins, E. M. (1987). Evidence on the compression of morbidity. *Gerontologica Perspecta, 1,* 45–48.

Demeny, P. (1984). A perspective on long term care population growth. *Population Development Review, 10,* 103–126.

Dilman, V. M. (1984). Three models of medicine (an integrated theory of aging and age-associated diseases). *Medical Hypotheses, 15,* 185–208.

Economos, A. C. (1982). Rate of aging, rate of dying and the mechanism of mortality. *Archives of Gerontology and Geriatrics, 1,* 3–27.

Faber, J. F. (1982). *Life tables for the United States 1900–2050.* (Actuarial Study No. 87). (DHHS Publication No. SSA 11-11534). Washington, DC: U.S. Government Printing Office.

Friedman, G. D. (1979). Decline in hospitalization for coronary health disease and stroke: The Kaiser-Permanente experience in Northern California, 1971–1977. In R. J. Havlik & M. Feinleib (Eds.), *Proceedings of the Conference on the Decline in Coronary Heart Disease Mortality* (NIH Publication No. 79–1610, pp. 116–118). Washington, DC: U.S. Government Printing Office.

Fries, J. F. (1980). Aging, natural death, and the compression of morbidity. *New England Journal of Medicine, 303,* 130–136.

Fries, J. F. (1983a). The compression of morbidity. *Milbank Memorial Fund Quarterly/Health and Society, 61*(3), 397–419.

Fries, J. F. (1983b). Toward an understanding of patient outcome measurement. *Arthritis and Rheumatism, 26,* 697–704.

Fries, J. F. (1984a). Aging, natural death, and the compression of morbidity. *New England Journal of Medicine, 310*(10), 659–660.

Fries, J. F. (1984b). The compression of morbidity, Benjamin Gompertz, the two types of chronic disease, and health policy. *Proceedings: Exploring New Frontiers of U.S. Health Policy,* Rutgers.

Fries, J. F. (1984c). The compression of morbidity: Miscellaneous comments about a theme. *Gerontologist, 24,* 354–359.

Fries, J. F. (1987). An introduction to the compression of morbidity. *Gerontologica Perspecta, 1,* 5–8, 54–64.

Fries, J. F., & Crapo, L. M. (1981). *Vitality and aging.* New York: W. H. Freeman.

Fuchs, V. R. (1984). Though much is taken. *Milbank Memorial Fund Quarterly/Health and Society, 62,* 143–156.

Gillum, R. F., Folson, A., Luepker, R. V., et al. (1983). Sudden death and acute myocardial infarction in a metropolitan area, 1970–1980: The Minnesota heart survey. *New England Journal of Medicine, 309,* 1353–1358.

Goldberg, R. J., Gore, J. M., Alpert, J. S., et al. (1986). Recent changes in attack and survival rates of acute myocardial infarction (1975–1981). The Worcester

Heart Attack Study. *JAMA: Journal of the American Medical Association,* *255,* 2774–2779.

Goldman, L., & Cook, E. F. (1984). The decline in ischemic heart disease mortality rates: An analysis of the comparative effects of medical interventions and changes in lifestyle. *Annals of Internal Medicine, 101,* 825–836.

Goldman, R. (1984). Normal human aging: A theoretical context. In C. K. Cassel & J. R. Walsh (Eds.), *Geriatric medicine* (Vol. 1, pp. 13–22). New York: Springer-Verlag.

Gruenberg, E. M. (1977). The failure of success. *Milbank Memorial Fund Quarterly/Health and Society, 55,* 3–24.

Gurewitsch, E. C. (1984). Reduced requirements for long term institutional care: Results of a retrospective study. *Gerontologist, 24,* 199–204.

Healthy people: The Surgeon General's report on health promotion and disease prevention. (1979). (DHEW Publication No. 79–55071). Washington, DC: U.S. Government Printing Office.

Holmes, O. W. (1908). The deacon's masterpiece, or the wonderful "one-hoss shay." From the autocrat of the breakfast table, 1857–1858. In *The complete poetical works of Oliver Wendell Holmes.* Boston: Houghton Mifflin.

Horm, J. W., & Kessler, L. G. (1986). Falling rates of lung cancer in men in the United States. *Lancet, 1,* 425–426.

Katz, S., Branch, L. G., Branson, M. H., et al. (1983). Active life expectancy. *New England Journal of Medicine, 309*(20), 1218–1224.

Kohn, B. L. (1982). Causes of death in very old people. *JAMA: Journal of the American Medical Association, 247,* 2793.

Kovar, M. G. (1987). Some comments on measuring morbidity. *Gerontologica Perspecta, 1,* 49–51.

Lane, N. E., Bloch, D. A., Jones, H. H., et al. (1986). Long-distance running, bone density, and osteoarthritis. *JAMA: Journal of the American Medical Association, 255,* 1147–1151.

Lane, N. E., Bloch, D. A., Wood, P. D., et al. (1987). Aging, long-distance running, and the development of musculoskeletal disability: A controlled study. *American Journal of Medicine, 82,* 772–780.

Langer, E. J., Rodin, J., and Beck, P. (1979). Environmental determinants of memory improvement in late adulthood. *Journal of Personality and Social Psychology, 37,* 2003–2013.

Larson, E. B., & Bruce, R. A. (1986). Exercise and aging. *Annals of Internal Medicine, 105,* 783–785.

Lipid Research Clinic coronary primary prevention trial results: I. Reduction of incidence of coronary heart disease. (1984). *JAMA: Journal of the American Medical Association, 251,* 351–364.

Loftus, E. F., & Loftus, G. R. (1980). On the permanence of stored information in the human brain. *American Psychologist, 35,* 408–420.

Manton, K. G. (1982). Changing concepts of morbidity and mortality in the elderly population. *Milbank Memorial Fund Quarterly/Health and Society, 60*(2), 183–244.

Manton, K. G., & Soldo, B. J. (1985). Dynamics of health changes in the oldest old: New perspectives and evidence. *Milbank Memorial Fund Quarterly/ Health and Society, 63,* 206–285.

Multiple Risk Factor Intervention Trial Research Group. (1982). Multiple risk factor intervention trial. *JAMA: Journal of the American Medical Association, 248,* 1465–1477.

Multiple Risk Factor Intervention Trial Research Group (1986a). Coronary heart disease death, non-fatal acute myocardial infarction and other clinical outcomes in the multiple risk factor intervention trial. *American Journal of Cardiology, 58,* 1–13.

Multiple Risk Factor Intervention Trial Research Group. (1986b). Relationship between baseline risk factors and coronary heart disease and total mortality in the multiple risk factor intervention trial. *Preventive Medicine, 15,* 254–273.

Myers, G. C., & Manton, K. G. (1984a). Compression of mortality: Myth or reality. *Gerontologist, 24,* 346–353.

Myers, G. C., & Manton, K. G. (1984b). Recent changes in the U.S. age at death distribution: Further observations. *Gerontologist, 24,* 572–575.

National Center for Health Statistics. (1965, 1968, 1974, 1978). *Inpatient utilization of short-stay hospitals by diagnosis: United States* (Series 13, Nos. 6, 12, 26, 46). Washington, DC: U.S. Government Printing Office.

Nesselroade, J., Schaie, K., Baltes, P. B. (1972). Ontogenetic and generational components of structural and quantitative change in adult behavior. *Journal of Gerontology, 27,* 222–228.

Olshansky, S. J. (1985). Pursuing longevity: Delay vs elimination of degenerative diseases. *American Journal of Public Health, 75*(7), 754–789.

Olshansky, S. J. (1986). The fourth stage of the epidemiologic transition: The age of delayed degenerative diseases. *Milbank Memorial Fund Quarterly/Health and Society, 64,* 355–391.

Olshansky, S. J. (1987). The compression of mortality and morbidity: Comments on the debate. *Gerontologica Perspecta, 1,* 19–22.

Oster, G., Colditz, G. A., & Kelly, N. L. (1984). *The economic costs of smoking and benefits of quitting.* Lexington, MA: Lexington Books, D.C. Heath.

Oster, G., & Epstein, A. M. (1986). Primary prevention and coronary heart disease: The economic benefits of lowering serum cholesterol. *American Journal of Public Health, 76,* 647–656.

Paffenbarger, R. S., Hyde, R. T., Wing, A. L., et al. (1986). Physical activity, all-cause mortality, and longevity of college alumni. *New England Journal of Medicine, 314,* 605–613.

Palmore, E. B. (1978). When can age, period, and cohort be separated? *Social Focus, 57,* 282–295.

Palmore, E. B., (1986). Trends in the health of the aged. *Gerontologist, 26,* 298–302.

Palmore, E. B. (1987). Some errors and irrelevancies in the debate over compression of mortality. *Gerontologica Perspecta, 1,* 30–31.

Panush, R. S., Schmidt, C., Caldwell, J. F., et al. (1986). Is running associated with degenerative joint disease? *JAMA: Journal of the American Medical Association, 255,* 1152–1154.

Pell, S., & Fayerweather, W. E. (1985). Trends in the incidence of myocardial infarction and in associated mortality and morbidity in a large employed population, 1957–1983. *New England Journal of Medicine, 312*(6), 1005–1011.

Plemons, J. K., Willis, S. L., & Baltes, P. B. (1978). Modifiability of fluid intelligence in aging: A short-term longitudinal training approach. *Journal of Gerontology, 33*, 224–231.

Poterba, J. M., & Summers, L. H. (1985). *Public policy implications of declining old-age mortality*. Brookings Conference on Retirement and Aging.

Report of the Surgeon General: The health consequences of *smoking: Cardiovascular diseases*. (1983). Public Health Service, pp. 344–347.

Rockstein, M. (1958). Heredity and longevity in the animal kingdom. *Journal of Gerontology*, Supp. No. 2 *13*(3), 7–12.

Rodin, J., & Langer, E. J. (1977). Long term effects of a control-relevant intervention with the institutionalized aged. *Journal of Personality and Social Psychology, 35*, 897–902.

Roos, N. P., & Shapiro, E. (1981). The Manitoba longitudinal study on aging: Preliminary findings on health care utilization by the elderly. *Medical Care, 19*, 644–657.

Rosenberg, L., Kaufman, D. W., Helmrich, S. P., et al. (1985). The risk of myocardial infarction after quitting smoking in men under 55 years of age. *New England Journal of Medicine, 313*, 1511–1514.

Russell, L. B. (1986). *Is prevention better than cure?* Washington, DC: Brookings.

Salkever, D. S. (1986). *Morbidity costs: National estimates and economic determinants*. (DHHS Publication No. 86–3393). Washington, DC: U.S. Government Printing Office.

Schneider, E. L., & Brody, J. A. (1983). Aging, natural death, and the compression of morbidity: Another view. *New England Journal of Medicine, 309*(14), 854–856.

Schneider, E. L., & Guralnik, J. M. (1987). The compression of morbidity: A dream which may come true, someday! *Gerontologica Perspecta, 1*, 8–13.

Schneider, E. L., & Reed, J. D. (1985). Life extension. *New England Journal of Medicine, 312*, 1159–1168.

Schwenger, C. W., & Cross, M. J. (1980). Institutional care and institutionalization of the elderly in Canada. In V. M. Marshall (Ed.), *Aging in Canada: Social perspectives* (pp. 248–256). Don Mills, ON: Fitzhenry & Whiteside.

Seidell, J. C., Bak, K. C., Deurenberg, P., et al. (1986). The relationship between overweight and subjective health according to age, social class, slimming behaviour and smoking habits in Dutch adults. *American Journal of Public Health, 76*, 1410–1415.

Siegel, J. S., & Davidson, M. (1984). *Demographic and socioeconomic aspects of aging in the United States*. (Bureau of the Census, Series P-23, No. 138).

Soldo, B. J., & Manton, K. G. (1985). Health status and service needs of the oldest old: Current patterns and future trends. *Milbank Memorial Fund Quarterly/ Health and Society, 63*, 286–319.

Spirduso, W. W. (1980). Physical fitness, aging, and psychomotor speed: A review. *Journal of Gerontology, 35*, 850–865.

Stamler, J. (1985). Coronary heart disease: Doing the "right things." *New England Journal of Medicine, 312*(16), 1053–1055.

Steel, K., & Barry, P. P. (1985). Geriatrics. *JAMA: Journal of the American Medical Association, 254*(16), 2286–2287.

Stern, M. P. (1979). The recent decline in ischemic heart disease mortality. *Annals of Internal Medicine, 91*, 630–640.

Taeuber, C. M. (1983). *America in transition. An aging society.* (Bureau of the Census, Series P-23, No. 128).

Tarlov, A. (1984). *Henry J. Kaiser Family Foundation Annual Report.* Menlo Park, California.

Valliant, G. (1979). Natural history of male psychological health: Effects of mental health on physical health. *New England Journal of Medicine, 301*, 1249–1254.

Verbrugge, L. M. (1984a). A health profile of older women with comparisons to older men. *Research on Aging, 6*(3), 291–322.

Verbrugge, L. M. (1984b). Longer life but worsening health? Trends in health and mortality of middle-aged and older persons. *Milbank Memorial Fund Quarterly/Health and Society, 62*(3), 475–519.

Veterans' Administration Cooperative Study Group on Anti-Hypertensive Agents. (1970). Effects of treatment on morbidity in hypertension. *JAMA: Journal of the American Medical Association, 213*, 1143–1152.

Vital Statistics of the United States, 1982. Life Tables Volume II, Section 6. (1985). Hyattsville, Maryland: National Center for Health Statistics.

Williams, A. F., & Lund, A. K. (1986). Seat belt use laws and occupant crash protection in the United States. *American Journal of Public Health, 76*, 1438–1442.

2. The Dynamics of Population Aging and Health

LOIS M. VERBRUGGE

INTRODUCTION

The recent decline in mortality rates among older persons in the United States and other developed countries is being called a mortality revolution.[1] That label reflects the surprise of demographers and public health scientists, who believed that mortality rates had reached a bottom point in the 1950s and 1960s and would not drop farther, given that no major changes in contemporary lifestyle and medical expertise were foreseeable. In tandem with the mortality drops, there have been gains in life expectancy, whether counted from birth onward or from some older age onward. What caused the truly sudden improvement, starting in 1968 (U.S.) and continuing since then, has been widely discussed. There is no absolutely definitive answer, but most scientists agree it came about, and continues, through a combination of three factors: drug control of hypertension starting in the early 1970s (the largest mortality gains are for cardiovascular and cerebrovascular diseases); sizable changes in nutrition, fitness, and personal health practices (especially smoking and alcohol consumption) in the 1960s and after; and better access to health services for all population groups.

Mortality is easy to measure because it is an event which occurs just once to a person, and because a standardized system for recording the event is in place (the death certificate and vital statistics program). Not so easy to measure is morbidity—the numerous acute and chronic problems that course through an individual's life, that remit or repeat, worsen or stand still, simply accumulate in number or interact synergistically. Morbidity influences physical and social functioning across days and years of life. And it ultimately influences the timing and cause of death.

Aging and Health: Linking Research and Public Policy, © 1989 Lewis Publishers, Inc., Chelsea, Michigan 48118. Printed in U.S.A.

Common sense tells us that morbidity and mortality are linked, on an individual basis and also in the aggregate (population basis). Typically, we think about the relationship in a "forward" manner: how changes in morbidity increase or decrease risks for individuals (or rates for populations) of mortality. But a reverse question has been raised in recent years: Does greater longevity for older people have a pernicious consequence on the population's health, increasing the number and percentage of very ill, frail people, who require protracted and expensive medical care and whose well-being is severely compromised? If so, is the price for more years of life too high for society, and also for many individuals?

In this chapter, I first lay out demographic information about *population aging* and why it is happening. Next, *recent mortality trends* are reviewed. Then, I discuss the evidence about *recent trends in population health,* drawn from real-world health surveys and also from formal theoretical work. Lastly, we look toward the future. How can we think sensibly about *health prospects* for future cohorts of older adults? What assumptions about how people and medicine behave lie behind several scenarios being discussed?

AN AGING POPULATION

Aging occurs when the percentage of people aged 65 and over steadily increases over time. (Other indicators of population aging exist, but this is the most common one.) The populations of developed countries have been aging throughout this century, so it is not a recent phenomenon. But the pace of aging increased in mid-century: From 1950–1980, the older population grew on average 2.4% per year in developed countries (less during the baby boom, more after) (Torrey, Kinsella, & Taeuber, 1987). In the realm of demography, that is a sizable growth rate. In the 1980s, the growth rate of the older population slowed a little in those countries because of low birth rates in World War I, thus, smallish cohorts (relative to others before them) were entering their older years. The pace is now picking up again. There are still more fluctuations ahead, which will mirror fertility patterns in the 20th century: Around the year 2000, there will be another dip in the aging pace due to low Depression era birth rates, and then another surge forward as the baby boom cohort arrives at age 65.

Thus, fertility peaks and troughs have echo effects through a society's age distribution for many years. They are not reflected perfectly at older ages, being muted because some deaths have occurred to a cohort's members before age 65. It is important to remember that, despite these fluctuations (some already behind, and some ahead) in growth *rates,* the older population will be growing *numerically* from one year to the next; the numbers will not diminish (Taeuber, 1983; Figure 1).

Many developing countries have also started to age (Torrey, Kinsella, &

Taeuber, 1987). Those with very rapid fertility declines, due to widespread use of modern contraception and abortion, are aging the fastest. This points to an important principle: *Fertility* is the main factor that influences age structure (Hermalin, 1966; Siegel & Davidson, 1984). Continuing high fertility rates bring in successively larger birth cohorts each year, creating a society with only a small percentage of elderly people. Protracted fertility declines have the opposite effect. And, short-term variations in fertility—5 to 10 years of unusually large or small birth cohorts—can promptly alter the relative size of age groups.

Mortality is a secondary factor. Mortality improvements are usually distributed across many age groups, so the relative size of age groups is not affected much. (There is variation to this theme: Mortality gains accrue somewhat more to children and youth in high mortality societies, and more to older adults in low mortality ones.) *Immigration* can also affect age structure, because typically young adults and their children are the newcomers; thus, immigration tends to damp aging processes. But since immigrant numbers are usually small relative to births and deaths, this is a minor factor in age-structure dynamics.

Through most of this century in developed countries, and currently in developing ones, aging has come about largely because of secular (long-term) fertility declines. But in the past two decades, mortality is taking a larger role, because the mortality gains have been concentrated at older ages. That is unprecedented in human history. And it fuels population aging with uncommon energy.

In sum, the forces behind the generally fast pace of aging in the late 20th century are both *distant* (unusual sizes of some birth cohorts during the century who now, or shortly, enter late life) and *proximate* (current low fertility rates and ongoing mortality declines focused at older ages). The current and projected percentages of older people (Figure 1) are the residue of powerful momentums of births and deaths.

Two oft-noted features of contemporary aging populations bear repeating: First, the older population is itself aging. In other words, the average age of persons 65 and over is increasing over time. Most striking is the numerical and percentage growth of the old-old (ages 85 and over). In the United States, they constituted 4% of the older population in 1920 and 9% in 1980, and this will rise markedly to 19% in 2040 (Taeuber, 1983). The social, cultural, and economic consequences of this *aging-within-aging* are immense: Boys and girls will have not only grandparents alive, but several great grandparents as well. The stretch of historical perspectives, the wealth of wisdom, and the persistence of political and moral opinions will grow in society. The costs of supporting society's older dependents will rise in proportion to other social expenditures, and the financial burden of illnesses of old age will rise dramatically.

Second, *feminization of the elderly* (increasing percent female) has been

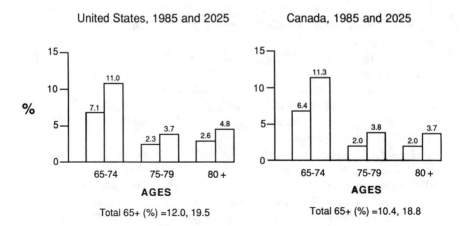

Figure 1. Aging of the total population, United States and Canada, 1985 and 2025. Percentage of population in older ages. (From Torrey, Kinsella, & Taeuber, 1987.)

occurring for many decades. Because of the persistent mortality gap between males and females, with generally higher mortality for males, the percent female tends to rise from one age group to the next. The sex mortality differential widened throughout the century, causing ever increasing disparity in the numbers of men and women at a given age. This phenomenon has its greatest expression at older ages, where the cumulative toll of mortality has removed notably more males than females. In the United States, females comprise 55% of the 65 and over age group, and 68% of the 80 and over age group (Torrey et al., 1987). In Canada, the corresponding figures are 54% and 65%. In coming years, the pace of feminization of the elderly will slow considerably, because the sex mortality differential has stabilized and may even narrow (i.e., relatively more improvement for males than females) and because of relatively few male deaths due to war for cohorts who will be entering older ages. But, now or 40 years from now, there will be a preponderance of older women, especially at the most advanced ages.

Will population aging stop? Yes, but neither abruptly nor soon. It is reasonable to assume that fertility rates in the United States will remain low (Westoff, 1986), and that mortality rates at older ages will continue to fall for some decades but then stabilize. Holding these rates constant for a long time will produce a "stable population," the demographic term for a population with a constant growth rate and fixed age structure. The latter feature means that aging (or any other age shift) ends. In real life, there are year-to-year variations in fertility and mortality, but if these are relatively small, a population will indeed approach a stable state.

Low and essentially stable fertility and mortality rates will likely be achieved sometime between 2000–2050. As this occurs, aging will slow down and eventually stop. By the end of the 21st century, the United States and other developed countries will be "aged," but not aging.

MORTALITY TRENDS

Life expectancy is a convenient summary of mortality rates in a given year. In the United States and other developed countries, increases in life expectancy at age 65 are now outpacing increases in life expectancy at birth (Table 1). That means the percentage gain in average remaining years is larger now for older adults than for newborns. For example, from 1950 to 1980 in the United States, life expectancy at age 85 rose 13% for males, compared to just 7% at birth. (In Table 1, look at the percentages in parentheses along a row. This compares change in life expectancy for different index ages, over the time interval.) This is exactly opposite to what happened for decades before 1950, when gains for children and young adults exceeded those for older people. Any future gains in mortality virtually *must* occur at older ages (Table 2). There is almost no room for improvement at other ages. For example, a person now age 20 who asks how many years of the next 25 (up to age 45) s/he can expect to live gets a remarkable answer: 24.4 for men, 24.8 for women. By contrast, someone age 65 asking about the next 20 years learns that the expectation is 12.8 for men, 15.5 for women (see also Crimmins, 1981, 1984; Fingerhut, 1982, 1984; Rosenwaike, 1985: Chap. 9).

Table 1. Life Expectancy at Birth and Older Ages, United States

	Years from Age x Onward People Can Expect to Live[a]			
	e_0	e_{65}	e_{75}	e_{85}
Male				
1900	46.4	11.3	6.8	3.7
	(41%)	(13)	(16)	(22)
1950	65.6	12.8	7.9	4.5
	(7)	(9)	(11)	(13)
1980	69.9	14.0	8.8	5.1
	(7)	(17)	(20)	(25)
2020	74.7	16.4	10.6	6.4
Female				
1900	49.0	12.0	7.2	4.0
	(45%)	(26)	(25)	(25)
1950	71.1	15.1	9.0	5.0
	(9)	(22)	(28)	(26)
1980	77.5	18.4	11.5	6.3
	(6)	(17)	(25)	(33)
2020	82.2	21.6	14.4	8.4

Source: Faber and Wade (1983).
[a]Shown in parentheses: Percent change in life expectancy at age x from earlier year to later year.

Table 2. Bounded Life Expectancy for Older and Young Adults, United States

	Years from Age 65 to 85, or from 20 to 45, People Can Expect to Live	
	e_{65-85}	e_{20-45}
Male		
1900	10.9	22.6
1950	11.9	24.3
1980	12.8	24.4
2020	14.1	24.5
Female		
1900	11.4	22.7
1950	13.6	24.6
1980	15.5	24.8
2020	16.7	24.8

Source: Olshansky and Ault (1986).

As life expectancy among older people increases, are they bumping up against some biological limits to life? After their newly added years of life, do they die swiftly in a small band of ages, rather than gradually leaving? This can be visualized, and answered, in Figure 2. It shows the distribution of ages at death for people 40 years old and over in three years: 1960 before the new mortality revolution, 1970 after it started, and 1980 in its midst. For both men and women (but easier to see for women), the distribution shifted to the right. This signals a change in timing, or average age, of death. There is no sign of reaching a limit; the distribution tapers off as before, and even stretches to more advanced ages at the far right for women. (If instead we saw a pronounced narrowing and peaking of the age band of deaths, and no sign of extension of ages at the far right, this would indicate "compression of mortality," or reaching a limit.) The female population is more important to watch than the male one on this issue, because women are closer to any intrinsic limit that may exist (see also Manton, 1982; Manton & Soldo, 1985; Myers & Manton, 1984a, 1984b; Olshansky & Ault, 1986.) In short, there has been a shift in timing of death, and no sound evidence that some maximum is being reached.

HEALTH TRENDS

Do more years of life mean more years of chronic illness, and of sensory and orthopedic impairments?

If the recent declines in mortality have come about by rescuing ill people from death (in other words, by reducing case fatality), then these survivors contribute prominently to measures of chronic disease prevalence and disability. The rescued people gain some time, but many are in a debilitated and

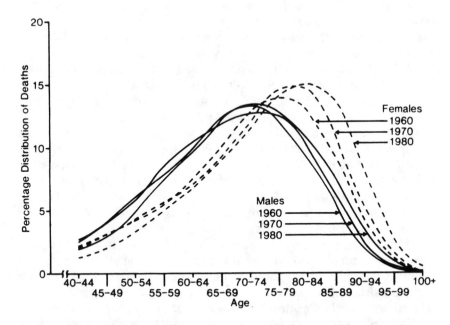

Figure 2. Shifting the age at death, United States, 1960–1980. Percentage distribution of deaths from all causes for the U.S. population aged 40 and over, by sex. (From Olshansky & Ault, 1986. Reprinted with permission of Milbank Memorial Fund.)

frail state. On the other hand, if recent mortality declines have come about because older people are healthier up-front, having prevented the onset of key killer diseases (in other words, by reducing disease incidence), then health of the older population should be improving. Smaller fractions of them should be in a perilous state. Because the skill of modern medicine lies in secondary and tertiary care (managing diseases after diagnosis and slowing their progression, and preventing death by heroic measures), and because recent lifestyle changes among older cohorts are more likely to have helped control diseases than prevent them entirely, it is widely believed that the mortality declines entail a greater social burden of illness. Ill people have been saved, rather than well people being rewarded by disease absence across their lifetimes.

What do the health data themselves tell us? Some scientists have turned to the U.S. National Health Interview Survey (NHIS), conducted continuously since 1957, for an answer. Consistently, they find evidence that short-term disability (days of cutting down regular activities and days in bed due to illness or injury) has increased for middle-aged and older people, largely since 1970 (Colvez & Blanchet, 1981; Verbrugge, 1984a; Ycas, 1987,

1988). The trends are bouncy, not smooth enough to make sense for some observers (Wilson & Drury, 1984), but strongly suggestive nonetheless to others. Measures of long-term disability also show pronounced increases among middle-aged men and women, and less obviously for older people (Baily, 1987; Chirikos, 1986; Feldman, 1983; and references just above). These rises occur at all levels of disability (complete limitation in major activity, partial limitation in same, limitation in secondary activities) (Rice & LaPlante, 1988). For older people, the sharpest rises are at mild levels.

Prevalence rates of specific diseases are not available for each year. But the sparse time series shows that morbidity has increased for most fatal diseases (leading causes of death such as diseases of heart, diabetes, cerebrovascular disease, and so on) and also for some prominent nonfatal diseases (especially arthritis and other musculoskeletal conditions) (Verbrugge, 1984a). Looking just at disabling diseases (this is an effort to control for severity), prevalence rates have also increased for many, including heart disease, hypertension, and arthritis (Feldman, 1983; Rice & LaPlante, 1986). Some people doubt these rises mean anything at all, citing changes in survey methodology and uncertain validity of self-reports. Still, the trends are so consistent across numerous diseases, they suggest that something quite general and socially important has occurred (see also Verbrugge, 1989).

What lies behind these signs of worsening health? Rapid mortality declines are certainly a candidate; many sick people have been rescued from early death. But other reasons figure as well: People are now more aware of their chronic diseases than before due to improved diagnostic techniques, more frequent visits to physicians (sharp rise in the 1960s, then leveling off), and more candor from physicians toward patients. This greater awareness leads to higher reporting in surveys and thus higher prevalence rates. (The higher rates are not "false" or artifactual, but actually truer than before.) Also, people may be more willing and able to adopt the sick role, both for short periods and long ones, than several decades ago. There are ampler social supports for disability, and public attitudes about long-term disability have become more gracious. Thus, increases in disease prevalence and disability rates can reflect these factors, as well as lowered mortality. Neither the data nor the explanations are completely surefooted. Still, the NHIS is virtually the best information we have, and shows quite consistent patterns of change toward worsening population health.

FORMAL MODELS OF MORTALITY AND FRAILTY

Let me end with the power of theory. Vaupel, Manton, and colleagues have developed a formal model of mortality which incorporates the notion of heterogeneity among individuals—simply put, that people vary in their robustness, or frailty (Manton, 1982; Vaupel, Manton, & Stallard, 1979).

More-frail individuals in a cohort die sooner, and over time the cohort contains individuals strongly selected for robustness; the selection is especially strong at older ages. When the force of mortality for the cohort is lowered, due to better medical care or improved lifestyles or fewer environmental hazards, the frailty of the cohort increases. This offsets gains of improved health; the offsetting effect is stronger at older ages than younger ones (Poterba & Summers, 1987). Stated as aphorism rather than formal model: " 'The rising tide lifts all ships equally', including those that might otherwise be resting at the bottom of the harbor" (Avorn, 1986).

The original model assumes that marginal survivors, once saved, are as likely to die as before; their individual frailty stays constant across life. But some scientists have noted the likelihood that rescued people not only have current illnesses, but also are especially susceptible to developing new ones. This additional feature, called insult accumulation, has been incorporated into the model (Alter & Riley, 1988). Whenever a person becomes ill, his/her frailty is elevated permanently; the more illnesses, the more one's susceptibility to death and further morbidity rises. Thus, marginal survivors, who suffer more illnesses, are in very special jeopardy. In sum, the models show the relations between declining mortality and increasing frailty explicitly and convincingly.

Frailty is a rather ethereal notion. The makers of formal models do not tell us where we will find the best indicators of frailty in medical or health survey data. Thus, although we can be absolutely sure that frailty has increased in the older population in the past few decades, we do not know exactly "where" it is to be found. This is a great challenge for population health surveys.

FUTURE HEALTH PROFILES

What can we say about future health of older adults—how levels of disease and disability of coming cohorts will differ from those of current cohorts?

Every forecast about future health makes some assumptions about predictors, the factors that drive population morbidity up or down. These assumptions, whether simple or sophisticated, must be explicit. Forecasts based on unspecified models and vague assumptions are prophecy; those springing from clear models and assumptions are science.

A CONCEPTUAL MODEL OF MORBIDITY AND DISABILITY

I shall lay out a rudimentary conceptual model for morbidity and disability, simply to guide our thinking about future health. Population health— past, present, or future—depends on six key causal factors:

1. *Genetic risks.* Populations with greater average intrinsic frailty are likely to manifest higher morbidity as well as reduced longevity.
2. *Personal behaviors and exposures* to violence and noxious environments that cause disease or impairment. The older a person is, the more such risks s/he has accumulated.
3. *Medical skill* in preventing, diagnosing, managing, and curing diseases, and in keeping people alive at the precipice of death. Modern medicine does best in diagnosis and all points beyond. Disease prevention is a lesser forte, largely because the key risk factors for most diseases are not well known.
4. Efficacy of *rehabilitation* techniques and special aids. These interventions aim at disability, not disease. Their purpose is to blunt disease impact without affecting disease process. They are a major aspect of chronic disease care.
5. *Social attitudes and economic incentives* about disease and disability. We know relatively little about historical changes in "sick role" attitudes in society, though there is wide consensus that people's predispositions for being disabled have changed in recent decades (that is, increasing acceptance of disability for oneself and others, and also greater incentives to become disabled).
6. *Age distribution* of the population. Older populations have a larger aggregate burden of illness, impairment, and dysfunction.

Is there a seventh cause: mortality changes? Mortality improvements do have immediate, and also perpetuating, *implications* for population morbidity, retaining ill people in the population who otherwise would have died. But, figuring out how they were rescued, why they were "healthy enough" to survive, brings us back to the six factors named above. In short, mortality changes are an outcome, not a cause, of morbidity changes.

The causal factors work their way into four aspects of population morbidity: *incidence* of diseases and impairments, their *duration,* their *severity,* and levels of *comorbidity.* Together, incidence and duration determine prevalence rates. This is shown schematically in Figure 3. The pool of *morbidity* at any point in time, represented by the ellipse, is composed of those four aspects. People exit from morbidity by *recovery* or *remission* or by *death.* When the first gateway widens (e.g., by lower disease incidence), population morbidity declines. It also declines when the second gateway widens by increased death rates. Statements about the exits that increase population morbidity can also be easily made.

Disability forms one section of morbidity; some ill or impaired people are disabled, and some are not. Disabled people can change their status by *restoring function* (back to morbidity alone) or *death.*

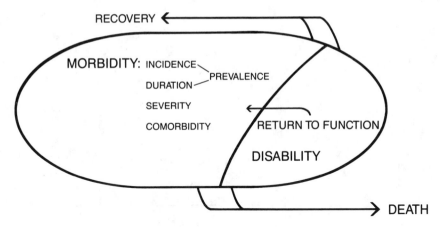

Figure 3. The pool of morbidity. (Modified from Johansson, 1987.)

APPLYING THE MODEL

Let us put this conceptual structure of causal factors and morbidity/disability/mortality outcomes to use. Various possible scenarios of future population health can be laid out if we make overt and sensible assumptions about the causal factors.

To envision changes, we use the device of survival curves (Figure 4). The horizontal axis is age, and the vertical one is the percentage of people (or the probability for an individual) of surviving the "event" to a given age. The events of interest are morbidity, disability, and mortality. Morbidity typically enters life first, disability later, and lastly, death.

The area under a curve represents years free of the event.[2] For U.S. females aged 70, the probability of being free of significant morbidity is about .65, and of having no significant disability, .83 (denominator for both is women alive at age 70) (Manton & Soldo, 1985). Of the initial birth cohort, chances of being alive at age 70 are about .75.

The curves can shift in shape over time. How do we interpret such shifts? The more a curve moves inward, the smaller the free zone becomes (meaning the sooner in life the unwanted event occurs). When a curve moves outward, that particular health or mortality situation becomes better. (The curves can tell us about incidence, duration, and prevalence, and also case fatality, but not about severity, comorbidity, and recovery or return to function. We must think through these last aspects without the benefits of a visual aid.)

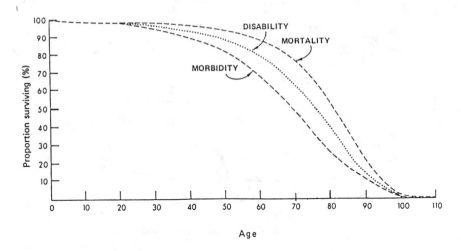

Figure 4. Survival curves for morbidity, disability, and mortality. Percentage surviving to given age without the event. (From Manton & Soldo, 1985. Reprinted with permission of Milbank Memorial Fund.)

THREE PREVENTION SCENARIOS

There are three basic (or "pure") futures, hinging on where disease prevention happens:

Tertiary Prevention

This is saving people at the brink of death by costly medical measures, either by maintaining basic life processes or by curing or averting fatal complications of certain diseases. Death is deterred without influencing the principal disease process. Tertiary prevention affects relatively few people in a population, so changes in the curves are slight. Population mortality improves just a little, while population morbidity and disability on average worsen just a little. In the diagram, the mortality curve stretches a bit to the right, and the other two curves to the left.

Progress in heroic medical care has occurred in the past few decades. Thus, the impact of tertiary prevention on morbidity and disability has already been felt; it is history more than future. Public and medical resistance to heroic care is increasing, and there may be a standstill in further development of ways to keep dying people alive.

Tertiary prevention is discussed with examples by Gruenberg (1977), and noted briefly in Kramer (1980).

Secondary Prevention

Controlling fatal chronic diseases so they advance less rapidly is a cardinal feature of contemporary medical care. People survive "better" (lower case fatality), but then have a disease more years of their lives. People are just as likely to acquire diseases in the first place—incidence does not change. As a consequence, disease and disability prevalences rise, because larger percentages of people are ill. But the symptoms and consequences are generally less severe than before. Comorbidity rates rise because people's longer lives give them more chance to develop diseases of all kinds. The more successful and widespread secondary prevention is, the more the mortality curve shifts outward, and the morbidity and disability curves inward.

This is the situation of "longer life but worsening health" for the population (Verbrugge, 1984a). We are certainly in the midst of this scenario now, with 20 years behind us and more to come. It has a strange but very important feature: Individual gains (less discomfort, less disability, longer life) are not paralleled in population health statistics, which show worsening on many dimensions.

What is happening to health and disability under conditions of chronic disease management is discussed in a number of articles (Brody, 1985; Brody, Brock, & Williams, 1987; Chapman, LaPlante, & Wilensky, 1986; Feldman, 1983; Manton, 1982, 1985; Schneider & Brody, 1983; Verbrugge, 1983, 1984a, 1984b).

Primary Prevention

Assume that striking changes in lifestyle and medicine have the marvelous outcome of reducing the clinical incidence of fatal diseases for most people. Incidence, duration, and prevalence rates of chief killers would fall rapidly. People who did become ill would typically have nonsevere cases, since what prevents onset deters progression as well. Comorbidity would diminish; as chances of each disease fall, so do chances of their co-occurrence. All three curves would shift outward, giving people more years free of morbidity, disability, and death.

The curves may be able to stretch outward for decades, but not forever. When the mortality curve approaches limits of maximum life expectancy and life span, then it will slow its outward motion. Continuing prevention behavior will then move the morbidity and disability curves closer to it, reducing the number of years spent between illness and death. This ultimate scenario, involving the "compression of morbidity," has been discussed by Fries (1980, 1983, 1984, 1987; Fries & Crapo, 1981).

Something very important has been forgotten in all of these scenarios: Concentrating on direct links between morbidity and mortality, and the fatal diseases that travel between them, the scenarios completely ignore *nonfatal conditions*. Where is arthritis, hearing impairment, or chronic low back pain? What is the future for such diseases and impairments? The most conservative view is to say that age-specific incidence of nonfatal conditions will remain constant in all scenarios, and that disability levels for them will also be constant. This especially affects the ebullient third scenario; people may remain free of fatal diseases, but they do acquire nonfatal conditions as readily as before. The outward stretching of morbidity and disability is drawn back somewhat, so a substantial gap remains between onset of morbidity-disability and death.

Furthermore, in all three scenarios, *population frailty* increases. Death becomes less selective, and intrinsically nonrobust people stay in the living population. It seems counterintuitive, but population frailty increases the least in Scenario 1 and most in Scenario 3. For Scenarios 1 and 2, increasing frailty puts additional inward pressure on disease-specific and disability curves. For Scenario 3, it damps any outward momentum of the morbidity-disability curves that may be happening. Whether it completely cancels or just partially reduces that momentum depends on the strength of health gains versus the increases in average frailty.

In all three scenarios, the most frail people do die sooner than the most robust, but the reasons begin to change. As diseases become less powerful propellers of death (from Scenarios 1 to 3), "natural aging" processes surface and become prominent. Increasingly, people will die from overall losses of physiologic reserve, and the frailest will do so sooner.

Which of the scenarios is right? They all are. Advances in tertiary, secondary, and primary prevention are occurring, though to different degrees. For example, recent decades have seen new techniques of resuscitation and life prolongation (Scenario 1), progress in surgery and drugs (2), and changes in lifestyle behaviors (3). At any given time, there are *mixed* forces acting to change morbidity, disability, and mortality.

The decades ahead hold not just one health future, but several futures sequenced in time. They will shift slowly from one to the next, as the three forces of prevention ascend and descend in absolute and relative importance. The *near future* will probably be much like the second scenario, with secondary prevention the lead actor. This will offer gains in mildness (disease progression and impact) but little change in incidence or comorbidity. Somewhat *later,* there may be an intermediate zone with powerful pushes from both medical control and primary prevention. We may then see larger proportions of older people in very poor health and vigorous health, thus, an increase at both poles of health. Secondary and primary prevention have compatible impact on the mortality curve, but competing impact on the morbidity and disability curves. It is hard to say how the average picture of illness and disability will shift. The *far future* may indeed entail delay of disease onset until near life's end for many people. But the compression of morbidity is not near at hand; it is too far off for any cohorts now alive to anticipate (see also Manton, 1987; Schneider & Brody, 1983; Schneider & Guralnik, 1987).

CONCLUSION

In coming decades, the dual forces of an *aging population* with *increasing morbidity, disability, and frailty among the elderly* will necessitate ample medical and home care services. But the per-person needs will probably decline; though there is a subgroup of very frail people, the majority of older people will have well-managed diseases. And on average, older individuals will be living more comfortable and functional lives as well as simply longer ones.

To see such changes in health statistics, surveys must monitor "minor" aspects of health (symptoms, botheration, changes in hobbies and other discretionary activities) as well as "major" ones, and private as well as public health behaviors. Only then will we be sure to track the full set of health trends that are individually and socially significant, rather than have them happen far from scientific and policy view.

ACKNOWLEDGMENT

Preparation of this chapter was facilitated by a Special Emphasis Research Career Award (K01 AG00394) to the author from the National Institute on Aging. Further discussion of health trends and futures appears in Verbrugge (1989).

NOTES

1. It is, in fact, a second or "new" mortality revolution. From the late 1800s to about 1950, the United States experienced a transition from high mortality rates to low ones. The declines that began in the late 1960s are fundamentally different from the earlier ones, occurring for chronic diseases and the older population. They signal a very different kind of demographic transition (Olshansky & Ault, 1986).
2. Where is the "pool of morbidity"? It sits above the morbidity curve and is bounded by the mortality curve. We are now focusing on the period before one enters that pool.

REFERENCES

Alter, G., & Riley, J. C. (1988). *Frailty, sickness, and death: Models of morbidity and mortality in historical populations.* Paper presented at the Population Association of America meetings. (Dept. of History, Indiana University, Bloomington, IN 47405)

Avorn, J. L. (1986). Medicine: The life and death of Oliver Shay. In A. Pifer & L. Bronte (Eds.), *Our aging society: Paradox and promise* (pp. 283–297). New York: W.W. Norton and Co.

Baily, M. N. (1987). Aging and the ability to work: Policy issues and recent trends. In G. Burtless (Ed.), *Work, health, and income among the elderly* (pp. 59–102). Washington, DC: The Brookings Institution.

Brody, J. A. (1985). Prospects for an aging population. *Nature, 315,* 463–466.

Brody, J. A., Brock, D. B., & Williams, T. F. (1987). Trends in the health of the elderly population. In L. Breslow, J. E. Fielding, & L. B. Lave (Eds.), *Annual review of public health* (Vol. 8, pp. 211–234). Palo Alto, CA: Annual Reviews Inc.

Chapman, S. H., LaPlante, M. P., & Wilensky, G. R. (1986). Life expectancy and health status of the aged. *Social Security Bulletin, 49*(10), 24–28.

Chirikos, T. N. (1986). Accounting for the historical rise in work-disability prevalence. *Milbank Quarterly, 64,* 271–301.

Colvez, A., & Blanchet, M. (1981). Disability trends in the United States population 1966–76: Analysis of reported causes. *American Journal of Public Health, 71,* 464–471.

Crimmins, E. M. (1981). The changing pattern of American mortality decline, 1940–77, and its implications for the future. *Population and Development Review, 71,* 229–254.

Crimmins, E. M. (1984). Life expectancy and the older population. *Research on Aging, 6,* 490–514.

Faber, J. F., & Wades, A. H. (1983). Life Tables for the United States: 1900–2050. *Actuarial Study* (No. 89). (SSA Publication No. 11–11536). Washington, DC: Social Security Administration, Office of the Actuary.

Feldman, J. J. (1983). Work ability of the aged under conditions of improving mortality. *Milbank Memorial Fund Quarterly/Health and Society, 61,* 430–444.

Fingerhut, L. A. (1982, 1984). Changes in mortality among the elderly: United States, 1940–78. *Vital and Health Statistics* (Series 3, No. 22 and 22a, Supplement). (DHHS Publication No. PHS 82–1406 and 84–1406a). Hyattsville, MD: National Center for Health Statistics.

Fries, J. F. (1980). Aging, natural death, and the compression of morbidity. *New England Journal of Medicine, 303,* 130–135.

Fries, J. F. (1983). The compression of morbidity. *Milbank Memorial Fund Quarterly/Health and Society, 61,* 397–419.

Fries, J. F. (1984). The compression of morbidity: Miscellaneous comments about a theme. *Gerontologist, 24,* 354–359.

Fries, J. F. (1987). An introduction to the compression of morbidity. Reduction of the national morbidity. *Gerontologica Perspecta, 1,* 5–8 and 54–64.

Fries, J. F., & Crapo, L. M. (1981). *Vitality and aging.* San Francisco, CA: W.H. Freeman and Co.

Gruenberg, E. M. (1977). The failures of success. *Milbank Memorial Fund Quarterly/Health and Society, 55,* 3–24.

Hermalin, A. I. (1966). The effect of changes in mortality rates on population growth and age distribution in the United States. *Milbank Memorial Fund Quarterly, 44,* 451–469.

Johansson, S. R. (1987). (Unpublished diagram used in presentation at the University of Michigan.)

Kramer, M. (1980). The rising pandemic of mental disorders and associated chronic diseases and disabilities. *Acta Psychiatrica Scandinavica, 62* (Supplement 285), 382–397.

Manton, K. G. (1982). Changing concepts of morbidity and mortality in the elderly population. *Milbank Memorial Fund Quarterly/Health and Society, 60,* 183–244.

Manton, K. G. (1985, November). Future patterns of chronic disease incidence, disability, and mortality among the elderly. *New York State Journal of Medicine,* 623–633.

Manton, K. G. (1987). Response to Fries, and to Schneider and Guralnik. *Gerontologica Perspecta, 1,* 23–30.

Manton, K. G., & Soldo, B. J. (1985). Dynamics of health changes in the oldest old. New perspectives and evidence. *Milbank Memorial Fund Quarterly/Health and Society, 63,* 206–285.

Myers, G. C., & Manton, K. G. (1984a). Compression of mortality: Myth or reality? *Gerontologist, 24,* 346–353.

Myers, G. C., & Manton, K. G. (1984b). Recent changes in the U.S. age at death distribution: Further observations. *Gerontologist, 24,* 572–575.

Olshansky, S. J., & Ault, A. B. (1986). The fourth stage of the epidemiologic transition: The age of delayed degenerative diseases. *Milbank Quarterly, 64,* 355–391.

Poterba, J. M., & Summers, L. H. (1987). Public policy implications of declining old-age mortality. In G. Burtless (Ed.), *Work, health, and income among the elderly* (pp. 19–58). Washington, DC: The Brookings Institution.

Rice, D. P., & LaPlante, M. P. (1986). *The burden of multiple chronic conditions: Past trends and policy implications.* Paper presented at the American Public Health Association meeting. (Institute for Health and Aging, University of California-San Francisco, San Francisco, CA 94143-0646)

Rice, D. P., & LaPlante, M. P. (1988). Chronic illness, disability, and increasing longevity. In S. Sullivan & M. E. Lewin (Eds.). *Ethics and economics of long-term care.* Washington, DC: American Enterprise Institute.

Rosenwaike, I. (1985). *The extreme aged in America.* Westport, CT: Greenwood Press.

Schneider, E. L., & Brody, J. A. (1983). Aging, natural death, and the compression of morbidity: Another view. *New England Journal of Medicine, 309,* 854–856.

Schneider, E. L., & Guralnik, J. M. (1987). The compression of morbidity: A dream which may come true, someday! *Gerontologica Perspecta, 1,* 8–14.

Siegel, J. S., & Davidson, M. (1984). Demographic and socioeconomic aspects of aging in the United States. *Current Population Reports* (Series P-23, No. 138). Washington, DC: U.S. Bureau of the Census.

Taeuber, C. M. (1983). America in transition: An aging society. *Current Population Reports* (Series P-23, No. 128). Washington, DC: U.S. Bureau of the Census.

Torrey, B. B., Kinsella, K., & Taeuber, C. M. (1987). An aging world. *International Population Reports* (Series P-95, No. 78). Washington, DC: U.S. Bureau of the Census.

Vaupel, J. W., Manton, K. G., & Stallard, E. (1979). The impact of heterogeneity in individual frailty on the dynamics of mortality. *Demography, 16,* 439–454.

Verbrugge, L. M. (1983). Women and men: Mortality and health of older people. In M. W. Riley, B. B. Hess, & K. Bond (Eds.), *Aging in society: Selected reviews of recent research* (pp. 139–174). Hillsdale, NJ: Lawrence Erlbaum Associates Inc.

Verbrugge, L. M. (1984a). Longer life but worsening health? Trends in health and mortality of middle-aged and older persons. *Milbank Memorial Fund Quarterly/Health and Society, 62,* 475–519.

Verbrugge, L. M. (1984b). A health profile of older women, with comparisons to older men. *Research on Aging, 6,* 291–322.

Verbrugge, L. M. (1989). Recent, present, and future health of American adults. In L. Breslow, J. E. Fielding, & L. B. Lave (Eds.). *Annual review of public health* (Vol. 10). Palo Alto, CA: Annual Reviews Inc.

Westoff, C. F. (1986). Fertility in the United States. *Science, 234,* 554–559.

Wilson, R. W., & Drury, T. F. (1984). Interpreting trends in illness and disability: Health statistics and health status. In L. Breslow, J. E. Fielding, & L. B. Lave (Eds.), *Annual review of public health* (Vol. 5, pp. 83–106). Palo Alto, CA: Annual Reviews Inc.

Ycas, M. A. (1987). Recent trends in health near the age of retirement: New findings from the Health Interview Survey. *Social Security Bulletin, 50*(2), 5–30.

Ycas, M. A. (1988). Are the eighties different? Continuity and change in the health of older persons. In *Proceedings of the 1987 Public Health Conference on Records and Statistics* (pp. 57–61). (DHHS Publication No. PHS 88–1214). Hyattsville, MD: National Center for Health Statistics.

3. *Hip Fracture Trends in Saskatchewan, 1972–1984*

ALAN D. MARTIN
KELLY G. SILVERTHORN
C. STUART HOUSTON
ANDRE WAJDA
LESLIE ROOS

INTRODUCTION

Osteoporosis is the progressive loss of bone with age to the extent that fractures may occur with little trauma. The most common fractures are those of the proximal femur (hip), distal radius (wrist), and vertebrae. These are observed predominantly but by no means exclusively in women, due in part to the rapid bone loss associated with the low-estrogen postmenopausal state. Wrist and vertebral fractures are seen in this middle-aged group, while hip fracture incidence dominates in the elderly (Cummings et al., 1985). While it is clear that osteoporosis is at epidemic proportions in many western countries, little is known about its incidence in Canada. Bone density measurements are costly and give limited information, thus fracture incidence is currently the best indicator of the prevalence of osteoporosis. We have selected hip fracture because it is the most serious and costly manifestation of osteoporosis, and virtually all cases require a lengthy hospital stay and will therefore be found in hospital records. We have used hospital discharge data from the Saskatchewan Hospital Services Plan (SHSP) over the period 1972 to 1984 to investigate two general questions: What is the incidence of hip fractures in the province of Saskatchewan by age and sex? How is this incidence changing with time?

Aging and Health: Linking Research and Public Policy, © 1989 Lewis Publishers, Inc., Chelsea, Michigan 48118. Printed in U.S.A.

METHODS

After a three-month residence period, all those living in the Canadian province of Saskatchewan are covered without premiums by a comprehensive provincial health care plan. We obtained computerized data on hospitalizations for hip fracture from SHSP. Hip fracture cases from 1972 through 1984 were identified from diagnosis codes. Estimated date of fracture was calculated as discharge date minus length of hospital stay. Associated data included sex, date of birth, and residential region. Data from 1985 were used to ensure inclusion of all patients who were discharged in 1985 but whose fractures occurred in 1984. We minimized case duplication arising from hospital transfers by excluding any case within seven days following a prior diagnosis for that individual. Fractures in those under 50 years of age were excluded as nonosteoporotic.

In addition to hospital records, SHSP has comprehensive demographic data on the covered population. We obtained annual midyear population broken down by sex and 5-year age groups. These were used to calculate sex- and age-specific incidences for each year from 1972 to 1984.

RESULTS

The population of Saskatchewan in 1972 was 934,607, of which 233,196 were age 50 years and over. In 1984, the last year of the study period, the total population had risen to 1,028,965, a 10.1% increase, while the number of men and women 50 years old and over had risen by 7.6% and 17.8%, respectively. These increases were not uniform across the 5-year age groups (Figure 1). Women showed greater increases than men, peaking in the 90 and over age group, which almost doubled from the 1972 population. The number of hip fractures occurring in 1984 would thus be expected to be substantially greater than in 1972 based on these changes in the population age distribution. Hip fractures in those aged 50 and over increased from 146 for men and 353 for women in 1972 to 252 and 627 respectively, and in 1984, increases of 72.6% and 77.6% respectively (Figure 2).

The percentage increase over the study period was calculated for each 5-year age group, then compared to the percentage increase in the population of that age group (Figures 3 and 4). In virtually all age groups and for each sex, the hip fracture increases were greater than would be expected from the observed changes in population age distribution alone.

This result was examined more closely by calculating the incidence of fractures within each 5-year group for each year of the study. These age-specific fracture rates, calculated per 1000 population for each 5-year age group, for men and women, are shown in Figures 5 and 6. An increasing trend can be seen clearly in each age group.

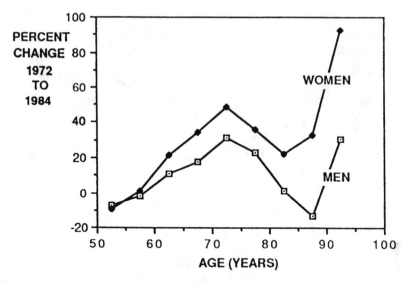

Figure 1. Percent change in Saskatchewan population by 5-year age groups, 1972–1984.

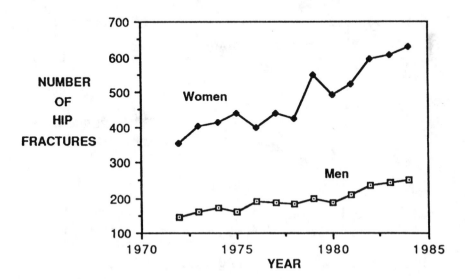

Figure 2. Crude rate of hip fractures in Saskatchewan, 1972-1984.

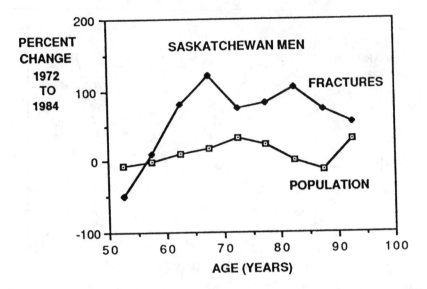

Figure 3. Percent change in population and crude rate of hip fractures by 5-year age groups, 1972–1984, Saskatchewan men.

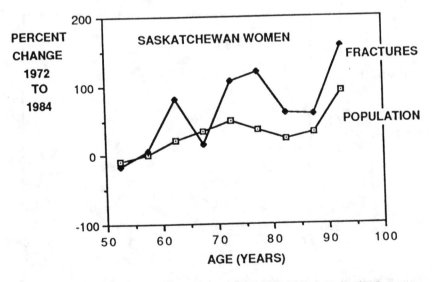

Figure 4. Percent change in population and crude rate of hip fractures by 5-year age groups, 1972–1984, Saskatchewan women.

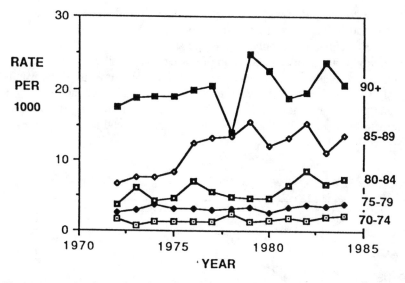

Figure 5. Age-specific hip fracture rates, 1972–1984, Saskatchewan men.

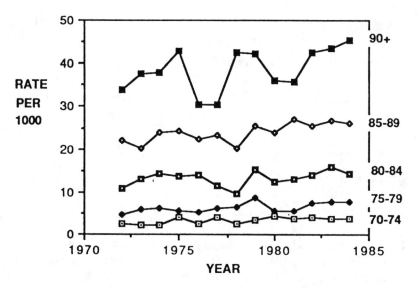

Figure 6. Age-specific hip fracture rates, 1972–1984, Saskatchewan women.

In order to compare incidence in populations with different age-specific rates for each 5-year age group, epidemiologists use age-adjusted values. These are calculated by applying the age-specific rates for the population under study to a reference population of known age distribution. In this way a single value is arrived at for each sex and year. We have used the Manitoba, 1984, population as the reference. Annual age-adjusted incidences for men and women are shown in Figure 7. Again, a clear increasing trend can be seen in both sexes, with a 53.6% increase in men and a 28.7% increase in women from 1972 to 1984.

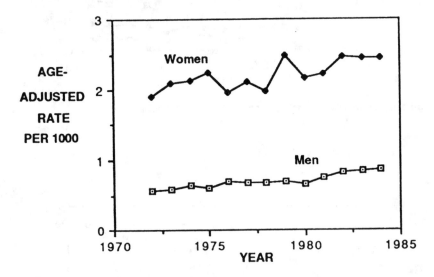

Figure 7. Age-adjusted hip fracture rate, 1972–1984 (adjusted to the Manitoba 1984 population).

DISCUSSION

Changes in Age-Specific Rates

Population changes in Saskatchewan have followed the general trend observed in western countries toward an increasing proportion of the elderly. This has important implications for those planning health care services. Osteoporotic fractures, already at an epidemic level, occur almost exclusively in those over 50 years of age. Hip fractures, the most serious and costly manifestation of osteoporosis, occur in the largest numbers in those over 75 years of age, a rapidly increasing segment of the population. Thus on the basis of population changes alone, hip fracture rates would be expected to increase substantially over the study period and should continue to increase in keeping with population age trends. In Saskatchewan, the fracture rate increased 75% from 1972 to 1984, an average of 5.6% per year, while the increase in the numbers of men and women over 50 years of age averaged only about 1% per year. When we examined the percentage growth of populations of separate 5-year age groups in relation to the percentage increase in fracture rates within each group (Figures 3 and 4), more fractures were found in 1984 for almost every age group, in men as well as in women, than could be explained by population age changes.

The age-specific rates (Figures 5 and 6) confirmed this. Despite the year-to-year variability, age-specific rates showed an increasing trend throughout the study period. This confirms reports from Scandinavia (Nilsson & Obrant, 1978; Zetterberg & Andersson, 1982) and Britain (Lewis, 1981; Wallace, 1983; Swanson & Murdoch, 1983) of rising age-specific rates in Western Europe and provides the clearest evidence to date that this phenomenon also occurs in North America. The Rochester, Minnesota study at first reported unchanging age-specific rates (Melton et al., 1982), but a recent reanalysis of their data suggested that age-specific rates in men, but not in women, were increasing (Melton, O'Fallon, & Riggs, 1987). Their study, with only 1701 hip fractures spread over more than 50 years, may not have been sensitive enough to detect the trends we have observed in Saskatchewan, with 7965 fractures over 13 years. In studies of this kind, population size is an important factor, because the total number of fractures must be broken down by year, sex, and 5-year age group; some age groups might have insufficient fractures for a trend to be observed.

The age-adjusted rates in Saskatchewan (adjusted to the Manitoba, 1984 population) reached values close to 2.5 per 1000 women over 50 years of age. For men over 50 years of age, the age-adjusted rate was close to 0.85, about one-third of the women's rate.

Mortality, Costs, and Projections

Hip fractures typically require a 21-day hospital stay, though this increases with the age of the patient. In-hospital mortality is high and also increases with age (particularly after age 70), reaching 22.8% for men 95 years of age and 15.7% for women of similar age (Figure 8). Mortality for men is higher than for women at all ages. Our data did not permit analysis of mortality after hospital discharge.

The lengthy hospital stay makes hip fracture the most expensive manifestation of osteoporosis. Reports on several Canadian hospitals summarized by Narod and Spasoff (1986) show a range of $5,000.00 to $9,465.00 in 1983/1984 Canadian dollars for acute care costs.

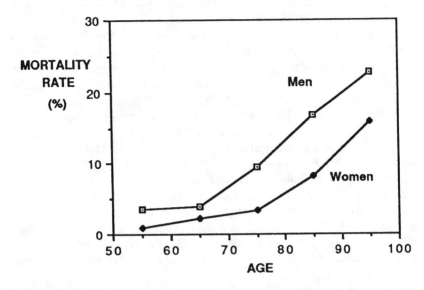

Figure 8. In-hospital mortality rates from hip fracture, by 5-year age groups, Saskatchewan, 1972–1984.

Statistics Canada's projection of percentage increases in each of the 5-year age groups over the period 1987 to 2006 are shown in Figure 9. These are particularly significant for hip fracture trends, because the greatest increases (80% to 125%) are seen in those over 80 years of age, where more than half of all hip fractures occur. The number of hip fractures in Canada in the years 1987 to 2006 can be estimated by applying the age-specific rates from Saskatchewan, 1984, to the projected Canadian populations for those two years. On this basis we have estimated that in 1987 there were 19,372 hip fractures in Canada of which 4,842 (25%) were in men and 14,530 (75%) in women. The projected total for 2006 is 33,795. The increases over the 20-year period from 1987 to 2006 are 69% for men and 76% for women.

These projections assume that the age-specific rates for Canada will remain the same as those for Saskatchewan in 1984. However, we have already observed a steady increase in these rates over the years 1972 to 1984. A second, more speculative approach, is to linearly project the age-specific rates as well as the population's age distribution. This assumption, that the trend in age-specific rates will continue at the same rate, results in estimations for Canada of 12,874 hip fractures in men and 34,035 in women in the year 2006, for a total of 46,909.

Despite previous reports of an increasing trend in the age-specific rates of hip fractures (Jensen, 1980; Johnell et al., 1984; Boyce & Vessey, 1985), there has only been speculation as to the causes. These include secular trends

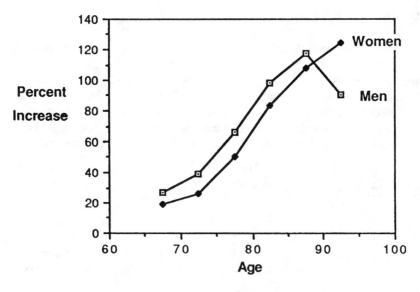

Figure 9. Projected percent increase in the Canadian population, by 5-year age groups, 1987–2006.

in calcium consumption or absorption, physical activity, tobacco or alcohol consumption, and hormonal changes such as those related to earlier meno-pause (Melton et al., 1987). It is also possible that increasing use of drugs in the elderly may result in more frequent falls. Any explanation should take into account that the increases seem to be more marked in men than in women, since age-adjusted rates in Saskatchewan increased almost twice as fast in men as in women from 1972 to 1984 (Figure 7).

CONCLUSIONS

The data reported here have important implications for those responsible for health care planning. Our projections based on Statistics Canada's popu-lation projections should be reasonably accurate, since all those who will suffer an osteoporotic hip fracture in the year 2006 have already been born. Assuming no change in age-specific rates from the Saskatchewan 1984 val-ues, the 69% (men) and 76% (women) increases in hip fractures from 1987 could seriously overburden hospital resources. If, as is also possible, age-specific rates continue to increase and trends for Canada as a whole are similar to those observed in Saskatchewan, 47,000 fractures are projected annually by the year 2006, almost 2.5 times the 1987 total.

ACKNOWLEDGMENT

The authors gratefully acknowledge the help of the Saskatchewan Hospital Services Plan, the Manitoba Health Services Commission, and the Saskatchewan Health Research Board. Research was supported in part by National Health Research and Development Project No. 6607–1197–44 and by Career Scientist Award No. 6607-1314–48 (L. L. Roos). Interpretations and viewpoints contained in this chapter are the authors' own and do not necessarily represent the opinion of any of the supporting agencies.

REFERENCES

Boyce, W. J., & Vessey, M. P. (1985). Rising incidence of fracture of the proximal femur. *Lancet, 1,* 150–151.

Cummings, S. R., Kelsey, J. L., Nevitt, M. C., & O'Dowd, K. J. (1985). Epidemiology of osteoporosis and osteoporotic fractures. *Epidemiology Review, 7,* 178–208.

Jensen, J. S. (1980). Incidence of hip fractures. *Acta Orthopaedica Scandinavica, 51,* 511–513.

Johnell, O., Nilsson, B., Obrant, K., et al. (1984). Age and sex patterns of hip fractures—changes in 30 years. *Acta Orthopaedica Scandinavica, 55,* 290–292.

Lewis, A. F. (1981). Fracture of neck of the femur: Changing incidence. *British Medical Journal, 283,* 1217–1220.

Melton, L. J., Ilstrup, D. M., Riggs, B. L., et al. (1982). Fifty year trend in hip fracture incidence. *Clinical Orthopaedics and Related Research, 162,* 144–149.

Melton, L. J., O'Fallon, W. M., & Riggs, B. L., (1987). Secular trends in the incidence of hip fractures. *Calcified Tissue International, 41,* 57–64.

Narod, S., & Spasoff, R. A. (1986). Economic and social burden of osteoporosis. In H. K. Uhtoff (Ed.), *Current concepts of bone fragility* (pp. 391–402). New York: Springer-Verlag.

Nilsson, B. E., & Obrant, K. J. (1978). Secular tendencies of the incidence of fracture of the upper end of the femur. *Acta Orthopaedica Scandinavica, 49,* 389–391.

Swanson, A. J. G., & Murdoch, G. (1983). Fractured neck of femur: Pattern of incidence and implications. *Acta Orthopaedica Scandinavica, 54,* 348–355.

Wallace, W. A. (1983). The increasing incidence of fractures of the proximal femur: An orthopaedic epidemic. *Lancet, 1,* 1413–1414.

Zetterberg, C., & Andersson, G. B. (1982). Fractures of the proximal end of the femur in Göteborg, Sweden, 1940–1979. *Acta Orthopaedica Scandinavica, 53,* 419–426.

4. *Late Onset Rheumatoid Arthritis*

DONALD M. MITCHELL†
PAT I. KRUTZEN
JOHN T. SIBLEY

INTRODUCTION

Rheumatoid arthritis (RA) is a common disorder in adults, affecting 1.5% of females and 0.75% of males. The disease frequently causes serious disability and shortened survival (Mitchell et al., 1986). Peak onset is from age 30 to 50 years and RA arising in the elderly was once thought to be uncommon and mild. We examined a large cohort of RA patients to determine the incidence and health consequences of late onset RA.

PATIENTS AND METHODS

Between 1966 and 1974, a cohort of 912 consecutive patients was entered into a prospective study at the University of Saskatchewan Rheumatic Disease Unit and followed long-term. All patients had definite or classic RA (Ropes et al., 1958). As of early 1988, mean follow-up of patients was 13.6 years. For the purpose of this study, the cohort was divided into late onset (age 60 years or older) and early onset (age less than 60 years) RA. All comparisons were made using a two-tailed Student's t-test or a chi-square test.

---

† Shortly after CONNECTIONS '88 we were saddened to learn of the untimely death of Dr. Don Mitchell, an honored friend and colleague to the research and clinical communities in Saskatchewan and elsewhere. Dr. Mitchell was unable to present his paper at the conference, and in his stead his co-author, Mrs. Pat Krutzen, ably presented their findings; she is listed at the end of this volume as the contributor to whom any correspondence should be addressed.

RESULTS

Mean age of onset of RA in all patients was 41.6 years. In 101 (11%) patients, disease onset occurred at or after age 60. The features of patients at entry into the study are shown in Table 1. Patients with late onset RA presented to a rheumatologist after shorter disease duration (3.8 vs 10.6 years, $p \leq 0.001$). However, despite the shorter disease duration, the late onset group had equal disability as defined by the American Rheumatism Association (ARA) Functional Class III (patient limited to few or no activities or self-care) and Functional Class IV (patient largely incapacitated, bedridden or confined to wheelchair and has little or no self-care) (Steinbrocker, Traeger, & Batterman, 1949). In addition, the late onset group presented with a greater number of active (i.e., swollen, tender) joints and a higher Lansbury clinical index, a composite measurement of disease activity (Lansbury, 1958).

Table 1. Features at Entry

	Early Onset n = 811) <60 yr	Late Onset (n = 101) ≥60 yr
Female (%)	63	68
Disease duration (yr)	10.6	3.8***
ARA criteria (#)	6.5	6.8
Active joints (#)	13.7	15.8*
Lansbury index	69	77 *
Ara Functional Class III–IV (%)	10.6	12.8

Note: ARA = American Rheumatism Association.
  *p < 0.05.
***p < 0.001.

Table 2 shows that a similar proportion of patients in both groups were rheumatoid factor positive and developed joint erosions. Fewer late onset RA patients developed rheumatoid nodules (34% vs 59%, $p \leq 0.001$), but this may simply reflect the shorter disease duration and follow-up in the late onset group. Despite this shorter disease duration, a similar proportion of patients in both groups (>50%) developed disability. In spite of the high proportion of disabled patients in both groups, significantly fewer late onset patients were treated with remittive agents (31.3% vs 62.9%, $p < 0.001$).

Table 3 reveals that disability occurred after much shorter disease duration in late onset patients (3.7 vs 11.9 years, $p \leq 0.001$), despite similar low incidence of serious comorbid diseases in both groups at the time disability first developed (Table 4). The majority (94%) in both groups had no apparent reason for disability other than RA. Death occurred a mean of 9.5 years after

Table 2. Features During Course

	Early Onset n = 811) <60 yr	Late Onset (n = 101) ≥60 yr
Disease duration (last visit %)	24.8	12.8***
Follow-up (yr)	14.2	9.0***
Rheumatoid nodules (%)	59	34 ***
Rheumatoid factor positive (%)	90	90
Joint erosions present (%)	89	81
ARA Stage III & IV (last visit %)	73.5	48.3***
ARA Functional Class III & IV (%)	56.8	51.0

Note: ARA = American Rheumatism Association.
***p < 0.001.

Table 3. Features of Patients with Functional Class III & IV

	Early Onset (n = 461) <60 yr	Late Onset (n = 52) ≥60 yr
Age at initial disability (yr)	50.6	70.7***
Disease duration to disability (yr)	11.9	3.7***
Death (%)	40.9	60.7***
Age at death (yr)	67.0	80.2***

Note: Approximately 50% in each group developed disability.
*** p < 0.001.

Table 4. Possible Contributing Comorbid Diseases to Initial Disability

	Early Onset (n = 466) <60 yr	Late Onset (n = 51) ≥60 yr
Cardiovascular (%)	0.8	1.9
Pulmonary (%)	3.0	3.9
Neurologic (%)	0.4	—
Psychiatric (%)	0.6	—
Cancer (%)	0.4	—
Fractures (%)	0.4	—
Total (%)	5.6	5.8

the development of disability in late onset RA and 17 years after the development of disability in early onset RA.

DISCUSSION

RA is a common disease in the elderly. In addition, because of the chronic nature of RA, there is an inevitable accumulation in the elderly. That RA can cause significant disability was confirmed in the present study. Late onset patients developed disability at a substantially faster rate than early onset counterparts. Despite the apparent aggressiveness of the disease, the late onset RA patients lived an average of 9.5 years after the onset of their disability. Thus, not only is disability common, it is prolonged and it appears that late onset RA is poorly tolerated.

The late onset of disease appears to be an important risk factor for the rapid onset of disability in RA. Thus, even though the elderly may be at increased risk of toxicity from antirheumatic drugs, including nonsteroidal antiinflammatory drugs, remittive agents, and corticosteroids (Collier & Pain, 1985; Kean, 1982), patients with late onset RA may be candidates for more, not less, aggressive therapy. However, in the present study significantly fewer patients received remittive agents (such as gold therapy). The explanation for this is not clear, but it may in part reflect some bias in the way the attending rheumatologists viewed the needs and therapeutic concerns in these patients. In light of the devastating functional impact of RA in the elderly, the potential risk-benefit ratio of all available therapy must be reassessed. As well, awareness of the rapid development of disability in late onset RA is crucial when considering health care policy decisions for this age group.

REFERENCES

Collier, D. St. J., & Pain, J. A. (1985). Non-steroidal anti-inflammatory drugs and peptic ulcer perforation. *Gut, 26,* 359–363.

Kean, W. F. (1982). Efficacy and toxicity of d-penicillamine for rheumatoid disease in the elderly. *Journal of the American Geriatrics Society, 30,* 94–100.

Lansbury, J. (1958). Report of a three-year study in the systemic and articular indexes in rheumatoid arthritis—theoretical and clinical considerations. *Arthritis and Rheumatism, 2,* 505–522.

Mitchell, D. M., Spitz, P. W., Young, D. Y., et al. (1986). Survival, prognosis and causes of death in rheumatic arthritis. *Arthritis and Rheumatism, 29,* 706–714.

Ropes, M. W., Bennett, G. A., Cobbs, et al. (1958). 1958 revision of diagnostic criteria for rheumatoid arthritis. *Bulletin of the Rheumatic Diseases, 9,* 175–176.

Steinbrocker, O., Traeger, C. H., & Batterman, R. C. (1949). Therapeutic criteria in rheumatoid arthritis. *JAMA: Journal of the American Medical Association, 140,* 659–662.

5. Hospital Utilization by Elderly Rheumatoid Arthritis Patients

JOHN T. SIBLEY
KENNETH L. N. BLOCKA

INTRODUCTION

Rheumatoid arthritis (RA) is a common disorder that may affect up to 1–2% of the adult population. It is a disease with profound health implications in a significant majority of patients who are faced with the prospect of increasing disability, frequent hospitalizations, and decreased life expectancy (Mitchell et al., 1986; Wolfe et al., 1986). RA was once regarded as uncommon in the elderly; however, approximately 11% of new cases arise after age 60 (Mitchell, Krutzen, & Sibley, 1989). Moreover, because of its chronic nature, there is a natural accumulation of RA in the elderly. We examined our RA population to determine whether there are differences in the hospitalization pattern between the elderly (age 65 or older) and nonelderly (age less than 65), looking in particular for any possible differences in admission rates, reasons for admission, and length of stay.

PATIENTS AND METHODS

Our Rheumatic Disease Unit (RDU) represents a four-physician university-based rheumatology practice. To determine our RA population base, and therefore the population at risk for admission to hospital, we reviewed the diagnoses of all outpatients seen in the rheumatology clinic from June 1985 to December 1986. Since it is our practice to reassess RA patients at least every six months, we felt that an 18-month survey would miss very few RA patients followed in our RDU.

The charts of all RA patients admitted to hospital under the rheumatology service from January 1986 to December 1986 were then reviewed and clinical and laboratory data of the elderly and nonelderly compared. In the nonelderly group, three patients were admitted twice and one patient admitted three times during the study period. For purposes of analysis, data from only the first admissions of these patients were used. Patients admitted for a concurrent, unrelated clinical study were excluded from analysis. All comparisons were based on either a two-tailed Student's t-test or a chi-square test.

RESULTS

From June 1985 to December 1986, 747 different RA patients were seen at least once in the rheumatology outpatient clinic. In 1986, there were 107 RA admissions to hospital under the rheumatology service, all of whom had attended the rheumatology outpatient clinic at least once within six months prior to admission. As seen in Table 1, the mean age was older in patients admitted to hospital than for patients seen in the outpatient clinic and a higher than expected proportion of patients admitted were age 65 or older.

Table 1. Rheumatoid Arthritis Population

	Outpatient (June/85–Dec/86)	Inpatient (Jan/86–Dec/86)
Patient number	747	107
Mean age (yr)	55.2	58.2*
Patients ≥ 65 yr (%)	31	39 *

*p < 0.05.

Among those patients admitted to hospital, mean age was 72.4 (range 65–88) for the elderly and 48.1 (range 24–64) for the nonelderly. Average duration of RA was longer in the elderly (18.4 vs 10.3 years, p < 0.01), as was average length of follow-up in the RDU (11.7 vs 5.6 years, p < 0.001). As one might expect, the elderly averaged more previous admissions to hospital under the rheumatology service (3.6 vs 1.5 admissions), although this difference did not reach statistical significance. However, when the number of previous admissions was corrected for duration of RA, the elderly averaged significantly fewer admissions per year of disease (0.39 vs 0.68, p < 0.05). There were few differences on admission in laboratory findings or in the use of antirheumatic drugs in the two groups (Table 2).

The major indication for admission in both groups—approximately 70% of cases—was therapy of the underlying disease (Table 3), generally physiotherapy, occupational therapy, and adjustment of drug regimens. In the eld-

Table 2.   RA Admissions—Entry Data

	Age <65 yr (n = 65)	Age ≥65 yr (n = 42)
NSAID[a] use (%)	76	78
DMARD[b] use		
Entry (%)	80	88
Ever (%)	63	45
Prednisone use (%)	36	50
Hb (gm/L)	113	111
WBC (cells/mm³)	7,100	7,000
Platelets (cells/mm³)	374,000	371,000
ESR (mm/hr)	50	70**
RF positive[c] (%)	87	95

[a]Nonsteroidal antiinflammatory drugs.
[b]Disease modifying antirheumatic drugs.
[c]Serum rheumatoid factor, latex agglutination titer >1/80.
** $p < 0.01$.

erly, all but two other admissions were for complications arising from RA (e.g., vasculitic skin ulcers) or from the therapy of RA (e.g., drug-induced peptic ulcer disease). In contrast, in the nonelderly only six admissions (9.2%) were for medical problems secondary to RA or RA therapy, whereas 11 (16.9%) were for unrelated medical problems (e.g., nonvasculitic cardio-vascular disease, $p < 0.05$). The average length of stay was significantly longer in the elderly (Table 3). Moreover, none of the elderly, but 24.6% of the nonelderly patients were admitted to our minimal supervision ward, the Hostel Unit ($p < 0.001$).

The Hostel Unit is in the main hospital building. It is available for admissions from all medical and surgical services. Coverage under universal provincial government medical insurance is identical to that of patients admitted to the regular hospital ward, but Hostel Unit patients must be independent.

Table 3.   RA Admissions—Entry Criteria and Hospital Course

	Age <65 yr (n = 65)	Age ≥65 yr (n = 42)
Reason for admission (%)		
RA therapy	76.9	66.7
Complication of disease or therapy	6.2	28.5
Other	16.9	4.7*
Mean length of stay (days)		
(RA therapy only)	16.2	20.9*
Hostel unit admission (%)		
(RA therapy only)	24.6	0 ***

* $p < 0.05$.
*** $p < 0.001$.

There is no nursing service available. Prescribed medications are paid for, but the patients are responsible for self-administration. Meals are paid for, but eaten in the hospital staff cafeteria (approximately 100 meters from the patients' rooms). Similarly, patients are responsible for getting to the correct hospital location for services such as physiotherapy, phlebotomy, and radiology. The regular hospital rheumatology ward is shared by cardiology and nephrology patients. Staff coverage for the Hostel Unit and regular hospital ward is outlined in Table 4.

Table 4. Personnel Cost in Hours per Patient per Week in the Hostel Unit and Hospital Rheumatology Ward

Hostel unit (32 beds)		
Ward clerk	168 hr	
Housekeeping	40	
Food services	20	
	228 hr	→ 7.1 hr/patient/wk
Hospital ward (35 beds)		
Ward clerk	80.75 hr	
Housekeeping	40	
Unit manager[a]	40	
Unit coordinator[a]	40	
Ward nurses[a]	570	
Nurse assistants	168	
Ward aide	84	
Food services	96	
	1118.75 hr	→ 31.9 hr/patient/wk

[a]Registered nurses.

Note: Both groups of patients were felt to have equal access to and use of services such as physiotherapy, occupational therapy, phlebotomy, diagnostic laboratory, pharmacy, and physicians. In determining cost per patient, full occupancy was assumed.

DISCUSSION

Although the peak onset of RA occurs between ages 30 and 50, a substantial proportion of cases (11%) begin after age 60. Because of the chronic nature of this disorder, the prevalence of RA typically increases in the elderly. As well, RA is poorly tolerated by the elderly, and many become disabled very quickly following their diagnosis, independent of any comorbid diseases (Mitchell et al., 1989). In the present study, the elderly were overrepresented among admissions to the rheumatology service, suggesting that age and disease duration are risk factors for hospitalization in RA. When corrected for disease duration, the elderly averaged significantly fewer admissions per year of disease. That is, although the nonelderly as a group averaged fewer admissions, of those patients who are hospitalized, it is the nonelderly who are admitted more frequently. Thus, previous admission to a rheumatology service appears to represent a more significant risk factor for subsequent admission in the nonelderly than in the elderly.

Although a similar proportion of patients in both groups were admitted primarily for therapy of joint symptoms, admissions for complications arising from the disease or its therapy accounted for 28.5% of admissions in the elderly but only 6.2% in the nonelderly. This may suggest that the elderly tolerate RA less well, and may be more susceptible to complications arising from the disease or its treatment.

In an attempt to compare homogeneous populations for length-of-stay analysis, only data from those patients admitted for therapy of joint symptoms were used. Not only was the average length of stay longer for the elderly (20.9 vs 16.2 days, $p < 0.02$), but no elderly patients were admitted to the Hostel Unit. It is not clear from this study whether this finding reflects the increased morbidity that RA imposes on the elderly, or whether there may also be some bias in how the four rheumatologists view the needs of the elderly RA patient. Regardless of the causes for the differences in disposition and length of stay of the elderly, the economic costs are profound and bear scrutiny. As is seen in Table 4, the regular hospital ward is labor intensive and therefore costly. This cost would perhaps be reduced by having specialized nursing units for more homogeneous patient populations. For example, RA patients would generally not require the same intensity of nursing care as would patients with cardiac, renal, or other serious medical illnesses. As well, where units with differing levels of care are available (as with our regular hospital ward and Hostel Unit), entry and exclusion criteria for those units should be defined to assist in appropriate placement of patients. Finally, outcome criteria are necessary in order to follow the day-to-day patient progress and to ensure an optimum length of hospital stay. These concerns apply to all RA patients, but particularly to the elderly with their increased health service requirements.

REFERENCES

Mitchell, D. M., Krutzen, P. I., & Sibley, J. T. (1989). Late onset rheumatoid arthritis. In this volume, Chapter 4.

Mitchell, D. M., Spitz, P. W., Young, D. Y., et al. (1986). Survival, prognosis and causes of death in rheumatoid arthritis. *Arthritis and Rheumatism, 29,* 706–714.

Wolfe, F., Kleinheksel, S. M., Spitz, P. W., et al. (1986). A multicenter study of hospitalization in rheumatoid arthritis: Frequency, medical-surgical admissions and charges. *Arthritis and Rheumatism, 29,* 614–619.

6. Alzheimer's Disease: Research and Public Policy

IRMA M. PARHAD
GINA ROHS

BIOMEDICAL ASPECTS OF ALZHEIMER'S DISEASE

Alzheimer's disease (AD) is the most common form of dementia in the industrialized countries. Dementia can be broadly defined as a generalized cognitive decline. Many disorders can produce dementia. Over half of dementias are primary degenerative dementias (60%); 20% are multistroke dementias; and the rest are related to alcohol, depression, vasculitis, metabolic and infectious disorders, tumors, or other causes. Some of these disorders, such as strokes, alcoholism, or depression, are relatively common. A minority of these disorders are treatable or reversible. It is mostly to rule out these dementias that are often difficult to distinguish from AD, that every patient with a dementia warrants a full medical evaluation, before the diagnosis of AD is made. AD is a progressive dementia that occurs in middle to late life, and is a diagnosis of exclusion.

Until recently the prevalence of AD could only be estimated from statistics on dementia. Approximately 7% of the population over the age of 65, and 20% of the population over the age of 85 have a dementia. Approximately 30–50% of the elderly population in nursing homes have a dementia, and it is stated that dementia is the fourth cause of death in the elderly. Within the last few years, studies have looked at the prevalence of AD, using strict criteria to distinguish it from other causes of dementia. These studies have shown that 0.1% of the population between the ages of 55–65, 5% of the population over the age of 65, and 10% of the population over the age of 85 have AD (Hutton & Kenny, 1985; Mas, Alperovitch, & Derouesne, 1987; Reisberg, 1983; Schoenberg, 1986). These figures will increase dramatically by the year 2000, because the older population is increasing relative to the

Aging and Health: Linking Research and Public Policy, © 1989 Lewis Publishers, Inc., Chelsea, Michigan 48118. Printed in U.S.A.

general population. For example, in Alberta in 1985, 7% of the population was older than 65, but it is projected that in year 2000, 9% of the population will be older than 65 years (Alberta Population Projections Update 1984–2011, 1984). In addition, the relative increase is greatest in the oldest group. For example, the demographics of Maryland show that between the years 1985–2000 there will be a 34% increase in the population between the ages of 65–74, a 97% increase in the population between the ages of 75–84, and a 165% increase in the population 85 and older (Reichel, 1986).

Although we do not know what causes AD, some factors that contribute to the process have been identified. These include: (1) increasing age, (2) positive family history, and (3) sex of the affected. The chances of developing AD increase with age, although some studies have suggested that this may plateau after 80. A positive family history, especially when a first-degree relative (sibling or parent) is affected, increases the chance by three- to fourfold. Women have approximately a 50% greater chance of developing AD. This difference between the sexes is age adjusted and cannot be accounted for by the fact that women live longer than men (Hutton & Kenny, 1985; Reisberg, 1983).

Other factors that have been associated with AD but are not satisfactorily documented include head trauma and aluminum. Retrospective studies have shown that head trauma is increased in all dementias, including AD as well as other neurological disorders, although such studies related to AD should be critically examined. One prospective study could not verify this finding. Aluminum has been associated with AD mostly due to a study that evaluated aluminum in Alzheimer brains as compared to age-matched controls. This study could not be reproduced. More recently, using a different technique, excess aluminum has been found in some neurons in AD brains. The main problem with these studies is that they cannot address the issue of whether aluminum is a causative factor in AD or simply an epiphenomenon, since degenerating neurons may have difficulty eliminating aluminum or other substances (Hutton & Kenny, 1985).

AD was first described by Alois Alzheimer, a German neuropsychiatrist, in 1906, in a 51-year-old woman with symptoms of dementia and a rapidly progressive course that led to her demise. Alzheimer evaluated her brain using the then newly developed silver stains, and defined for the first time some of the pathological hallmarks of AD (Reisberg, 1983).

The symptoms of AD that bring the patient to medical attention can be one or more of the following: difficulty with memory, concentration, and orientation; changes in mood and personality; focal symptoms such as aphasias, apraxias, and agnosias. Later in the course of the disorder, the patient develops abnormalities of posture and muscle tone, and may become incontinent and generally debilitated. The patient often succumbs to pneumonia or urinary tract infections (Reisberg, 1983).

There are no peripheral markers or tests to diagnose AD. For many years, it was difficult to diagnose AD with any assurance. Two developments within the last two decades have helped make the diagnosis more secure: (1) more sophisticated brain imaging techniques, such as computerized axial tomography (CAT) and nuclear magnetic resonance (NMR); and (2) clearer definition of AD, using specific standardized tests for evaluation of mental status function and strict standardized criteria for the diagnosis of AD.

The diagnosis of AD can be made at three levels of assurance. First, the diagnosis of *definite AD* can only be made if tissue from a brain biopsy or autopsy is examined. Second, the diagnosis of *probable AD* can be made with an approximately 90% assurance if the patient fulfills specific criteria (McKhann et al. [1984] or the University of Calgary Dementia Research Clinic). Third, the diagnosis of *possible AD* can be made if it is clinically suspected that the patient has AD despite not fitting the standardized criteria for the diagnosis (McKhann et al., 1984).

McKhann et al. (1984) reported criteria for clinical diagnosis of probable AD as follows:

1. dementia established by clinical exam and documented by Mini-Mental test or similar test and confirmed by neuropsychological tests
2. deficits in two or more areas of cognition
3. progressive worsening of memory and other cognitive functions
4. no disturbance of consciousness
5. onset between 40–90, most often after age 65
6. absence of systemic disorders or other brain diseases that in and of themselves could account for the progressive deficits in memory and cognition

The University of Calgary Research Clinic criteria for probable AD are:

1. insidious onset and worsening of dementia syndrome
2. Mini-Mental test score less than 24
3. neurological exam normal (except for dementia) for the first 3 years
4. modified ischemia score less than or equal to 3
5. no significant psychiatric disorder
6. no mental retardation (except Down's syndrome)
7. hematology, chemistry, serology, normal or nonspecific
8. CAT scan of brain normal or shows atrophy
9. EEG normal or diffusely slow

A patient presenting with a dementia should have a full physical and neurological evaluation. The evaluation should carefully examine evidence for vascular disease and strokes, other neurological disorders, and depression or psychiatric disorders. The examination should include some standardized tests for mental functioning which should be easy to administer, valid, specific, and reproducible. One such widely used test is the Mini-Mental State Examination (MMSE). This test evaluates recall, orientation, abstract problem solving, aphasia, apraxia, agnosia, and constructional abilities. It is simple to administer, short, and reproducible. It has also been tested repeatedly in dementia evaluation. Laboratory studies obtained from the patient should include serum chemistry (SMA-6, SMA-12), complete blood count and sedimentation rate, serology (VDRL or a comparable test), thyroid function tests, B_{12} and serum folate levels, chest X-ray, electrocardiogram, electroencephalogram, and CAT or NMR scans (McKhann et al., 1984).

AD patients progress through various stages of the disorder. The progress varies between individuals, from a rapidly progressive to an indolent course. The severity of dementia can be broadly classified into three stages (Table 1). In the first or *forgetfulness stage*, the patient starts having problems with recall and concentration. It is important to realize that most elderly individuals may have some difficulty with recall, which is not dementia but a benign forgetfulness that does not progress. In the second or *confusional stage*, the person frequently becomes disoriented even in familiar surroundings. In the third or *dementia stage*, the patient needs some assistance from another individual in order to survive (Reisberg, 1983).

The neuropathology of AD consists of presence of neuritic plaques and neurofibrillary tangles, accumulation of amyloid, neuronal loss in various regions (hippocampus, nucleus basalis of Meynert, locus ceruleus, neocortex, and others), and gliosis. All these changes are seen to a certain degree in the normal aging brain. The difference between AD and normal brains is a matter of degree, and not the simple presence or absence of a specific lesion (Reisberg, 1983).

The neurochemical changes in AD vary between regions. The neocortex is the region that is, at present, best studied neurochemically. The changes in the neocortex show a marked decrease in acetylcholine marker and somatostatin. Other neurotransmitters decreased in the neocortex include the monoamines (dopamine, serotonin, and norepinephrine). There are variations between these neurochemical changes in AD cases. The younger AD

Table 1. Clinical Phase, Mini-Mental Score (MMS), and Global Deterioration Score (GDS) in AD

Clinical Phase	MMS	GDS
Forgetfulness	>24	1
Confusional		
mild	20–24	2
moderate	15–20	3
severe	10–15	4
Dementia		
mild	5–10	5
moderate	0–5	6
severe	0	7

Note: See also Reisberg, 1983.

patient may have a more severe monoamine deficit, whereas the older AD patient may have a more severe cholinergic deficit. Many but not all neurotransmitters are decreased in the AD cortex (Radouco-Thomas et al., 1986).

acetylcholine (ACh) ↓ ↓ ↓
dopamine (DA) ↓ or ↓ ↓
5-hydroxytryptamine (5HT) ↓ or ↓ ↓
norepinephrine (NE) ↓ or ↓ ↓
γ-aminobutyric acid (GABA) ↓
somatostatin (SS) ↓ ↓ ↓
substance P (SP) ↓

Therapy in AD can be categorized as definitive, symptomatic, and management of patient and support to caregiver. Definitive therapy at present involves therapeutic trials, and is mostly based on replacing various neurotransmitters (Table 2). Metabolic enhancers (e.g., piracetam) produce a generalized increase in many neurotransmitters simultaneously. Enhancing specific neurotransmitters has also been tried at either presynaptic, synaptic, or postsynaptic levels. Although neurotransmitter enhancement in AD is a logical approach and has worked favorably for another neurodegenerative disorder, Parkinson's disease, it has to date not resulted in any definitive improvement in AD patients (Radouco-Thomas et al., 1986).

It is not known why the replacement therapy is not working in the treatment of AD, but some possibilities include (Radouco-Thomas et al., 1986):

1. There may be more than one type of AD—as discussed earlier, the neurotransmitter deficit pattern varies amongst cases.

Table 2. Some Therapeutic Trials Performed on AD Patients

		Presynaptic	Synaptic	Postsynaptic
	ACh	lecithin choline	bethanecol	physostigmine; tetrahydroaminoacridine (THA)
Metabolic enhancers (ergoloids, piracetam)	DA	L-dopa	bromocriptine Ergoloid	tricyclic antidepressants
	5HT NE		zimeledine clonidine	
	GABA		muscimol benzodiazepine	
	SS		SS analogue	

Note: Also see Radouco-Thomas et al., 1986. ACh = acetylcholine; DA = dopamine; 5HT = 5-hydroxytryptamine; NE = norepinephrine; GABA = γ-aminobutyric acid; SS = somatostatin.

2. Many neurotransmitter systems are affected in AD and replacement of one neurotransmitter may not have an obvious effect.
3. Since the diagnosis of AD is often not secure unless the patient has a certain degree of dementia, the replacement may be given too late in the course, when there is already a high degree of neuronal loss.
4. It is also assumed in these therapeutic trials that the postsynaptic neuron functions normally when it is quite possible that in its denervated state it may not do so.
5. Finally, an improvement on a specific neuropsychological test does not translate into a real-life functional improvement.

Symptomatic therapy in AD should be directed at treating the symptoms of depression, anxiety in the early and intermediate stages, and hallucinations at later stages of the process. Depression is a very common symptom in the early stages and responds somewhat to antidepressant medication. Anxiety occurs at all stages and often responds to anxiolytic medication. Hallucinations are common in the late stages and antipsychotic medications are often helpful. It is noteworthy that none of these psychopharmacologic agents are specifically tailored to the demented or AD patient. Symptomatic medication that is developed specifically for the AD patient could theoretically produce fewer untoward side effects.

Education of the caregiver and the family is extremely important for the welfare and management of the AD patient. The demented individual will become totally dependent on his or her caregiver, and the caregiver must appreciate what dementia actually implies to the patient. Often, very simple suggestions from the physician or therapist as to the management of the patient may avert a crisis. In addition, if the caregivers know what to expect, they can plan ahead and avert a crisis. The therapist or physician must aim to help the patient and the caregiver in their daily lives. In order to do so, a realistic but positive attitude by the therapist is necessary.

While overall future research trends in AD are difficult to predict, some will continue to be very enlightening within the next decade. Among these are genetic studies on AD patients who have a family history. Evidence at this time indicates that some familial AD victims have a genetic marker on chromosome 21, whereas others may not. It is reasonable to suggest that AD may be heterogeneous and more than one chromosomal abnormality may result in AD. Neurochemical studies started in the early 1970s on AD brains continue to shed light on the neurochemistry of this complicated disorder. Therapeutic trials both to develop definitive as well as symptomatic therapy tailored to the needs of the AD patient are important research trends.

BURDEN OF AD TO THE PATIENT, FAMILY, AND SOCIETY

AD is a long-term burden to the individual, the caregiver, the family, and society. It is a psychological burden that often produces depression in the individual and the caregiver. Because the patient often undergoes a personality change, the caregiver and the family become confused and apprehensive. In addition, the family is concerned about the genetic implications of AD in a direct family member.

AD is a social burden. The two aspects singled out as the most difficult for the caregiver are (1) isolation of the individual and caregiver, since most of their friends and some of their family seem to desert them; and (2) the lack of leisure time the caregiver has, given the need to be almost constantly with the demented individual. This becomes an even greater problem when the patient's sleep-wake cycle is altered and the caregiver remains awake at night to watch over the patient.

AD is a financial burden to the family of the afflicted as well as to society. The financial loss to the family can be due to the early forced retirement of the patient, or to the caregiver who has to stop working to care for the AD victim. In addition, there are caregiving costs such as hiring a companion to relieve the caregiver; paying for transportation, since the AD victim cannot drive; and costs for modifying the home to make it safe for the patient.

Public resources spent on caregiving in Canada vary in different provinces, but most have home care services or day care centers, lodges, nursing homes, or auxiliary hospitals, and sometimes special units for AD patients. The special units for AD patients become very important at later stages of the disorder when the patient wanders out of a less supervised environment (Gwyther & George, 1986).

PUBLIC POLICY RECOMMENDATIONS FOR AD

Recently some public policy recommendations for AD were developed in the State of Maryland (Reichel, 1986). An adaptation of these recommendations follows:

Service resources
1. Develop a pool of respite caregivers.
2. Assist nursing homes and hospitals to be receptive to short respite stays.
3. Expand and extend adult day care centers.
4. Extend network of mutual help support groups.
5. Provide legal and financial counseling.
6. Improve diagnostic services.
7. AD should be considered a physical illness, in order to access certain services.

Education and training
1. Develop dementia training centers.
2. Incorporate dementia content in all professional medical education.
3. Engage the local AD society to conduct informational and educational activities.

Financial relief
1. Furnish financial incentives to families, averting institutionalization costly to the system.

Data
1. Develop provincial data on dementia: its extent, demography, epidemiology, and services.

Follow-through and coordination
1. Charge a provincial agency with coordinating and monitoring progress of these recommendations.

To date they are the only published recommendations of this kind. Our experience in Alberta shows us that the needs for dealing with AD are very similar to those developed in Maryland. Unless some public policy for dealing with AD is implemented soon, AD will become a public burden that will not be easily contained.

REFERENCES

Alberta population projections update 1984–2011. (1984). Edmonton: Alberta Treasury Bureau of Statistics.

Gwyther, L. P., & George, L. K. (1986). Symposium caregivers for dementia patients: Complex determinants of well-being and burden. *Gerontologist, 26*, 245–278.

Hutton, J. T., & Kenny, A. D. (Eds.). (1985). *Senile dementia of the Alzheimer type.* New York: Alan R. Liss.

Mas, J. L., Alperovitch, A., & Derouesne, C. (1987). Epidemiology of Alzheimer's type dementia. *Revue Neurologique (Paris), 143*, 161–171.

McKhann, G., Drachman, D., Folstein, M., Katzmann, R., Price, D., & Stadlan, M. (1984). Clinical diagnosis of Alzheimer's disease: Report of the NINCDS-ADRDA Work Group under the auspices of Department of Health and Human Services Task Force on Alzheimer's Disease. *Neurology, 34*, 939–944.

Reichel, W. (1986). Survey research guiding public policy making in Maryland: The case of Alzheimer's disease and related disorders. *Experimental Gerontology, 21*, 439–448.

Reisberg, B. (Ed.). (1983). *Alzheimer's disease—The standard reference.* New York: The Free Press, A Division of Macmillan, Inc.

Radouco-Thomas, C., Gottfries, C. G., Amaducci, L., Reisberg, B., Garcin, F., & Coyle, J. T. (Eds.). (1986). Senile dementia and Alzheimer's disease etiopathogenesis, diagnosis and pharmacotherapy. *Progress in Neuro-Psychopharmacology and Biological Psychiatry, 10*(3–5), 9–665.

Schoenberg, B. S. (1986). Epidemiology of Alzheimer's disease and other dementing illnesses. *Journal of Chronic Diseases, 39,* 1095–1104.

7. A Method to Examine Confusion-Potentiating Medications in Studies of the Institutionalized Elderly

NORMA J. STEWART
J. STEVEN RICHARDSON

INTRODUCTION

Clinical intervention studies are often difficult to interpret because several interventions other than the one selected for study may coexist and confound results with alternative explanations. This problem is not unique to studies of the elderly in long term care facilities, but is rather a central issue in the evaluation of clinical approaches in general. Valid conclusions are possible only when confounding variables are taken into account.

In studies of the institutionalized elderly, medication use is often ignored rather than controlled. On the one hand, it is often difficult in such studies to have direct experimental control over medication administration. On the other hand, the development of statistical methods of examining medications tends to be rejected because of the large number of different medications in use and the wide variability in the dosages of medications prescribed. While in some instances the medication profile may be irrelevant, any study investigating brain function must pay close attention to the effects of the drugs taken by the subjects.

Medications with anticholinergic side effects are especially relevant to studies of the cognitively impaired elderly. Neurons using acetylcholine as a neurotransmitter are found in many areas of the brain. These cholinergic

Aging and Health: Linking Research and Public Policy, © 1989 Lewis Publishers, Inc., Chelsea, Michigan 48118. Printed in U.S.A.

neurons participate in emotional reactions, sensory processing, hormonal and cardiovascular regulation, and motor control, and are especially important in memory and thought processes. While cognitive impairment may be a direct result of dementia or depression, it may also be an iatrogenic side effect of anticholinergic medications such as: (1) major tranquilizers used to manage agitation associated with dementia; or (2) antidepressants used as treatment for depression.

Existing assessment tools, such as mental status questionnaires, provide an indication of the degree of cognitive impairment of the individual, but are not helpful in identifying its underlying cause. For example, the widely used Mini-Mental State Examination (Folstein, Folstein, & McHugh, 1975) does not differentiate between the irreversible impairment of dementia (e.g., multiple infarct dementia or dementia of the Alzheimer's type) and the impairment seen in delirium, which can result from reversible causes such as medications. Kane and Kane (1981) conclude that we do not as yet have an adequate assessment instrument to differentiate depression from dementia. In cases of combined dementia, depression *and* drug-induced delirium, the assessment issue becomes both more difficult and more important.

These assessment problems underscore the importance of documenting the potential for anticholinergic toxicity as a confounding variable in studies of the cognitively impaired elderly or building in medication effect as an experimental variable. One possible hypothesis is that cognitive impairment attributed to irreversible dementia is partly or completely due to reversible drug-induced delirium—that is, an acute confusional state related to the interaction of drugs taken by a particular patient.

THE ELDERLY AND ANTICHOLINERGIC MEDICATION

Many psychotropic drugs have an unintended side effect of blocking brain muscarinic acetylcholine receptors. With some drugs, the anticholinergic effect is rather mild. But other drugs, such as amitriptyline and thioridazine, are very potent muscarinic blockers. However, the mild blockade of individual drugs is additive, and a patient taking two or more of these compounds may develop serious cognitive impairment due to the summation of anticholinergic effects. In addition to the psychotropic drugs, strong anticholinergic activity is found in over 100 other prescription and over-the-counter drugs, as well as in numerous cultivated and wild plants (Johnson, Hollister, & Berger, 1981).

The elderly are particularly sensitive to the deleterious effects of muscarinic blockade because of their relative cholinergic deficit at the outset, due to progressive degeneration of cholinergic neurons with advancing age (Bartus et al., 1982). This predisposition, combined with the summative and potentiating effect of polypharmacy (i.e., multiple drugs with anticholinergic side effects) can lead to parasympathetic blockade with peripheral effects, such as dry mouth and urinary retention, and central effects that may mimic the cognitive and emotional impairments seen in Alzheimer's disease and other dementias.

As the adverse effects due to direct receptor blockade are increased, the therapeutic effects due to changes in the number of receptors tend to be slower in the elderly, due to a reduced metabolic rate and slowed receptor regulation. For example, antidepressants that normally act in three to four weeks in a younger adult may take much longer in the elderly. The risk of anticholinergic toxicity to drugs given to the elderly in doses appropriate for younger adults is further increased due to slower excretion of drugs with advancing age (Pagliaro & Pagliaro, 1983). Given these changes associated with aging and the specific properties of anticholinergic agents, elders who need these medications are at greater risk for deleterious side effects than younger adults.

Patients with Alzheimer's disease are even more susceptible to the anticholinergic side effects of drugs than the normal elderly. The neuropathology of Alzheimer's disease includes a rather massive loss of cholinergic neurons such as those with cell bodies in the nucleus basalis of Meynert and synaptic terminals in the cortex, hippocampus, and other limbic structures (Coyle, Price, & DeLong, 1985). Due to the death of these acetylcholine neurons, even the drug-free Alzheimer's brain has a major reduction in cholinergic neural activity. Giving the Alzheimer's patient drugs with potent anticholinergic side effects, such as amitriptyline or thioridazine, would further disrupt cholinergic neural activity in the brain and exacerbate the cognitive and emotional impairments in the patient.

DEVELOPMENT OF THE MEDICATION MEASURE

The Study Context

The method to examine confusion-potentiating medications described in this chapter was developed for a study of predictors of cognitive impairment in the institutionalized elderly. The purpose of the study was to attempt to separate out the reversible component of cognitive impairment, such as that attributable to environmental variables, in elders with mild to severe cognitive impairment in long term care settings. Medication effect and other possible predictors of reversible cognitive impairment were examined using a regression analysis. To conduct this analysis, it was necessary to express the medications which could potentiate confusion (i.e., cognitive impairment) as a single numerical score.

Background

Our method refined an earlier clinical approach (Summers, 1978) which classified drugs from patient records in terms of relative potential for causing delirium, and incorporated a weighting system based on daily therapeutic drug dosage levels. The advantage of this clinical approach was that it could be used retrospectively and in situations where it was not possible to use more invasive procedures, such as measures of anticholinergic activity (Richardson et al., 1985) in serum or cerebrospinal fluid.

The problem with Summers' scoring method is that the "drug risk number" (p. 1514) has been derived from a qualitative, categorical system (Class I to III) of delirium potential combined with a quantitative system (Dosage levels 1 to 3). Although Summers argued that the delirium gradient relates to underlying anticholinergic activity, the mechanism of action for some drugs so classified (e.g., antihypertensives) is clearly *not* blockade of the muscarinic receptor sites.

The Anticholinergic Score

Our method created two scores: a general confusion-potentiating score and an anticholinergic score, which was a subset of the general score. The rationale for this approach was that, while there are many ways that medication can disrupt cognitive function, perhaps the most common mechanism involves the blockade of muscarinic acetylcholine receptors in the hippocampus. Hippocampal cholinergic neurons are crucially involved in memory processes (Brito et al., 1983), and any drug that gets into the brain and blocks the postsynaptic muscarinic receptors of these neurons will produce cognitive impairment.

All psychotropic drugs enter the brain very readily, and the concentration of the drug in the blood closely parallels the drug concentration in the brain. Although we did not do it in this study, it is possible, using a competitive radioligand binding assay, to quantify accurately and correlate serum anticholinergic activity in the blood with cognitive function (e.g., Miller et al., 1988). Drugs such as diuretics may contribute to confusion through altering the ion concentrations surrounding the brain cells. Cognitive impairment produced by diuretics and antihypertensive drugs could also be due to a reduction in the delivery of oxygen and glucose to the brain due to lowered blood pressure and blood volume. As yet, we do not have accurate ways of quantifying ion, oxygen, or nutrient abnormalities in the brain.

The anticholinergic score used here was obtained by recording all medications with anticholinergic side effects administered for seven days prior to the study day. We recorded actual administrations on the nurses' medication charts rather than physicians' orders because many of these drugs were given as needed under the nurses' discretion. Because of the cumulative effects of these medications, we arbitrarily chose one week as an interval that would give an indication of the anticholinergic activity that summates across drugs and over time. We have not yet correlated this method with serum anticholinergic values to see how closely this chart-based measure corresponds to actual serum anticholinergic activity.

Each anticholinergic drug was coded in 24-hour dosage, then weighted as *less than* (weight = 1), *greater than* (weight = 3), or *within recommended dosages* (weight = 2) for the elderly. Where no guidelines for the elderly were available, we used recommended adult doses. The final score was the sum of the weighted scores over seven days. For example, if the resident was given thioridazine within the recommended dose daily, plus low-dose amitriptyline daily at bedtime, the score would be:

[thioridazine (2 × 7) = 14] + [amitriptyline (1 × 7) = 7] = 21.

General Confusion-Potentiating Score

Although our original plan was to analyze only anticholinergic medication, we found that numerous medications were given that can have confusion as a side effect but which do not have direct effects on the muscarinic receptors. The anticholinergic subset (Table 2) of the confusion-potentiating drugs (Table 1) included only agents with demonstrated affinity for muscarinic receptors. In Table 2, the affinity of a particular drug for brain muscarinic receptors is compared to the classical anticholinergic drug atropine. In general, the closer a particular drug is to atropine, the greater the potential for cognitive impairment. The drugs with a low number under anticholinergic potency in Table 2 need very few molecules of drug to block the receptors. Although the benzodiazepines, such as diazepam, are very effective disrupters of memory formation (indeed, the amnesic effect of diazepam is an advantage when used prior to certain medical procedures), the benzodiazepines do not have affinity for muscarinic receptors and so do not appear in Table 2.

In conclusion, the proposed method can be used to score confusion-potentiating medication, with an anticholinergic subscore, in quantitative analyses where multiple factors may contribute to cognitive impairment. An assumption underlying the use of a dose-related score is that therapeutic effect and side effect potential are equivalent. This assumption needs validation in further research to compare the anticholinergic clinical measure with laboratory analysis of antimuscarinic activity in serum and cerebrospinal fluid. Other methods have been developed (e.g., Pepper, 1985) to examine anticholinergic side effects more directly, but until the necessary laboratory studies of the full range of anticholinergic agents have been completed, an interpolation process is still needed for some drugs.

The present measurement approach provides a useful first step in examin-

Table 1.   Confusion-Potentiating Medications

General Class	Subclass or Specific Examples
Parasympatholytics	atropine, propantheline, ipratropium, pirenzepine

Cardiovascular system
  Antihypertensives
  Antiarrhythmics
	clonidine, propranolol quinidine

Central nervous system	analgesics (narcotic and nonnarcotic), hypnotics, anxiolytics, antidepressants, antipsychotics, anti-Parkinson drugs
Electrolyte, caloric, and water balance	diuretics, diabetes preparations
Gastrointestinal	cimetidine, other noncholinergic antiulcer drugs
Hormones and substitutes	thyroid preparations, estrogens, glucocorticoids, etc.
Spasmolytics	noncholinergic smooth muscle relaxants, antiasthma drugs

Table 2.   Drugs with Demonstrated Affinity for Brain Muscarinic Cholinergic Receptors

Drug	Trade Name (Originator)	Anticholinergic Potency[a]
Anticholinergics		
scopolamine	—	0.3
atropine	—	0.4
trihexyphenidyl	Artane	0.6
benztropine	Cogentin	1.5
Antidepressants		
amitriptyline	Elavil	10
doxepin	Sinequan	44
nortriptyline	Aventyl	57
imipramine	Tofranil	78
desipramine	Pertofrane	170
trazodone	Desyrel	>100,000
phenelzine	Nardil	>100,000
Antipsychotics		
thioridazine	Mellaril	150
chlorpromazine	Largactil	1,000
perphenazine	Trilafon	10,000
trifluoperazine	Stelazine	13,000
haloperidol	Haldol	48,000

Source: Data based on Snyder et al., 1974, and Snyder & Yamamura, 1977.
[a]IC_{50}: concentration of drug in nanomolars needed to inhibit, by 50%, the specific binding of 0.06 nanomolar of the radioligand QNB to rat brain muscarinic receptors.

ing the risk of drug-induced cognitive impairment where invasive procedures, such as taking blood samples, are not feasible in a given study. It may be used to detect reversible drug effects that mimic irreversible dementia such as that of Alzheimer's disease or that are superimposed on a dementing process. Treatment measures, such as reduction of total anticholinergic medication intake, may reduce cognitive impairment and improve function even in a dementia that is normally considered untreatable. Further clinical research is needed to examine current medication practices in the cognitively impaired elderly to compare drugs of choice from two perspectives: (1) therapeutic benefit, such as reduction of agitation in residents with Alzheimer's disease; and (2) side effects, such as anticholinergic toxicity or brain electrolyte imbalance, which may accentuate another dimension of the original problem and lead to increased cognitive impairment.

The approach to measurement used here has focused on application of the existing pharmacological knowledge on underlying mechanisms of confusion induction. As laboratory studies improve measurement of other drug effects that disrupt cognitive function, such as sedation and ion concentration mechanisms, the general score identified in this chapter may be further subdivided into measurable components that can be validated in studies that compare medication administration with serum levels of the composite of drugs with a similar underlying mechanism. This measurement work is needed to achieve a valid and reliable score that predicts the degree of a given side effect as well as therapeutic effects.

REFERENCES

Bartus, R. T., Dean, R. L., Beer, B., & Lippa, A. S. (1982). The cholinergic hypothesis of geriatric memory dysfunction. *Science, 217,* 408–417.

Brito, G. N. O., Davis, B. J., Stopp, L. C., & Stanton, M. E. (1983). Memory and the septo-hippocampal cholinergic system in the rat. *Psychopharmacology, 81,* 315–320.

Coyle, J., Price, D., & DeLong, M. (1985). Alzheimer's disease: A disorder of cortical cholinergic Innervation. In P. H. Abelson, E. Butz, & S. H. Snyder (Eds.), *Neuroscience* (pp. 418–431).

Folstein, M. F., Folstein, S. E., & McHugh, P. R. (1975). "Mini-Mental State": A practical method for grading the cognitive state of patients for the clinician. *Journal of Psychiatric Research, 12,* 189–198.

Johnson, A. L., Hollister, L. E., & Berger, P. A. (1981). The anticholinergic intoxication syndrome: Diagnosis and treatment. *Journal of Clinical Psychiatry, 42,* 313–317.

Kane, R. A., & Kane, R. L. (1981). *Assessing the elderly: A practical guide to measurement.* London: Johns Hopkins U. Press.

Miller, P. S., Richardson, J. S., Jyu, C., Lemay, J. S., Hiscock, M., & Keegan, D. L. (1988). Association of low serum anticholinergic levels and cognitive impairment in elderly presurgical patients. *American Journal of Psychiatry, 145,* 342–345.

Pagliaro, L. A., & Pagliaro, A. M. (Eds.). (1983). *Pharmacologic aspects of aging.* Toronto: Mosby.

Pepper, G. A. T. (1985). *Central and peripheral anticholinergic adverse drug effects in the institutionalized elderly.* Unpublished doctoral dissertation. University of Colorado Health Sciences Center.

Richardson, J. S., Miller, P. S., Lemay, J. S., Jyu, C. A., Neil, S. G., Kilduff, C. J., & Keegan, D. L. (1985). Mental dysfunction and the blockade of muscarinic receptors in the brains of the normal elderly. *Progress in Neuro-Psychopharmacology and Biological Psychiatry, 9,* 651–654.

Snyder, S. H., Greenberg, D., & Yamamura, H. I. (1974). Antischizophrenic drugs and brain cholinergic receptors. *Archives of General Psychiatry, 31,* 58–61.

Snyder, S. H., & Yamamura, H. I. (1977). Antidepressants and the muscarinic acetylcholine receptor. *Archives of General Psychiatry, 34,* 236–239.

Summers, W. K. (1978). A clinical method of estimating risk of drug induced delirium. *Life Sciences, 22,* 1511–1516.

8. Age and Sensitivity to Light: Implications for Depression, Sundowning, and Lighting Standards

JO SEGGIE
SUSAN TAINSH

INTRODUCTION

A possible relationship between the process of entraining biological rhythms and the circadian dysregulation seen in depression was highlighted as an area of interest during the 1980s (Wehr & Goodwin, 1983). Indeed, considerable effort has been expended on understanding the physiological (Turek, 1985), biochemical (Siever & Davis, 1985), pharmacological (Goodwin, Wirz-Justice, & Wehr, 1982; Kripke, Mullaney, & Gabriel, 1986), and hormonal (Seggie, 1988a) aspects of such relationships. Endogenous periodic systems depend on environmental events for entrainment. Numerous stimuli in the environment have the capacity to serve as a *zeitgeber* (i.e., time cue, synchronizer, entraining agent). Such stimuli as light/dark, feeding, social interactions, temperature, sound, and gravitational and magnetic forces have been observed to influence the temporal order of biological events (Weitzman, 1982; Winget et al., 1984). However, there appears to be a definite hierarchy of potency among stimuli in their ability to serve as time cues for entrainment of biological rhythms. For rhythms with a period of about 24 hours (circadian rhythm), light and dark are the most potent stimuli under normal conditions.

Melatonin, the pineal hormone, is well recognized as the biological signal which provides information about light and dark to all cells of the body via circulation in the blood. Melatonin levels are low in light and high in dark-

Aging and Health: Linking Research and Public Policy, © 1989 Lewis Publishers, Inc., Chelsea, Michigan 48118. Printed in U.S.A.

ness. The physiology of the system which regulates melatonin secretion, namely the retinal-hypothalamic-pineal axis, is best understood in animal models (Armstrong et al., 1985). However, a similar role for melatonin is now suspected in the human (Arendt & Broadway, in press).

It has been proposed that both the pathophysiology of depression and the mechanism of action of antidepressants involve alteration of the intrinsic rhythm for circadian regulation and the sensitivity of the eye to light (Wehr & Wirz-Justice, 1982). Indeed, patients with affective disorder have increased supersensitivity to light as measured by the ability of light to suppress melatonin levels (Lewy et al., 1981) or ophthalmological procedures that assess sensitivity to light at the level of the retina (Seggie, 1988b; Seggie et al., in press).

Brown et al. (1985) have reported attenuated nocturnal levels of serum melatonin in depressed patients, manifested in a flattened 24-hour rhythm. Age-related changes in serum melatonin level have also been found in all species studied (Tang, Hadjiconstantinou, & Pang, 1984; Touitou et al., 1984; Nair et al., 1986), including the human. Characteristically, older individuals exhibit reduced nocturnal melatonin levels, resulting in a flattened circadian rhythm. The "clock" hypothesis of aging (Everitt, 1980) shares much conceptually with the rhythm hypothesis of depression. It has been suggested that a common defect in the regulation of circadian rhythms may underlie the observed changes in melatonin rhythms in both the elderly and depressed (Nair, Hariharasubramanian, & Pilapil, 1985).

Therefore, we questioned whether aged individuals, in whom melatonin patterns parallel those seen in depression, might also exhibit supersensitivity to light. The present study was undertaken to determine the effects of age on serum melatonin rhythms in the sheep model and to see if age modifies the ability of light to suppress nocturnal melatonin levels. A report on this project appeared in Seggie, Brown, and Rollag (1986). Portions of these data are currently discussed and interpreted more specifically with respect to behavioral pathology in aging. It is suggested that circadian dysregulation in aging may be a common pathology underlying behavioral disturbances such as wandering, noisemaking, and sundowning (Dawson & Reid, 1987; Evans, 1987; Ryan et al., 1988).

METHODS

Subjects

Five young and seven old female sheep of the Dorset X Suffolk breed, free of gross eye and retinal pathology, were used in the present study. They were housed in pens with free access to feed and water under a lighting regime of 10 hours light/14 hours dark (10L:14D) supplied by incandescent light at an intensity of 20–40 μw/cm^2. Data were collected in December and January.

Blood Sampling Procedure

Blood was sampled from the jugular vein using the Vacutainer system. This procedure took less than a minute. All dark time samples were taken under low-intensity red light, which has no effect on serum melatonin levels.

Assays

Dr. Gregory M. Brown assayed serum melatonin by RIA using antibody R158 (13/9/76) from CIDtech Research Inc. Parallelism of various aliquots of sheep serum was found. Recovery of labeled melatonin added to sheep serum was 91 ± 1%. Intra- and interassay coefficients of variation were 7 and 14%. Least detectable concentration in serum was 10 pg/mL and mid-range of the assay was 50 pg/mL.

Study 1: Effect of Age on Resting Melatonin Levels

Resting blood samples were taken at three times in the 10L:14D cycle, corresponding to 3 hours after light onset and 8 and 11 hours after dark onset.

Study 2: Effect of Age on Nocturnal Melatonin Response to Bright Light

During the second half of the dark phase, animals were individually subjected to bright light. The intensity at the level of the sheep eye was 500–800 μw/cm^2. Blood samples were taken prior to and 5, 10, 15, and 20 minutes after exposure to bright light.

RESULTS

Data were analyzed using repeated measures ANOVA. In study 1, resting melatonin levels were low in the light and high in the dark. Young animals, with a mean age of 1.2 ± 0.2 years, exhibited a significant diurnal rhythm ($F = 9.05$; df 2, 5; $0.10 < p > 0.05$). Melatonin levels in old animals with a mean age of 8.6 ± 0.8 years did not evidence significant variation over the three times ($F = 3.19$; df 2, 6; $p > 0.05$); however, there was the expected light/dark difference. Data are shown in Figure 1. The absolute level of nocturnal melatonin in old animals was significantly less than that of young animals ($F = 10.2$; df 1, 9; $p < 0.01$) at the two time points in the dark phase of the lighting cycle, and this effect was not apparent during the

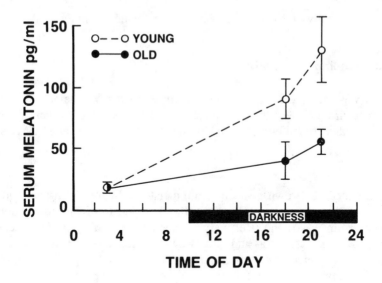

Figure 1. Circadian pattern of resting levels of serum melatonin in young and old sheep.

light. A linear regression analysis was done on nocturnal melatonin levels as a function of age. Data are shown in Figure 2. Melatonin levels were negatively and significantly correlated with age with a regression coefficient of -0.75($t = 3.41$; df 9, $p < 0.01$).

In response to exposure to bright light in the middle of the dark, young sheep exhibited a rapid fall in melatonin levels ($F = 9.22$; df 4, 11; $p < 0.01$). Data are shown in Figure 3. This absolute decline reached significance 5 minutes after the start of light ($F = 8.1$; df 1, 6; $p < 0.05$), but did not decline any further during 20 minutes of continued exposure to light ($F = 1.6$; df 3, 7; $p < 0.05$). Old sheep, in contrast, evidenced a significant decline from resting melatonin levels only after 20 minutes exposure to bright light ($F = 6.96$; df 1, 7; $p < 0.05$).

Because of the difference in nocturnal resting levels between the old and young group prior to bright light stimulation, data were also expressed as a percentage of the resting level for each animal. Expressed this way, the data show that the magnitude of the response of the young sheep during 5–20 minutes of exposure to bright light was significantly larger than in the old sheep ($F = 11.3$; df 1, 20; $p < 0.01$). On average, young sheep suppressed melatonin levels to $25.6 \pm 2.6\%$ of resting values, while old sheep suppressed to $52.6 \pm 7.6\%$ of resting levels.

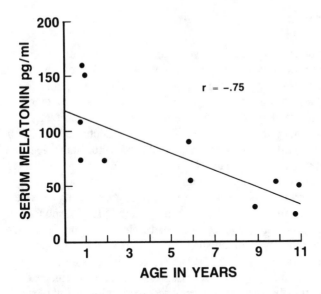

Figure 2. Age and resting nocturnal melatonin. Regression analysis of resting levels of nocturnal melatonin as a function of age in sheep (r is significant at p < 0.01).

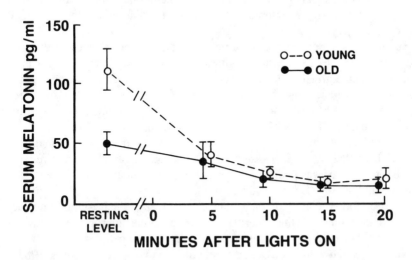

Figure 3. Nocturnal response to bright light. Melatonin levels in young and old sheep following exposure to bright light during the middle of the dark portion of an alternating light/dark lighting schedule.

DISCUSSION

Under an alternating lighting cycle, female sheep exhibited the expected diurnal rhythm in serum melatonin levels, with low levels during the light and higher levels during the dark. Old sheep had significantly lower levels of nocturnal melatonin than young sheep and exhibited a flattened circadian rhythm similar to that observed in aged humans (Nair et al., 1986) and depressed patients (Brown et al., 1985). Resting nocturnal melatonin levels and age were significantly negatively correlated to the same degree as elsewhere reported for aged humans (Nair et al., 1986). In response to exposure to bright light, nocturnal melatonin levels were dramatically suppressed. However, the pattern of the response differed significantly between young and old sheep. Both in terms of latency and magnitude of response, old sheep were less sensitive than young sheep to bright light. Insofar as the sheep exhibited the same type of changes in circadian melatonin levels as aged humans, these data do not support the suggestion of Nair et al. (1985) that circadian abnormalities in aging and depression share a common defect. Nor does the present observation of decreased sensitivity to light in aged individuals concur with the findings of increased sensitivity to light in young depressed patients (Lewy et al., 1981; Seggie et al., in press). However, the present data do support the idea that aging is accompanied by circadian dysregulation, which may be due to altered sensitivity to light. We have observed significant aberration in function of the retinal-hypothalamic-pineal axis, whose integrity is essential for normal circadian entrainment in aged vs young subjects.

Sundowning syndrome, characterized by late afternoon or early evening increase in levels of confusion, agitation, or motor restlessness, is a phenomenon well known to institutional caregivers. It has been formally described in an elderly institutionalized population (Evans, 1987). Noisy behavior as a form of agitation has also been described in one third of institutionalized elderly (Ryan et al., 1988); however circadian distribution of these behaviors has yet to be determined. The severity of sundowning was significantly correlated with factors known to play a role in circadian entrainment, and light intensity was posited as a potentially important factor in the induction of sundowning (Evans, 1987).

The possibility that light may play a significant role in optimizing circadian entrainment in the elderly and hence in the appropriate temporal ordering of behavior deserves further study. Depressed patients are supersensitive to light and exhibit circadian dysregulation (Wehr & Goodwin, 1983). Increased sensitivity to light in depressed patients is normalized by antidepressant medication (Seggie, 1988b; Seggie et al., in press). Although bright light therapy for depression in the elderly has not yet been documented, the antidepressant effectiveness of bright light therapy in young depressed patients is dependent on the eye and not the skin (Wehr et al., 1987). The present animal model data suggest that the physiological substrate of the biological clock is less sensitive to light in the elderly. Recently it was demonstrated that patients with Alzheimer's disease, who exhibit many of the behavioral disturbances characteristic of circadian dysregulation, have a significant peripheral visual field loss (Steffes & Thralow, 1987) that would seriously compromise their ability to detect light/dark cues and hence their ability to be appropriately behaviorally entrained to their caregiving environment.

The characteristics of the lighting environment most suitable for aged individuals have yet to be ascertained. The significant variables include not only the intensity, but also the duration and wavelength composition of light. It may be that decreased sensitivity to light and consequent circadian dysregulation could be alleviated with drugs or attention to the physical characteristics of the light in the caregiving environment. Affective disorders in the aged and pathological behavior patterns seen in dementia may be improved by attention to the augmentation of impaired perception of light/dark cues by the elderly, and to the lighting environment.

ACKNOWLEDGMENT

This study was supported in part by funds from the Ontario Mental Health Foundation (OMHF) and the Medical Research Council of Canada. Jo Seggie is an OMHF Research Associate. Thanks to Dr. G. M. Brown for assistance with the RIA.

REFERENCES

Arendt, J., & Broadway, J. (in press). Light and melatonin as zeitgebers in man. *Chronobiology International.*

Armstrong, S. M., Cassone, V. M., Chesworth, M., Redman, J., & Short, R. (1985). Synchronization of mammalian circadian rhythms by melatonin. In R. J. Wurtman & F. Woldhausen (Eds.), *Melatonin in humans.* Cambridge, MA: Center for Brain Sciences and Metabolism Charitable Trust.

Brown, R., Kocsis, J., Caroff, S., Amsterdam, J., Winokur, A., Strokes, P. & Frazer, A. (1985). Differences in nocturnal melatonin secretion between melancholic depressed patients and control subjects. *American Journal of Psychiatry, 142,* 811–816.

Dawson, P., & Reid, D. W. (1987). Behavioural dimensions of patients at risk of wandering. *Gerontologist, 27,* 104–107.

Evans, L. K. (1987). Sundown syndrome in the institutionalized elderly. *Journal of the American Geriatric Society, 35,* 101–108.

Everitt, A. (1980). The neuroendocrine system and aging. *Gerontology, 26,* 108–123.

Goodwin, F. K., Wirz-Justice, A., & Wehr, T. A. (1982). Evidence that the pathophysiology of depression and the mechanism of action of antidepressant drugs both involve alterations in circadian rhythms. *Advances in Biochemical Psychopharmacology 32*, 1–11.

Kripke, D. F., Mullaney, D. J., & Gabriel, S. (1986). The chronopharmacology of antidepressant drugs. In A. Reinberg, M. Smolensky, & G. Labrecque (Eds.), *Annual Review of Chronopharmacology*, (Vol. 2, pp. 275–289). Oxford: Pergamon Press.

Lewy, A. J., Wehr, T.A., Goodwin, F.K., Newsome, D. A., & Rosenthal, N. E. (1981). Manic-depressive patients may be supersensitive to light. *Lancet, 1*, 383–384.

Nair, N. P. V., Hariharasubramanian, N., & Pilapil, C. (1985). Circadian rhythm of plasma melatonin and cortisol in endogenous depression. *Advances in the Biosciences, 53*, 339–345.

Nair, N. P. V., Hariharasubramanian, N., Pilapil, C., Isaac, I., & Thavundayil, J. X. (1986). Plasma melatonin—an index of brain aging in humans. *Biological Psychiatry, 21*, 141–150.

Ryan, D. P., Tainsh, S. M., Kolodny, V., Lendrum, B. L., & Fisher, R. H. (1988). Noisemaking amongst the elderly in long term care. *Gerontologist 28*, 369–371.

Seggie, J. (1988a). Melatonin, the retinal-hypothalamic-pineal axis and circadian rhythm regulation. In F. N. Johnson (Ed.), *Lithium and the endocrine system* (Lithium Therapy Monographs, Vol. 2, pp. 35–50). Basal, Germany: Karger.

Seggie, J. (1988b). Lithium and the retina. *Progress in Neuro-Psychopharmacology and Biological Psychiatry, 12*, 241–253.

Seggie, J., Brown, G. M., & Rollag, M. D. (1986). Effects of age on nocturnal melatonin levels at rest and following exposure to bright light in sheep. *Society for Neuroscience, 12*, abs. 233.6.

Seggie, J., Canny, C., Mai, F., McCrank, E., & Waring, E. (in press). Antidepressant medication reduces supersensitivity to light in depressed patients. *Progress in Neuro-Psychopharmacology and Biological Psychiatry*.

Siever, L. J., & Davis, K. L. (1985). Overview: Toward a dysregulation hypothesis of depression. *American Journal of Psychiatry, 142*, 1017–1031.

Steffes, R., & Thralow, J. (1987). Visual field limitations in the patient with dementia of the Alzheimer type. *Journal of the American Geriatric Society, 35*, 198–204.

Tang, F., Hadjiconstantinou, M., & Pang, S. F. (1984). Aging and diurnal rhythms of pineal serotonin, 5-hydroxyindoleacetic acid, norepinephrine, dopamine and serum melatonin in the male rat. *Neuroendocrinology, 40*, 160.

Touitou, Y., Fevre, M., Bogdan, A., Reinberg, A., De Prius, J., Beck, H., & Touitou, C. (1984). Patterns of plasma melatonin with aging and mental condition: Stability of nyctohemeral rhythms and differences in seasonal variations. *Acta Endocrinologica, 106*, 145.

Turek, F. W. (1985). Circadian neural rhythms in mammals. *Annual Review of Physiology, 47*, 49–64.

Wehr, T. A., & Goodwin, F. K. (1983). *Circadian rhythms in psychiatry*. Pacific Grove: Boxwood Press.

Wehr, T. A., Skwerer, R. G., Jacobsen, F. M., Sack, D. A., & Rosenthal, N. E. (1987). Eye versus skin phototherapy of seasonal affective disorder. *American Journal of Psychiatry, 144,* 753–757.

Wehr, T. A., & Wirz-Justice, A. (1982). Circadian rhythm mechanisms in affective illness and in antidepressant drug action. *Pharmacopsychiatry, 15,* 31–39.

Weitzman, E. D., (1982). Chronobiology of man: Sleep, temperature and neuroendocrine rhythms. *Human Neurobiology, 1,* 173–183.

Winget, C., Deroshia, C., Markley, C., & Holley, D. (1984). A review of human physiological and performance changes associated with desynchronosis of biological rhythms. *Aviation, Space, and Environmental Medicine, 55,* 1085–1096.

9. Increase in Hospital Discharge Rates by the Oldest Old Despite Changes in Reimbursement Mechanisms, Olmsted County, MN, 1970–1985

CYNTHIA L. LEIBSON
JAMES NAESSENS
MARY CAMPION
IQBAL KRISHAN
FRED NOBREGA

INTRODUCTION

Similar to many of the countries represented at this conference, the United States is experiencing an increase in both the total numbers and the relative proportion of elderly in the population. Accompanying this observation is the well-demonstrated association between aging and increased utilization of health care services (Davis, 1984). These two facts have been a source of concern for persons responsible for the planning, delivery, and financing of high quality health care which will be appropriate to the needs of an aging society.

Rice and Wicks (1985) have attempted to predict the demand for services which will occur as a result of the projected increases in numbers of elderly and shifts in the age structure. Based on age-sex specific health status and medical care utilization rates in 1980 applied to population estimates for

Aging and Health: Linking Research and Public Policy, © 1989 Lewis Publishers, Inc., Chelsea, Michigan 48118. Printed in U.S.A.

2000, they predicted a 24% increase in the days of hospital care in the United States between 1980 and 2000.

Point-in-time projections such as those by Rice and Wicks assume constant rates of utilization by the various age-sex specific subgroups. The data presented in this chapter suggest that predictions based on these assumptions may underestimate future needs by failing to consider changes in age-sex specific rates of utilization over time. Preliminary observations revealed increases in utilization have been especially dramatic for the older elderly, those aged 75 and older. As this is the fastest growing age group, further investigation into the source of these increases is essential for a full appreciation of future demands for health care services.

The present study examines hospital utilization rates by persons aged 65 and older within a geographically defined community. It compares hospitalization rates and length of stay for the years 1970, 1980, and 1985. Readmission rates, procedures, and diagnoses are compared for the years 1980 and 1985. The geographically defined community under study is Olmsted County, Minnesota, with 97,876 residents in 1985, 9.7% of whom were aged 65 or older. Between 1970 and 1985 there was a 32% increase in the number of persons aged 65 and older, which compares to a 16% increase for all ages over that time period. Olmsted County is located in southeastern Minnesota, 80 miles from Minneapolis/St. Paul. The relative isolation from a major metropolitan center and the presence of one of the world's largest medical centers, the Mayo Clinic, result in the finding that over 98% of hospitalizations by County residents occur in the three area hospitals (Elveback, 1988, 1975). All admissions by County residents can be tracked by a patient-based medical records system established in 1906 which links all hospitals in the County. The medical records system has been the data base for a series of health services utilization and cost analyses for the years 1970, 1976, 1980, 1985, and 1987 (ongoing) (Shaller & Gunderson, 1986). This series of studies is the basis of this report.

OBSERVATIONS

There were 2.47 inpatient days per County resident aged 65 and older in 1970. This number increased to 2.84 days in 1980 and over the next five years decreased to 2.44 days, a figure below that for 1970. This decline in utilization can be attributed to a drop in mean length of stay between 1980 and 1985 for all age categories 65 and older (Table 1).

The decline in length of stay was sufficiently greater among the older age groups that the association between age and length of stay reversed directions between 1980 and 1985. While number of days per admission was declining faster for the older elderly, the rate of admission was increasing more rapidly for this age category relative to younger elderly. The changing association

Table 1. **Mean Length of Hospital Stay in Days, Olmsted County, MN, Age 65 and Older, 1980 vs 1985**

Age	1980	1985	Decline
65–69	9.3	8.5	0.8
70–74	8.7	8.5	0.2
75–79	10.2	9.0	1.2
80–84	10.7	8.1	2.6
85+	10.4	7.8	2.6

between age and hospitalization rate is illustrated dramatically in Figure 1. The 10-year period 1970 to 1980 exhibited increased hospitalizations by all age groups, but the percentage increase in hospitalizations per 1000 persons was greater for both sexes in the older relative to younger age groups (24% for 65–74 vs 45% for 75 and older). Between 1980 and 1985 the number of hospitalizations per population declined 6.2% for persons aged 65–74 (1086/4702 in 1980 vs 1089/5027 in 1985). In contrast, no decline occurred among persons aged 75 and older (1407/3872 in 1980 vs 1688/4490 in 1985). In this five-year period, older males exhibited increased admission rates while female rates remained essentially unchanged in every age category.

PERSONS HOSPITALIZED/1,000 POPULATION ≥ 65 YEARS OLD, 1970-1985, OLMSTED COUNTY, MN

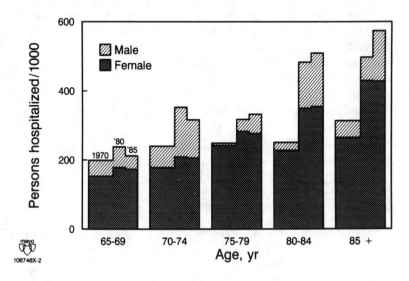

Figure 1. Persons hospitalized/1000 population ≥65 years old, 1970–1985, Olmsted County, MN.

SOME POSSIBLE EXPLANATIONS FOR INCREASED UTILIZATION

Readmissions

Why has the hospitalization rate increased for males 75 and older despite a decline in rate for males aged 65–74 between 1980 and 1985? As stated earlier, the drop in length of stay in 1980–1985 was greater among older age groups. A preliminary hypothesis suggested that shorter lengths of stay might result in patients leaving the hospital "quicker and sicker" and that such individuals, especially the frail elderly and the oldest old, would be at greater risk for readmission (Champlin, 1987). However, a comparison of both short- and long-term readmission rates for Olmsted County elderly in 1980 vs 1985 did not support this explanation (unpublished data). The increase in hospitalizations between 1980 and 1985 for persons aged 75 and older is not accounted for by increased hospitalizations per patient, which declined from 1.50 per patient per year (1980) to 1.44 (1985). Rather, the increase can be attributed to a significant increase ($p < 0.05$) in the number of males in the population who were hospitalized in 1985 vs 1980. This contrasts with a significant decline in the number of Olmsted County males aged 65–74 who were hospitalized in 1985 ($p < 0.05$) (Table 2).

Increased Ambulatory Care

Given that readmissions did not account for increased utilization, an alternate possibility was that procedures for which patients were hospitalized in 1980 were being performed on an ambulatory basis in 1985. This shift from an inpatient to an outpatient setting had occurred for Olmsted County residents aged 65–74, but not for residents aged 75 and older. It has been suggested that changes in the method of reimbursement for Medicare patients implemented in 1983 resulted in such a shift on the national level between 1980 and 1985 for the age group 65 and older (Heath, 1987).

Table 2.   Number of Persons Hospitalized per 1000 Population, Olmsted County, MN, Age 65 and Older, 1980 vs 1985

Age	1980	1985
65–74		
F	142 (396/2793)	135(401/2967)
M	213 (406/1909)	184(379/2059)
75+		
F	244 (650/2668)	248(769/3096)
M	268 (323/1204)	304(423/1393)

In order to examine this possibility in Olmsted County, the number of elderly hospital discharges with principal procedures defined as "outpatient" were compared for the various age-sex categories 1980 vs 1985. Principal procedures were coded according to the *International Classification of Diseases, 9th Revision, Clinical Modification* (ICD-9-CM) (Public Health Service and Health Care Financing Administration, 1980). The definition of a procedure as "outpatient" was based on the list of ambulatory/outpatient procedures—distributed by the Minnesota State Professional Review Organization (PRO) (Minnesota Professional Review Organization, 1984)—for which inpatient stays, as of 1984, would no longer be routinely reimbursed by Medicare.

The categorization of a particular procedure as "outpatient" in the present study was inclusive rather than exclusive. Various procedures on the Minnesota State PRO list are limited by the descriptors "simple" or "uncomplicated." Such procedures were defined as "outpatient" in all instances even when the ICD-9-CM code made no distinction as to complexity or severity. Similarly, decisions about which procedures should be classified as "outpatient" were based solely on the ICD-9-CM code and not on the appropriateness of a specific hospitalization. Consideration of appropriateness might bias the results in favor of the hypothesis, since complications and comorbidities that may legitimate a hospital stay are more frequent among the older age groups.

An example of a procedure that in 1984 was no longer routinely reimbursed on an inpatient basis is unilateral hernia repair. The number of hospital discharges/1000 residents for males aged 65–74 with unilateral hernia listed as a principal procedure declined from 15.2 in 1980 (29/1909) to 5.3 in 1985 (11/2059). For males aged 75 and older, this figure increased from 6.6/1000 residents (8/1204) in 1980 to 9.3/1000 (13/1393) in 1985. When the analysis was applied to all procedures defined as "outpatient," this distinction between age groups was again apparent (Table 3).

Table 3. Number of Hospital Stays per 1000 Population, Total and "Outpatient," Olmsted County, MN, Age 65 and Older, 1980 vs 1985

Age[a]	Total Hospitalizations/1000			"Outpatient" Hospitalizations/1000		
	1980	1985	Change	1980	1985	Change
65–74						
F (2793,2967)	193	188	−5	33	30	−3
M (1909,2059)	286	257	−29	64	38	−26
75+						
F (2668,3096)	345	348	+3	47	52	+5
M (1204,1393)	404	437	+33	65	84	+19

[a]Numbers in parentheses are 1980 and 1985 populations, respectively.

These findings support the hypothesis that the lack of decline (1980–1985) in total hospitalization rates by older relative to younger elderly reflects a tendency for older elderly to be hospitalized for procedures no longer performed on an inpatient basis for younger elderly. Table 3 also illustrates that the number of "outpatient" procedures being performed on an inpatient basis accounts for only some of the increase in total hospitalizations per population by males aged 75 and older.

Further examination focused on discharges with principal procedures not classified as "outpatient" and which fit the criteria for Class 1 surgical procedures as outlined by *Uniform Hospital Discharge Data* (National Committee on Vital and Health Statistics, 1980). As shown in Table 4, there was a significant increase in the rate of hospitalizations for Class 1 "not-outpatient" surgical procedures for males aged 65–74 ($p < 0.01$) and males aged 75 and older ($p < 0.01$). The increase among females was not significant in either age category. The differences over time between males and females are not readily explainable and require further investigation.

Table 4. Number of Class 1 Surgical Procedures per 1000 Population, "Outpatient" Procedures Excluded, Olmsted County, MN, Age 65 and Older, 1980 vs 1985

Age	1980	1985	Change
65–74			
F	59 (165/2793)	70 (208/2967)	+11
M	86 (164/1909)	114 (235/2059)	+28
75+			
F	78 (208/2668)	87 (269/3096)	+9
M	99 (119/1204)	137 (191/1393)	+38

Changes in Diagnostic Patterns

Hospitalizations occur for reasons other than surgical procedures. In order to investigate further the source of increased hospitalization rates by males aged 75 and older, individual discharges for 1980 and 1985 were assigned to one of the 470 diagnosis related groups *(Physician's DRG Working Guidebook,* 1984). Discharges were dichotomized as "medical" or "surgical" in accordance with the established medical/surgical subdivisions within each major diagnostic category of the diagnosis related groups (Table 5).

The data show the familiar pattern of a decline for males aged 65–75 and an increase for males aged 75 and older. The increase in medical discharges per 1000 persons for older males may partially be explained by a higher mean age for the 75 and older cohort 1985 vs 1980. The prevalence of cancer, and therefore the risk of hospitalization with this disease, increases with age (DeMaria & Cohen, 1987). Age-adjusted differences in health

Table 5. Number of Medical and Surgical Diagnoses per 1000, Olmsted County, MN, Age 65 and Older, 1980 vs 1985

Age	MDC Discharges/1000, Males		Change
	1980	1985	
	Medical		
65–74	162 (309/1909)	142 (292/2059)	−20
75+	272 (327/1204)	284 (396/1393)	+12
	Surgical		
65–74	125 (239/1909)	115 (237/2059)	−10
75+	132 (159/1204)	154 (214/1393)	+22

Note: MDC = major diagnostic category.

status for the 75 and older cohort over time cannot be ruled out, however. Findings for surgical discharges are essentially a restatement of the "outpatient" and "not-outpatient" results presented in Tables 3 and 4.

SUMMARY

1. The increase in hospitalization rate has been most dramatic for persons aged 75 and older. Between 1970 and 1980 this was true for both sexes. Between 1980 and 1985, a significant increase for males aged 75 and older contrasted with a significant decline for males aged 65–74.

2. The increased hospitalization rate for persons aged 75 and older was due to a greater percentage of the population being hospitalized, not a greater number of hospitalizations per individual.

3. The decline in hospitalizations for procedures defined as "outpatient" which occurred for younger elderly was not observed for older age groups.

4. Higher hospitalization rates occurred in both medical and surgical categories, but a majority of the increase in hospitalizations was attributable to a greater number of surgical procedures being performed on the older elderly over time.

IMPLICATIONS

The findings reported here may have repercussions beyond the geographically defined area of Olmsted County, Minnesota. The Mayo Clinic is an ambulatory care center with a long-standing historical emphasis on outpatient care. The conservative practice style that has characterized the Mayo Clinic has resulted in consistently lower rates of utilization for Olmsted County compared to U.S. figures. Age-sex adjusted hospitalization rates for Olmsted County residents aged 65 and older for 1970, 1980, and 1985 were 70%, 72%, and 79% of national rates for these respective years. Total Medicare expenditures per elder, including physician fees, after adjustments for area age, sex, and wage factors, were 24% less than the national average in 1982 (McClure & Shaller, 1985). Over the past decade, there have been efforts at both the national and local levels to control health care costs and contain utilization. These efforts have been followed by a decline in hospitalization rates at the national level (National Center for Health Statistics, *Recent Declines in Hospitalization: United States, 1982–86,* cited by Schmid, 1987). This decline between 1980 and 1985 was not mirrored in Olmsted County where, on the contrary, hospitalization rates increased for residents aged 75 and older. The concern is that the goal of providing ready access to high quality health care in an efficient manner will require methods other than those which have been traditionally successful if we are to meet the needs and demands of an aging society.

REFERENCES

Champlin, L. (1987). DRG's: Putting the squeeze on your older patients? *Geriatrics, 40,* 77–81.

Davis, K. (1984). Paying the health-care bills of an aging population. In A. Pifer & L. Bronte (Eds.), *Our aging society: Paradox and promise.* New York: Norton.

DeMaria, L. C., & Cohen, H. J. (1987). Characteristics of lung cancer in elderly patients. *Journal of Gerontology, 42*(5), 540–45.

Elveback, L. (1968, 1975). Special surveys conducted by Department of Epidemiology. By communication.

Heath, D. (1987, September 14). Surgery centers increasing their cut. *The News-Sentinel,* Fort Wayne, IN.

McClure, W., & Shaller, D. (1985). *Variations in Medicare expenditures per enrollee.* Center for Policy Studies, internal memorandum.

Minnesota Professional Review Organization. (1984). *Ambulatory/outpatient procedure list.* Unpublished.

National Committee on Vital and Health Statistics. (1980). *Uniform hospital discharge data. Minimum data set* (DHEW Publication No. PHS 80–1157). Hyattsville, MD: U.S. Dept. HEW.

Physician's DRG working guidebook. (1984). Louisville, KY: St. Anthony Hospital.

Public Health Service and Health Care Financing Administration. (1980, September). *International classification of diseases, 9th revision, clinical modification* (DHHS Publication No. PHS 80-1260). Washington, DC: U.S. Government Printing Office.

Rice, D., & Wicks, A. L. K. (1985). *Impact of an aging population on health care needs: State projections*. San Francisco: University of California, Institute for Health and Aging.

Schmid, R. E. (1987, October 4). Hospitalizations, length of stays decrease sharply. *St. Paul Pioneer Press Dispatch*.

Shaller, D., & Gunderson, S. (1986, October). Setting benchmarks for cost-effective care. *Business and Health*, 28–32.

10.   One-Stop Access for Senior Citizens: A Model of Integrated Service Delivery for Rural Areas

BRENDA FRASER
ANTHONY M. FULLER

INTRODUCTION TO ONE-STOP ACCESS

The Policy Framework

The concept of One-Stop Access as it is being introduced in the province of Ontario reflects the current policy orientations of the government toward services for the aged in the 1980s. With the growth in the population over the age of 65, there has been increasing recognition of the importance of supporting independence in the community and a subsequent reorientation in the thrust of programs and services for the elderly falling within the public domain.

This shift in the approach to services for the elderly is reflected in a report entitled *A New Agenda: Health and Social Service Strategies for Ontario's Seniors* (Minister for Senior Citizens Affairs, 1986). It states that "the central theme of [the Ontario Government's] proposals is to improve and/or maintain the health and functional status of the elderly (primarily through enhanced community care and services) and thereby, to significantly reduce preventable and inappropriate institutionalization" (p. vii). This document clearly outlines strategies designed to "lead to a more effective and affordable system of health and social services for the elderly" (p. vii). The need for

Aging and Health: Linking Research and Public Policy, © 1989 Lewis Publishers, Inc., Chelsea, Michigan 48118. Printed in U.S.A.

improved access and a more comprehensive approach to the delivery of community health and social services emerge as priorities. Simplification of access and coordination of service provision is seen as essential to address the fragmentation, duplication, and confusion often found in community-based services. **A One-Stop Access concept therefore proposes a system which would provide a single point of entry for community services, comprehensive functional assessments, and referral to appropriate services via a case management system.**

Despite the laudable objectives of simplified access and improved coordination, there is an inevitable degree of complexity involved in attaining such goals. Community-based programs and services span multiple government ministries and programs both provincially and locally, and affect many different organizations both public and private. The consultation process preceding the publication of *A New Agenda* (1986) determined that "at the present time, no single agency has the responsibility or the authority to plan, develop, and manage local services for the elderly. The result is an ad hoc approach, which cannot fully respond to the overall needs of our senior citizens" (p. 20).

Two approaches incorporated within the One-Stop Access concept address these issues. First, community health and social services are to be *integrated* and second, responsibility for the planning, development, and management of these services is to be devolved to a *local* authority. These two factors represent perhaps the most exciting, yet challenging, features of the One-Stop Access concept beyond the operational aspects of a comprehensive case management system. As policy initiatives, they signify an important shift in the way the Government of Ontario plans to fund and administer community-based programs in the years ahead. What is equally relevant and of particular interest is the ramifications of this proposed marriage of health and social services at the local municipal level, where agencies will be expected to implement this policy. An understanding of and sensitivity to the characteristics of the area where these initiatives will be introduced has implications for research and policy.

The Objectives of the One-Stop Access

The overall objectives of the One-Stop Access concept are (Office for Senior Citizens Affairs, 1987):

- to ensure an integrated approach to the delivery of community health and social services
- to take the first step toward the development of a more comprehensive approach, which can be expanded to include:
  - a broader range of services
  - other target groups

- to devolve responsibility for the planning and management of One-Stop Access to a local authority so that it is most responsive to local needs
- to make maximum use of existing and future administrative and program resources
- to strengthen and rationalize the role of service providers
- to avoid excessive professionalization and to enhance and supplement, not replace existing or potential family and volunteer support services

An extensive consultation was conducted to locate five pilot sites for One-Stop Access, all of which were required to have in place an integrated homemaking program in addition to a home care program and a range of home support services. Huron County, the Regional Municipality of Waterloo, and the District of Cochrane were the first three areas selected in 1987/88 as pilot sites.

In Huron County, the designated Local Authority, the Board of Health, sought the assistance of external consultants to help develop their proposal. The Gerontology Research Centre and the School of Rural Planning and Development at the University of Guelph were invited to collaborate to design a model of One-Stop Access for the County. Of particular interest to the research team was the prospect of developing a model of One-Stop Access in a predominantly rural area.

ISSUES RELATING TO RURALITY

Simplifying access to health and social services in a rural area is a daunting task, not only because of the issues of integrating "domains" of service, but also because of the physical and cultural aspects of rurality itself. Krout (1986) has noted "that the provision of services in rural areas must differ from service delivery in urban areas because of the ecological, organizational, and economic features of these places and the attitudes and characteristics of the rural elderly themselves" (p. 144).

Rural environments in Canada are invariably land extensive with low population densities and varying distances between communities. Community-based services must reconcile the requirements of small town locations, dispersed farm and rural nonfarm populations, and seasonal impediments to travel. Service models based on home delivery systems are faced with overcoming the difficulties resulting from these characteristics.

Other factors which influence the search for appropriate models in rural areas include the "undermanning" phenomenon (Wicker, 1979; Wolfe, 1987). Small rural populations understandably have only a limited number of leaders, professionals, and trained personnel, and these are often oversubscribed in their commitment to community service. This is especially true of the volunteer sector. Political idiosyncrasies of local government, traditional decisionmaking procedures, and strongly held views of "independence" often confound the economic rationality of models and programs (Coward et al., 1983). In matching public policy with these realities, the problems of model development and implementation are exacerbated.

Rural areas in Ontario have both positive and negative features that impinge on the question of improved service provision for senior citizens. By far the greatest density of the elderly reside in service centers of between 1000–5000 people (Hodge & Qadeer, 1983; Joseph & Fuller, 1987). This reflects an in-migration of farm and rural nonfarm retirees as well as seniors from more urban locations, which together with those who have aged in-place, produces average figures for small town elderly of 20% above the age of 65 (Martin-Matthews & Vanden Heuvel, 1986). The implication is that many older citizens have moved to places that are not only desirable in terms of residential preference, but also to have greater access to essential services. Nevertheless, such service centers are small and the distances between them are often large, posing the problem of how to service geographically disparate populations which generally lack the "critical mass" to justify permanent, specialized services.

The research question related to the development of a workable model is thus structured by three overriding considerations:

- the problems of integrating and accessing services
- the problems of service provision in rural areas
- the issue of introducing policy changes from "top down"

THE PROPOSED ONE-STOP ACCESS MODEL

The challenge for the research team was to develop a model that would allow for the incorporation of the "rural" strengths and limitations of the pilot site into the prescribed features of One-Stop Access. Direct research through the community consultation process guided much of the model development and proposed structure of One-Stop Access. Information was sought in four areas: services currently provided, interagency relationships, perceived gaps in service, and response to the One-Stop Access concept. Further information sharing and feedback was obtained at two public meetings and incorporated into the proposed structure for One-Stop Access.

In developing a model for One-Stop Access in a rural area, it was important to consider the organizational features of the system, case management functions, and locational features.

The primary components in the One-Stop Access model are the Local Authority, the Management Unit, a Citizens' Advisory Council, and the service providers.

The Local Authority

The *Local Authority* is that body which has to plan, develop, and manage a comprehensive system of community health and social services for the elderly. It is accountable for the planning and management of One-Stop Access. In a rural area this may be a local government or a special purpose body such as a Board of Health. The community consultation undertaken by the research team suggested that the Local Authority be independent, although with a reporting relationship to the County Council, and that it have a professional image and be seen to represent both health and social services. For these reasons, a special purpose committee of the Board of Health was recommended in Huron County.

The management function of the Local Authority is largely undertaken by the One-Stop Manager and the management staff. The Local Authority gives direction to the management unit, is accountable for all budgetary decisions, and hears appeals from consumers and service providers. The manager supervises the case managers and ensures that contracts and agreements with service providers are met. The manager also oversees the central recordkeeping and information system.

Fitting available resources to the immediate need is an important short-term operational planning function. Longer term planning (strategic planning) enables the One-Stop Access program to adjust to future needs in both supply and demand for services.

In order to ensure an effective planning function, the Local Authority requires information from local planning authorities, service providers, and representatives of the consumers themselves. Through the planning process, the rural area brings its resources together to represent all the sectors and interest groups involved and to determine the future systems of delivery and levels of provisions.

The Case Management System

The case management system approach is integral to the process of increasing the coordination and appropriateness of service delivery. Capitman, Haskins, and Bertstein (1986) suggest that case management can be considered as an administrative service that directs client movement through a series of phased involvement with the long term care system. It is also an advocacy service that attempts to integrate the formal long term care system with the caregiving provided informally by family members, friends, and community groups. There are five readily distinguishable components to the case management process: intake and screening, assessment and reassessment, care planning, service arrangement, and monitoring and counseling.

Decentralization

In determining the optimal location for the case management system, it is important to consider several interrelated factors. The choice of an alternative along a *centralized-decentralized continuum* must take into account the critical information, assessment, and referral aspects of the One-Stop Access system as well as the ongoing case management functions. It will be necessary to ensure that any alternative allows for the implementation of an information system and a One-Stop (single) Access point via a toll-free phone contact system. Equally, it must facilitate prompt in-home functional assessments and the delivery of multisource services within a comprehensive health and social services case management system.

Four factors were determined critical to the issue of centralization or decentralization: (1) community visibility and communication; (2) ease of contact among case manager, clients, and service providers; (3) peer interaction; and (4) cost. Each factor was evaluated from the perspective of consumers/clients, case managers, service providers, and the system as a whole.

Because each centralized/decentralized option entails distinct strengths and limitations, it was important to determine which factors held the greatest weight in the ultimate success of a One-Stop Access system. In many respects, the locational alternatives did not differ significantly in their ability to provide information, assessment, and referral for a range of community health and social services. This affirms the value of the One-Stop Access "management" that coordinates care on behalf of clients regardless of location. However, effective *delivery* is largely dependent upon knowledge and interaction among the resources and services on which One-Stop Access was reliant.

This latter point was perhaps the most critical in assessing the centralized/decentralized question. The prime objectives of One-Stop Access are to simplify access and coordinate service, objectives dependent in large degree upon communication and program visibility. Although centralization would not preclude communication, it was felt that a locally visible case management structure would afford greater sensitivity to local needs and to service opportunities, and *equally for One-Stop Access to become recognized as a local resource*. Consumer perception was deemed to be an important aspect of One-Stop Access. Given considerations of cost however, a partially decentralized model was proposed in the Huron County model.

IMPLICATIONS

Clearly, many of the ongoing issues related to the implementation of One-Stop Access represent inevitable reactions to change. Service providers and consumers retain a healthy degree of cynicism about the benefits of new government initiatives and are understandably reticent to embrace programs that at least initially represent increased workloads. Equally, policies directed toward reduction of service duplication may be perceived as threatening or intruding into areas of specific professional domains. Resistance to change, distrust of government, and territoriality are not new phenomena nor are they particularly rural. However, these aspects, when coupled with factors characteristic of rural environments, can have a significant effect on the success of government policy initiatives such as One-Stop Access.

As described in the One-Stop model, the system is reliant on committed individuals at all levels. The high-level skill of case managers, the specialized expertise of the provider network, and the commitment to and understanding of the importance of planning and management of members of the Local Authority are implicit in a model that seeks to plan, manage, and provide services in a simplified yet coordinated way. This is not to suggest that rural areas are without these individuals, merely that they may be in short supply or committed to other aspects of the community organizational structure. In a county such as Huron which is relatively isolated and distant from a major center, recruitment of professionals poses difficulties. Recruitment and staffing issues bear consideration when introducing programs into rural areas. Training and upgrading become critical support features for the system as a whole.

The undermanning phenomena referred to earlier also have implications for an initiative seeking to combine health and social services at the local level. Because One-Stop Access service provision is based on a fee-for-service model, some of the most knowledgeable and capable members of the system would be placed in conflict-of-interest positions by virtue of their contractual arrangements with One-Stop Access. In an area that can only support a small number of agencies, there is by association a limited resource pool upon which to draw. If government intends to devolve program and funding control to local authorities, residents need to be assured that the new decisionmakers will demonstrate capability and fairness based on their knowledge and experience related to health and social services. It is conceivable that in a rural area the most desirable candidates may be excluded de facto.

Another critical observation concerns the need for balance between providing integrated services at the community level and the cost of such provision. The strong sense of "locality," that is, the need to locate services within local communities and to use familiar personnel, is paramount. Here the challenge lies in utilizing new technology and management techniques to centralize and make cost-effective certain aspects of the system while maintaining community-based services wherever possible. This may create useful tension between centralizing and decentralizing forces in rural service areas. There may be some major gains, for example, through the use and adaptation of computer-based information and communications systems, which essentially can link service units (fixed or mobile) into highly functional networks. Such systems may help to overcome the problems of isolation and need for strong peer group and supervisory support for case managers, given the expanding nature of their roles and responsibilities.

Finally, our research demonstrated once more the difficulties that provincial agencies often have in prescribing program changes in local community services. The possibility of program rejection rests not necessarily on the merits of the proposition, but on the way that it is perceived. Rural service systems are often small, ongoing, and strained by lack of resources and are frequently confronted with efforts to coordinate, evaluate, and streamline.

We have yet to discover how best to introduce new ideas so that they are considered carefully by *all* the affected groups, and a process of decision-making such that whatever the outcome, it is the product of a genuine "community" decision. To this extent, the movement toward the provision of community services will require, at several levels, more attention to the processes of community development and to research that links the proposed solutions and the specific setting where they are to be introduced. In this way, new initiatives may come to be viewed as representative of "public" policy and their implementation at the local level will be grounded in an understanding of the organizational, institutional, and ecological context into which they must fit.

ACKNOWLEDGMENT

This chapter is based on the research of the University of Guelph team, which includes Dr. Anne Martin-Matthews (Director, Gerontology Research Centre); Dr. Jackie Wolfe (University School of Rural Planning and Development); and Dr. Alun Joseph (Dept. of Geography). The ideas presented here do not reflect the position of the provincial agencies or the Huron County Board of Health.

REFERENCES

Capitman, J. A., Haskins, B., & Bertstein, J. (1986). Case management approaches in coordinated community-oriented long term care demonstrations. *The Gerontologist, 26*(4), 398–404.

Coward, R. T., DeWeaver, K. L., Schmidt, F. E., & Jackson, R. W. (1983). Mental health practice in rural environments: A frame of reference. *The International Journal of Mental Health, 12,* 3–24.

Hodge, G., & Qadeer, M. (1983). *Towns and villages in Canada.* Toronto: Butterworths.

Joseph, A., & Fuller, A. M. (1987). Aging in rural communities: Interrelated issues in housing, services and transportation. *Papers on Rural Aging* (No. 3). University School of Rural Planning and Development and Gerontology Research Centre, University of Guelph.

Krout, J. A. (1986). *The aged in rural America*. New York: Greenwood Press.

Martin-Matthews, A., & Vanden Heuvel, A. (1986). Methodological issues in research on aging in rural versus urban environments. *Papers on Rural Aging* (No. 1). University School of Rural Planning and Development and Gerontology Research Centre, University of Guelph.

Minister for Senior Citizens Affairs. (1986). *A new agenda: Health and social service strategies for Ontario's seniors*. Toronto: Queen's Printer.

Office for Senior Citizens Affairs. (1987). *Guidelines for the development of one-stop access by the Huron County Board of Health*. Toronto: In-house document.

Wicker, A. W. (1979). The Theory of Manning. In *An introduction to ecological psychology* (chap. 5, pp. 70–80). Monterey: Brooks/Cole Publishing Company.

Wolfe, J. S. (1987). *Introducing community government in small northern territory towns*. Darwin: Australian National University, North Australia Research Unit, Seminar Series 1987.

11. The Impact of Health Education on the Use of Medications in Elderly Women

LAN T. GIEN
JOCK A. D. ANDERSON

INTRODUCTION

It has been well documented that the elderly, compared to the young, take more medicines, resulting in more drug reactions. They suffer from more chronic illnesses, and have longer and more frequent hospitalization periods (Greenblatt, Sellers, & Shader, 1982). Eighty-five percent of the ambulatory population over 65 years of age take, on average, three or four prescribed drugs each day, and medication errors occur more commonly in these older adults (Lamy, 1980, pp. 89–108). In addition to prescribed drugs, the elderly use over-the-counter (OTC) medicines. Many OTC medicines are multiple-ingredient products. Self-medication, which is a part of self-care, is not only practiced widely but is here to stay. Generally, nonprescribed medicines are used approximately twice as frequently as prescribed medicines, and this ratio has remained fairly constant during the last 20 years (Jefferys, Brotherston, & Cartwright, 1960; Wadsworth, Butterfield, & Blaney, 1971; Dunnell, 1973; Morrell & Wale, 1976; Crooks & Christopher, 1979). The risk of adverse drug reactions in older people is nearly double that of younger adults, and an alarming number of elderly patients are admitted to hospitals as a direct result of preventable drug reactions. Many have a second reaction during their hospital stay (Hurwitz, 1969; Frisk, Cooper, & Campbell, 1977; Steel et al., 1981). Furthermore, drug reactions in hospitalized patients double the length of their hospital stay (Seidl et al., 1966).

Aging and Health: Linking Research and Public Policy, © 1989 Lewis Publishers, Inc., Chelsea, Michigan 48118. Printed in U.S.A.

The causes of adverse drug reactions in the elderly are multiple. They include polypharmacy, self-medication, lack of compliance, lack of clear understanding of drug regimen, improper storage of drugs, doctors' lack of training in geriatric prescribing, poor supervision of the elderly, dual prescribing systems, and increased sensitivity of the elderly to drugs due to normal physiological change in aging (Gien & Anderson, in press).

Several authors have proposed guidelines for safe geriatric prescribing as well as suggested steps to promote comprehension of drug regimens and to increase compliance. The role of the nurse in patient teaching has been emphasized. However, research exploring this role is scarce. This study is designed to measure the effect of a health education brochure, given by the visiting nurse to a group of ambulatory elderly women in their own homes.

Although life expectancy is increasing for both men and women, women live, on average, seven years longer than men and account for a rising proportion of the older population as age increases (Fries, 1980; Stone & Fletcher, 1986). Women take more medications, both prescribed and nonprescribed (Law & Chalmers, 1976; May et al., 1982; Dunnell, 1973; Crooks & Christopher, 1979). They have a higher incidence of adverse drug reactions, and they visit the general practitioner (GP) more frequently than men (Hurwitz, 1969; Petersen & Thomas, 1975). Thus, elderly women will be the most important customers of the pharmaceutical industry and of the health care system in future years. Hence, they are the focus of this study.

SPECIFIC OBJECTIVES

The specific objectives of the study are:

1. to identify the types and amount of prescribed medicines regularly used by a sample of elderly women
2. to assess the degree of compliance in using these prescribed drugs
3. to identify the types, amount, and degree of appropriate use of self-medications in the sample
4. to assess the frequency of possible adverse interactions between prescribed and OTC medicines in the sample, and related degree of harm
5. to assess the impact of the health education program on the appropriate use of prescribed and OTC medicines and their possible adverse interactions in the study group, at one year after intervention
6. to explore the roles of the nurse in promoting the appropriate use of prescribed and OTC medicines, thus improving collaborative care

The study was designed as a randomized controlled trial to test three hypotheses: (1) that the health education program would decrease the number of prescribed medicines being *used* inappropriately; (2) that the health education program would decrease the number of prescribed medicines being *kept* inappropriately; and (3) that the health education program would reduce the risk of *adverse interaction* between prescribed and OTC drugs.

METHOD

The initial sample for the study consisted of 145 elderly women between 67 and 76 years of age who were on prescribed medicines, selected from the records of a group of participating general practitioners (GPs) providing medical care for a population of about 10,000 in a residential urban area. Baseline data on the types and amounts of medications used (prescribed and nonprescribed), the errors made, and their possible adverse interactions were obtained from the GPs' records and through guided interviews using an interviewer-administered questionnaire with an interrater reliability of 92%.

After the initial interview, the sample was allocated at random to the study and control groups. A self-care education brochure was introduced by the visiting nurse, and the content was discussed individually with each member of the study group. The purpose of the self-care education program was to help the elderly to safely use prescribed and OTC medicines and to deal effectively with some common minor ailments in this age group without risk. To allow the participants adequate time to read and to absorb the content of the self-care brochure, the visiting nurse returned the following week to answer any questions, to clarify any misunderstanding, or to discuss again the content of the brochure if necessary.

One year after the self-care education was introduced, the entire sample was reinterviewed, using the same questionnaire. Those who had moved, changed GPs, were deceased, or had dropped out of the study were excluded from the final analysis, which consisted of 62 women in the control group and 57 in the study group. Data obtained at this time together with the information from the GPs' records would indicate the changes in medication-taking behaviors of both control and study groups. The significance of these changes were measured by multiple regression analyses.

RESULTS

The baseline data of 119 individuals remaining in the sample were analyzed. The following sections present a pattern of medication-taking behaviors of the cohort in relation to their prescribed medicines, OTC products, possible adverse drug interactions, and the impact of the health education program on these behaviors. The relationships of the demographic variables such as age, marital status, social contact, and health status with medication-taking behaviors are being examined and will be reported in another paper.

Prescribed Medicines

The number of prescribed medicines ranged from 1 to 10, with an average of 3.37 for each person. Of these drugs, nearly 6% were prescribed by the hospital, and the remainder by the general practitioners. The most common neuroactive drugs prescribed were analgesics, major tranquilizers, and hypnotics, followed by diuretics and antihypertensive drugs (Table 1). This finding is consistent with that of several previous studies (Bowling, 1982; May et al., 1982; Wade & Finlayson, 1983). Table 1 lists classifications of prescribed medicines identified in the sample. Medicines prescribed for less than 5% of the sample were not included. An individual may have more than one prescribed medication. Therefore, the total percentage of the sample is more than 100.

More than 61% of the sample used from one to eight prescribed medicines inappropriately. More than 20% had incorrect knowledge about one or more of their prescribed drugs. Nearly 13% had no knowledge about some or all of their drugs.

The most common categories of inappropriate use involved complete omission of taking drugs or taking less than the prescribed dosage (45.8% of the sample) as well as keeping and using medicines after their prescribed period (also 45.8%).

Again, analgesics were the medication most commonly kept and used after their prescribed period, followed by hypnotics. Failure to have the prescrip-

Table 1.   Classification of Prescribed Medicines

Medication Categories	Percentage of Sample
Analgesics	46.2
Hypnotics, sedatives, tranquilizers	33.6
Diuretics	33.6
Antihypertensives	30.3
Nonsteroidal antiinflammatory drugs	23.5
Cardiac drugs (for arrhythmias, angina, ischemic heart)	16.8
Bronchospasm relaxants	15.1
Embrocations (drugs rubbed into the skin)	10.1
Expectorant, cough suppressants	8.4
Laxatives	8.4
Antiemetics	8.4
Topical steroid preparations	7.6
Vitamins	6.7
Muscle relaxants	6.7
Antidepressants	6.7
Thyroid, antithyroid	5.9
Antibiotics	5.0
Soothing, protective preparations	5.0
Others	

tion filled occurred in 24.6% of the sample (Tables 2 and 3). According to criteria suggested by Hansten (1985), nearly 40% of all medicines kept and used after their prescribed period would be considered potentially harmful, due to possible adverse drug interactions or contraindications for the pathological conditions of the cohort members at the time of the interview.

Over 65% of the sample kept from one to seven medicines inappropriately. Close to 40% had one or more medicines with incomplete labels or no label at all. Over 29% of the sample kept the prescribed medicines but did not use them (Table 3).

Over-the-Counter Medicines (OTC)

Nearly 49% of the sample used from one to five OTC products, which ranged from analgesics (most common), laxatives, vitamins, and cough suppressants to substances not assigned to any pharmaceutical category, such as garlic supplements, tea herbs, and olive oil (Table 4). Approximately 16% of the entire sample used OTCs inappropriately.

Table 2.   Inappropriate Use of Prescribed Medicines

Categories	Percentage of Sample
Underdosage; omission of medicines	45.8
Use of medicines after prescribed use was over	45.8
Failure to have prescription filled	24.6
Overdosage	7.6
Wrong purpose and wrong dosage	7.6
Wrong purpose but correct dosage	5.9

Note: An individual could use more than one medicine, which could be classified into more than one category.

Table 3.   Prescribed Medicines Kept Inappropriately

Categories	Percentage of Sample	Potentially Harmful (% of category)
Medicines kept and used after prescribed period, but within shelf-life	45.8	40
Presence of incompletely labeled or unlabeled medicine containers	39.5	
Medicines kept but not used	29.4	34
Medicines kept after expiry date	5.0	16
Medicines prescribed for someone other than the person interviewed	4.2	20

Table 4.   Over-the-Counter Products (OTC)

Categories	Percentage of OTC Users
Analgesics	72.4
Laxatives	17.2
Vitamins	13.8
Cough suppressants	6.9
Products not assigned to any pharmaceutical category	19.0

The results affirmed that self-medication is a vital part of self-care in elderly women. If the use of medicines kept beyond their prescribed period is considered as self-medication, then the prevalence of self-medication nearly doubles.

Of all the individuals who used OTCs, nearly 78% took them only when needed, and over 62% used them regularly. Approximately 40% took one or more OTCs inappropriately. Of the OTCs that were used inappropriately, over 42% were considered potentially harmful according to Hansten's criteria.

Possible Adverse Drug Interactions due to OTCs

Over 15% of the entire sample had from one to four possible drug adverse interactions due to OTCs, 71% of which were considered potentially harmful. The interactions among prescribed drugs were not examined in this study.

Impact of the Health Education Program

Of 119 women in the cohort, 62 were in the control group and 57 in the study group. The purpose of the analysis was to determine how much the change in the medication-taking behaviors differed between the control and the study group for the variables presented in Table 5.

Initial examination of the frequency distribution of the variables showed a decrease in the number of prescribed medicines kept inappropriately, the number of prescribed medicines used inappropriately, and the number of possible adverse interactions in the study group. After allowing for the difference due to time lapse between the preeducation and posteducation data collections, multiple regression analyses were done using each variable as the dependent variable. The decrease in the number of prescribed medicines kept and used inappropriately by the study group was statistically significant at $p < 0.01$. The decrease in the number of possible adverse drug interactions due to OTC failed to reach statistical significance. The number of medical consultations did not change significantly in the study group.

Table 5. The Impact of the Health Education Program

Variables	Control Group (n = 62)		Study Group (n = 57)		Significance of Change
	Preeducation Mean	Posted Preeducation Change (%)	Preeducation Mean	Posted Preeducation Change (%)	
1. No. of prescribed medicines kept inappropriately	1.323	+36.5	1.298	−12.2	p < 0.01
2. No. of prescribed medicines used inappropriately	1.419	+22.72	1.351	−23.37	p < 0.01
3. No. of possible adverse interactions	0.194	−41.6	0.281	−62.5	nonsignificant
4. No. of GP consultations	3.806	−0.84	4.018	+ 3.5	nonsignificant

Note: Multiple regressions using variables 1, 2, 3, 4 as dependent variables. Multiple regressions with transformation of variables using formula: square root (n + 0.5) gave almost identical results.

Multiple regression analyses done with transformation of variables using the formula square root (n + 0.5) where n was the frequency of each variable listed in Table 5, gave almost identical results to those discussed above.

Further analysis is being done to examine the relationship between the effect of the health education program and the demographic variables.

Discussion

This study demonstrated that written health education materials, given and reinforced by a visiting nurse, could have a positive impact on the medication-taking behaviors in ambulatory elderly women, by significantly decreasing the number of prescribed medicines kept and used inappropriately.

The study did not reveal a significant change in the number of medical consultations in the study group. It may indicate that the rate of medical consultations in elderly women depends on several critical factors such as loneliness, lack of confidence in self-care due to the presence of multiple chronic conditions, and availability of time to visit the physician's office. Moreover, the nursing intervention in this study was of short duration, which might have partly accounted for the small impact on the rate of medical consultations.

Further research may include elderly men in the sample, and a comparison of the impact of the health education program on both sexes could be useful.

As stated earlier, among the multiple causes for increased adverse drug reactions in the elderly are lack of compliance and improper storage of drugs (Gien & Anderson, in press). A decrease in the number of prescribed medicines kept and used inappropriately would contribute to reducing the risk of adverse drug interactions, reducing the unnecessary hospital admissions as a direct result (Hurwitz, 1969; Frisk et al., 1977; Steel et al., 1981).

The potential economic impact of this change would be of interest to the insurance companies and government officials, especially in the present fiscal restraint environment.

In a multicenter study of the incidence of adverse drug reactions in the elderly, Williamson and Chopin (1980) found that over 81% were receiving prescribed drugs at the time of hospital admission and adverse reactions occurred in over 15% of this group. If the positive change in the medication-taking behavior could shorten the hospitalization period by one day for each of these 15% of elderly patients with adverse reactions, the savings in Canada would be approximately $160 million annually, extrapolating from the present average Newfoundland daily hospital cost. This saving applies to a national 65 and older population base of 2.7 million; it would increase as the elderly population reaches nearly 4 million as the 21st century approaches. By 2021, this population will reach 6 million, and by 2031, 7.5 million (Stone & Fletcher, 1986).

In addition to financial savings, the reduction of unwarranted illnesses would optimize the level of health in this age group, and slow down or delay decline in functional capacity in the later years, thus improving the quality of life and overall self-satisfaction.

The results of this study also indicated that a policy for the promotion of self-care education in this age group is needed. Since the majority of the elderly are living in their own homes, the education program should not only be applied in long term care institutions and senior citizen housing complexes, but should reach every household of the elderly.

Ideally, health teaching should be a part of the role of every health care professional. Nurses, whether in acute care, long term care facilities, or in the community, are readily accessible to patients. By nature of their professional education and experience, they are well suited to advise the elderly about medicines in general. It may be necessary for the nurse to visit regularly not only the ill elderly, but also the well elderly in their own homes, to supervise their medical regimes and to provide other primary health care services. To provide the opportunity for the nurses to use their full potential in caring for the elderly may prove to be an innovative and cost-effective health care delivery practice that would better meet the needs of Canada's elderly.

Furthermore, to maximize the patient-teaching role of health care professionals, their educational curricula should include basic principles of teaching-learning, effective teaching strategies for groups and individuals, and opportunities for planning and implementing patient teaching in clinical practice.

In summary, this study has provided empirical support for greater utilization of nurses as primary health care service providers envisaged by the Alma-Ata Declaration (WHO, 1978) and currently supported by the Canadian Department of National Health and Welfare (Epp, 1986) as well as by the World Health Organization (Mahler, 1985). This service controls health care expenditure growth while maintaining and/or improving the quality of care to one of the high risk groups—the elderly.

ACKNOWLEDGMENT

We thank the many people who cooperated in this study: Professor P. Higgins, Department of GP Research, Guy's Hospital, London, England; Dr. V. Radclyffe and the partners in his medical practice; Dr. I. Eade for organizing and collecting data for the pilot study; Dr. C. I. Lee, Department of Mathematics and Statistics, Memorial University; and Dr. D. Bryant, Department of Epidemiology and Biostatistics, Faculty of Medicine, Memorial University, for advice on statistical analysis.

This research was supported in part by the Vice-President Research Grant, Memorial University, St. John's, Newfoundland, Canada and by the Overseas Research Student Award ORS 84904 administered by the Committee of Vice-Chancellors and Principals of the Universities of the United Kingdom.

REFERENCES

Bowling, A. (1982, January 23). Nurses for residential homes. *Lancet, 1,* 229.

Crooks, J., & Christopher, L. J. (1979). Use and misuse of home medicines. In J. A. D. Anderson (Ed.), *Self medication* (p. 33). Lancaster, England: MTP Press.

Dunnell, K. (1973). Medicine takers and hoarders. *Journal of the Royal College of General Practitioners, 23*(Suppl.), 2–9.

Epp, J. (1986). *Achieving health for all: A framework for health promotion.* Ottawa: Health and Welfare Canada.

Fries, J. F. (1980). Natural death and the compression of morbidity. *New England Journal of Medicine, 303,* 130–5.

Frisk, P. A., Cooper, J. W., & Campbell, N. A. (1977). Community-hospital pharmacist detection of drug-related problems upon patient admission to small hospital. *American Journal of Hospital Pharmacy, 34,* 738–742.

Gien, L. T., & Anderson, J. A. D. (in press). Medication and the elderly: A review. *Journal of Geriatric Drug Therapy*.

Greenblatt, D. J., Sellers, E. M., & Shader, R. I. (1982). Drug therapy: Drug disposition in old age. *New England Journal of Medicine, 306*(18), 1081–1088.

Hansten, P. D. (1985). *Drug interaction* (5th ed.). Philadelphia: Lea & Febiger.

Hurwitz, N. (1969). Predisposing factors in adverse reactions to drugs. *British Medical Journal, 1,* 536–539.

Jefferys, M., Brotherston, J. H. F., & Cartwright, A. (1960). Consumption of medicines on a working-class housing estate. *British Journal of Preventive and Social Medicine, 14,* 64–76.

Lamy, P. P. (1980). Health care expenditure and drugs. In *Prescribing for the elderly*. Littleton, MA: PSG Publishing.

Law, R., & Chalmers, C. (1976). Medicines and elderly people: A general practice survey. *British Medical Journal, 1,* 565–568.

Mahler, H. (1985). Nurses lead the way. *WHO Features, 97,* 1–3.

May, F. E., Stewart, R. B., Hale, W. E., & Marks, R. G. (1982). Prescribed and non prescribed drug use in an ambulatory elderly population. *Southern Medical Journal, 75*(5), 522–528.

Morrell, D. C., & Wale, C. J. (1976). Symptoms perceived and recorded by patients. *Journal of the Royal College of General Practitioners, 26,* 398–403.

Petersen, D. M., & Thomas, O. W. (1975). Acute drug reaction among the elderly. *Journal of Gerontology, 30*(5), 552–556.

Seidl, L. G., Thornton, G. F., Smith, J. W., & Cluff, L. E. (1966). Study on the epidemiology of adverse drug reactions: III. Reactions in patients on a general medical service. *Bulletin of the Johns Hopkins Hospital, 119,* 299–315.

Steel, K., Gertman, P. M., Crescenzi, C., & Anderson, J. (1981). Iatrogenic illness on a general medical service at a university hospital. *New England Journal of Medicine, 304,* 638–42.

Stone, L. O., & Fletcher, S. (1986). *The seniors boom.* (Statistics Canada Catalogue No. 89–515). Ministry of Supply and Services, Canada.

Wade, B., & Finlayson, J. (1983, May 4). Drugs and the elderly. *Nursing Mirror, 156*(18), 17–21.

Wadsworth, M. E. J., Butterfield, W. J. H., & Blaney, R. (1971). *Health and sickness: The choice of treatment.* London: Tavistock Publ.

Williamson, J., & Chopin, J. M. (1980). Adverse reactions to prescribed drugs in the elderly: A multicenter investigation. *Age and Ageing, 9*(2), 73–80.

World Health Organization. (1978). Declaration of Alma-Ata. *Primary Health Care* (Report of the International Conference on Primary Health Care, Alma-Ata, USSR. 6–12 September 1978). Geneva: World Health Organization, 2–6.

12. Policy as Significant Determinator of the Use of Physical Restraints

ERNA J. SCHILDER

INTRODUCTION

Rights of the patient are grounded in the ethical principle of autonomy. Patients are entitled to protection and to checks on those who have privileges and power over them. This entitlement imposes duties on others to enable the expression of human qualities, feelings, inclinations, and thoughts. Absolutely essential for the achievement of the human potential are health, free expression, self-determination—and life, liberty, and the pursuit of happiness.

The Honourable Jake Epp (1986), Canada's Minister of National Health and Welfare, has taken up the challenge in *Achieving Health for All: A Framework for Health Promotion* promising "the opportunity to make choices and to gain satisfaction from living" (p. 3). The framework for health promotion comes at a most opportune time in the development of public policy. In this context, discussion of confinement in health care settings is long overdue.

REVIEW OF LITERATURE

The use of restraint has come under judicial scrutiny since several accidents, some of them with fatal outcomes, have been reported. The recommendations from the various sources address the issue of proper use of the devices. Manufacturers are to improve the labeling, instructions, and warnings as well as modify the design to prevent patients from freeing themselves. Juries have urged closer surveillance, use of restraints by prescription

Aging and Health: Linking Research and Public Policy, © 1989 Lewis Publishers, Inc., Chelsea, Michigan 48118. Printed in U.S.A.

from a physician only, and better nursing practices and continuing educational programs to provide a safe environment (Canadian Government, 1981, 1982). However, none of the directives address the justified and legitimate use of restraint and what appropriate alternative measures could be tried prior to the curtailment of freedom of movement. "Any treatment that results in physical harm or mental suffering or deprivation of goods and services necessary to avoid physical harm or mental suffering" constitutes abuse in the eye of the law (The BRN Report, 1986).

In the absence of stringent standards and policies that protect human rights, the prevalence of use of restraints is not surprising. The magnitude of the use of physical restraint on patients has attained staggering proportions if the reports of some authors are indeed representative of hospitalized patients in general. McLean et al. (1982) have reported that 10% of patients in general hospitals and 50% of the residents of specialized institutions are restrained in some form or another for variable periods of time. Among four hospitals in Baltimore, where a patient classification system provided for the reporting of restraint as a category, between 5% and 40% of the patients were restrained at any given time (J. O'Shea, personal communications, July and August 24, 1983). However, there was no ready explanation for the widely divergent use of restraints.

In a survey conducted in a 400-bed community hospital, of the 279 patients 70 years or older whose functional abilities were assessed, 19% were found to be in either body or arm restraints or both (Warshaw et al., 1982). Newbern (1982; personal communications, August 11, 1983) reported the results of 162 interviews of nurses and other health care providers on the incidence of patient abuse. What she terms "socially acceptable" abuse, that is, "under- or overmedication, improper use of restraints, invasion of territory without permission," occurs most frequently among chronically ill or aggressive female patients. While she recommends restoring the locus of control to the patient and promoting self-care, from the clinician's perspective the issue is more complex.

Friedman (1983) reports nurses' responses to an inquiry on the value and application of restraints. While none advocated the use of restraints, most considered them a necessary evil. However, a number expressed "strong reservations about physically restraining patients in any but the most desperate circumstances" (p. 79). Others expressed their views that "it is kinder to restrain a patient than to risk serious injury or interruption of crucial treatment" (p. 88). While all agreed that restraints should be applied for the sake of the patient and not as a substitute for inadequate availability nor for the convenience of the staff, the perceived level of what constitutes danger that the patient might injure himself, another patient, or a staff member varied according to orientation and values of the caregiver.

Dewhurst (1970) draws attention to the reintroduction in "open door" hospitals of several reprehensible methods of restraint and advocates an undisguised locked door as preferable to the illusion of freedom. Curiously enough, in North America physical restraint seems never to have been abandoned as a method of intervention in the treatment of the mentally ill (Rosenblatt, 1984; Voineskos, 1976; Whaley & Ramirez, 1980). Each society throughout history has defined differently the boundaries of acceptable practices (Foucault, 1961; Illich, 1982).

During the Enlightenment, social leaders came to question solutions to all kinds of problems. Philippe Pinel first insisted that insanity was a functional disturbance, and unshackled the insane at the Bicetre asylum in Paris in 1793 (Pinel, 1806/1962). The animality in madness was considered evidence that the mad were not sick "persons," and therefore madness could be mastered only by discipline and brutality (Wilson, 1983). Pinel's humane treatment of the insane—and outrage over the "barbarous provocations of idle and unfeeling visitors ... and rude brutality of attendants" (Pinel, p. 67)—is considered one of the milestones of psychiatric history.

POLICIES ON THE USE OF RESTRAINT

The spread of the humane treatment by philanthropic and inspired citizens on both sides of the Atlantic Ocean 200 years ago seems to have been eroded. In spite of the reasonableness of the nonrestraint principle and the demonstrably marked improvements its application achieved in patients, the Association of Medical Superintendents of American Institutions for the Insane (which became the American Psychiatric Association) decided from its inception in 1844 to uphold the use of restraint (Bromberg, 1954, p. 100). As late as 1885, an extensive survey of American and Canadian institutions revealed that some of the superintendents and psychiatrists were stout defenders of mechanical restraint, including the crib bed (Tuke, 1885).

The debate over the use of seclusion and mechanical restraints has continued over the century and actions remain inconsistent (Voineskos, 1976). Guirguis and Durost (1978) surveyed 370 psychiatric facilities in Canada to examine the prevailing practices in the management of disturbed or violent patients. The vast majority of facilities (76.4%) were found to use mechanical restraints, most frequently within psychiatric hospitals (p. 213). The majority of facilities were found to lack a policy on the restraining practices, while citing the control of violent behavior as the main reason for their use (p. 214).

Morrison et al. (1987) essentially make the same claim as McLean et al. (1982), that the absence of an institutional policy and procedure can account for the discrepancies in approaches and treatments even for similar patient scenarios. Tuke (1885) had argued that the absence of a policy regarding the use of restraints led to their excessive use. From the figures he had extracted from the compendium of the Tenth Census of the United States, 1880, Tuke derived that 40,992 patients were in asylums and 2242 (5.4%) were under some form of restraints, with another 1444 restrained by personal attendants (p. 55).

Bannister and Moyer (1882) claimed that the debate on the topic of mechanical restraints was already voluminous, in their report of a survey of 50 mental institutions. Five of the institutions stated in their bylaws, "it is in most cases much better for one or two attendants to sit by a patient for some hours than to put on any restraining apparatus, though the latter may ultimately be necessary and even beneficial" (p. 473).

The adoption of a nonrestraint policy came from a conviction of its being a rational and humane method of treatment. However, in the intervening one to two centuries, we seem to have somehow forgotten the lessons that could be learned. Authors report that the gradual disuse of restraints was accompanied by a great improvement in the conduct of the patients, while attendants developed more tact and perceived less benefit from the use of restraints. Conolly (1856/1973) stated that "restraint and neglect are synonymous. They are a substitute for the thousand attentions needed by a disturbed patient."

Thus while the use of physical restraints and seclusion rooms have remained an embarrassing reality in the management of acutely disturbed and disruptive patients in the psychiatric field (Soloff, 1979), it would appear that the concerns had no bearing in the treatment of the "soma" branch of the discipline. At a workshop that arose from a growing concern about the widespread use of restraining as part of routine care, Cape (1979) pointed out that restraining devices are so widely accepted that no one questions their use on ethical or humanitarian grounds. He suggested rather than participants concerning themselves with policy or standards, the focus has to be on the inhumanity of restraints, and to bear in mind that unless we throw them away now, we may one day find ourselves in one of them. Blatt (1973) states that to observe sorrow untouched is to cause it to continue, and urges us to reconsider our legal or quasi-legal, sanctioned policies and practices that lead to and encourage the denial of human rights (p. 10).

ADVOCACY FOR THE ADOPTION OF POLICIES OF NONRESTRAINT

The use of physical restraints is primarily a nursing issue, because such intervention is most often initiated at the request of nurses to provide for the safety of the patient. From a legal perspective the basic rule is that "any nurse can apply as much restraint as is necessary to protect a patient from hurting himself" (Regan Report, 1983). Accordingly, rather than requiring a physician's order to apply restraints, one is needed *not* to do so. In the United States, court cases have resulted from accidental injuries when patients were not restrained (Regan Report, 1983), while in Canada, the court cases resulted from accidental deaths due to restraint or safety vests (Canadian Government, 1981, 1982). However, the opposing legal implications in the two countries do not seem to result in divergent practices (I. A. Brown, personal communication, January 26, 1983).

Although the use of physical restraints is a gray area of practice, studies have demonstrated that rather than preventing accidents or injury, the restriction of people's movements has an adverse effect (Bronstein & Zalar, 1982; Canadian Government, 1981; Cape, 1979; Creighton, 1982; Kulikowski, 1979; Morse, 1985; Morse et al., 1985; Schilder, 1987). Mitchell-Pedersen (1984) presented data on the beneficial effects of change to a nonrestraint policy, confirming findings of other investigators (Jacobi et al., 1958; Ramirez, Bruce, & Whaley, 1981; Stegne, 1978). Joel (1985) in a study of a change in policy to using restraint only as a last resort where all other measures tried for a week's duration had failed, found a significant reduction in morbidity, a 25% increase in functional ability in the nursing home residents, and a reduction of absenteeism among the staff.

L. Christman (personal communication, January 7, 1983) recounts an innovative approach to the abolition of restraint devices. He asked the staff to assemble for a special event on the hospital grounds and requested them to bring their favorite mechanical restraint as price of admission. After the restraints were in a large pile, he poured kerosene over them and lit it. None of the dire predictions came to pass as a result of nonrestraint due to the absence of such devices.

Jacobi et al. (1958) reported a study in nonrestraint after seven months. The program was directed toward boosting the patient's ego and self-respect, which required greater availability of the doctor to the patients as well as regular meetings with the staff to make them "feel the importance of their work" (p. 119). Patients who had been constantly in restraint were able to be sent home on overnight visits, and discharge rates increased by a factor of 9. Difficult patients transferred from other services usually quieted down within one to two days, and their destructiveness diminished markedly. Without changes in medication for their epilepsy, patients were having fewer seizures. Tube feedings were no longer necessary, and though quite common before, no double shifts were required since the program started. Thus, with an emphasis on permissiveness and a philosophy that punishment had no place in the treatment of mentally ill patients, the authors report how in a therapeutic milieu the 500 female patients in their sample, dispersed over 12 wards that previously averaged 40 patients in restraints each day, could be transformed without additional staff.

CONCLUSION

The most blatant shortcomings with regards to the use or nonuse of physical restraints center around the lack of knowledge of the effects of such intervention and alternative approaches that could be employed. Only some of the reviewed literature presented the patient's experience of being restrained, although it has been pointed out that "the last hours (of a person's life) are all too often spent in restraints" (Benner, 1984, p. 216). Blake (1969) speaks to the feelings of grief, rage, helplessness, fear of attack and bodily injury, abandonment, guilt, and despair of immobilized hospitalized youth. Schilder (1987) confirmed those findings in adults. While it is plausible that there are instances when physical restraints constitute a positive aspect of care (E. Bunch, personal communication, January 10, 1983; Schilder, 1984; P. Seabrooks, personal communication, March 20, 1984), the literature documents only rare and special instances where that applies (Favell et al., 1981; Hamad, Isley, & Lowry, 1983). The restraining will be perceived as punitive by most patients and damaging to the ill patient's self-concept (Blackwell, 1979). The nonrestraining of mentally ill was once called "absurd, speculative, the attempt of a theoretic visionary, a candidate of popular applause" (Hill, 1850, p. 355) and a "wild scheme of a philanthropic visionary" and "a breaking of the sixth commandment" (Bromberg, 1954, p. 99).

The standards of care, now required by court ruling, include not only food, shelter, clothing, and medical attention, but an overall quality of life that provides dignity, pleasure, and maximum freedom for the individual (Wortis, 1984). The apparent discrepancy between what we profess and what we do needs to be addressed.

REFERENCES

Bannister, H. M. & Moyer, H. N. (1882). On restraint and seclusion in American institutions for the insane. *Journal of Nervous and Mental Disease, 9,* 457–478.

Benner, P. E. (1984). *From novice to expert: Excellence and power in clinical nursing practice.* Menlo Park: Addison Wesley Publishing Co. Inc.

Blackwell, M. W. (1979). *Care of the mentally retarded.* Boston: Little, Brown.

Blake, F. (1969). Immobilized youth: A rationale for supporting nursing intervention. *American Journal of Nursing, 69,* 2364–2369.

Blatt, B. (1973). *Souls in extremes: An anthology on victims and victimizers.* Boston: Allyn and Bacon.

Bromberg, W. (1954). *Man above humanity.* Philadelphia: J. B. Lippincott.

Bronstein, J., & Zalar, M. K. (1982, November 20). *Reduced incidence of patient falls in acute care settings.* Paper presented at the Nursing Research Conference, San Francisco.

BRN Report, The. (1986). Abuse reporting responsibilities. *Official Publication of the California Board of Registered Nursing, 5*(1), 1.

Canadian Government. (1981). *Alert medical devices letter 32.* Health and Welfare Canada, Ottawa.

Canadian Government. (1982). *Information letter, 618.* Health and Welfare Canada, Ottawa.

Cape, R. D. (1979, April 20). Report on the panel presentations. In *Restraints: Necessity or convenience. Proceedings of a Workshop for the Ontario Psychiatric Association,* Queens Park, Toronto, Ontario.

Conolly, J. (1973). *Treatment of the insane without mechanical restraints.* London: Dawson of Pall Mall. (Original work published 1856)

Creighton, H. (1982). Are side-rails necessary? *Nursing Management, 13*(6), 45–48.

Dewhurst, K. (1970). The new methods of restraints. *Nursing Times, 66,* 749–751.

Epp, J. (1986). Achieving health for all: A framework for health promotion. *Canadian Nurse,* Supplement 1987, *83*(11), 3.

Favell, J. E., McGimsey, J. F., Jones, M. L., & Cannon, P. R. (1981). Physical restraint as positive reinforcement. *American Journal of Mental Deficiency, 85,* 425–432.

Foucault, M. (1961). *Madness and Civilization: A History Of insanity in the Age of Reason* (R. Howard, Trans.). London: Tavistock.

Friedman, F. B. (1983). Restraints: When all else fails, there still are alternatives. *RN, 46*(1), 79–88.

Guirguis, E. F. & Durost, H. B. (1978). The role of mechanical restraints in the management of disturbed behavior. *Canadian Psychiatric Association Journal, 23,* 209–218.

Hamad, C. D., Isley, E., & Lowry, M. (1983). The use of mechanical restraint and response incompatibility to modify self injurious behavior: A case study. *Mental Retardation, 21,* 213–217.

Hill, R. G. (1850). The modern treatment of the insane. Letter, *Lancet,* 355–356.

Illich, I. (1982). Vernacular gender and economic sex. Lecture series. University of California, Berkeley.

Jacobi, M. G., Babikian, H., McLamb, E., & Hohlbein, B. (1958). A study in non-restraint. *American Journal of Psychiatry, 115,* 114–120.

Joel, L. A. (1985). *Annual progress report. Teaching Nursing Home Project.* Rutgers University.

Kulikowski, E. S. (1979). A study of accidents in hospitals. *Supervisor Nurse, 10*(7), 44–58.

McLean, J., Shamian, J., Butcher, P., Parsons, R., Selcer, B., & Barrett, M. (1982). Restraining the elderly agitated patient. *Canadian Nurse, 78*(5), 44–46.

Mitchell-Pedersen, L. (1984, May 23). *Free from restraints.* Paper presented at the Second National Conference on Gerontological Nursing, Winnipeg, Manitoba.

Morrison, J., Crinklaw-Wiancko, D., King, D., Thibeault, S., & Wells, D. L. (1987). Formulating a restraint policy. *Journal of Nursing Administration, 17*(3), 39–42.

Morse, J. M. (1985). *Examination of patient falls* (Final Report). University of Alberta Hospitals, Edmonton.

Morse, J. M., Prowse, M., Morrow, N., & Federspiel, G. (1985). Patient falls: A retrospective analysis of patient falls. *Canadian Journal of Public Health, 76*(2), 116–118.

Newbern, V. B. (1982, November 18–20). *A study of patient abuse and patient abusers.* Paper presented at Nursing Research: Advancing Clinical Practices, San Francisco.

Pinel, P. (1962). *A treatise on insanity.* D. D. Davis, (Trans.). New York: Hofner. (Original work published in 1806)

Ramirez, L. F., Bruce, J., & Whaley, M. (1981). An education program for the prevention and management of disturbed behavior in psychiatric settings. *Journal of Continuing Education in Nursing, 12*(5), 19–21.

Regan Report on Nursing Law (1983). Restraints and bedfalls: Most frequent accidents. Case in point: Washington Hospital Center v. Martin (454 A.2d 306-D.C.), *23*(10), 4.

Rosenblatt, A. (1984). Concepts of the asylum in the care of the mentally ill. *Hospital and Community Psychiatry, 35,* 244–250.

Schilder, E. (1984). Interview data.

Schilder, E. J. (1987). *The use of physical restraints in an acute care medical ward.* Unpublished doctoral dissertation, University of California, San Francisco. (University Microfilms No. 8708453)

Soloff, P. H. (1979). Physical restraint and the non-psychotic patient: Clinical and legal perspectives. *Journal of Clinical Psychiatry, 40,* 302–305.

Stegne, L. R. (1978). A positive approach to negative behavior. *Canadian Nurse, 74*(6), 44–48.

Tuke, D. H. (1885). *The insane in the United States and Canada.* London: H.K. Lewis.

Voineskos, G. (1976). Locked wards in Canadian mental hospitals: The return to custodialism. *Canadian Medical Association, 114*(8), 689–691.

Warshaw, G. A., Moore, J. T., Friedman, W., Currie, C. T., Kennie, D. C., Kane, W. J., & Mears, P. A. (1982). Functional disability in the hospitalized elderly. *JAMA: Journal of the American Medical Association, 248,* 847–850.

Whaley, M. S., & Ramirez, L. F. (1980). The use of seclusion rooms and physical restraints in the treatment of psychiatric patients. *Journal of Psychiatric Nursing, 18*(1), 13–16.

Wilson, H. S. (1983). Presencing: Social control of "schizophrenics" in an antipsychiatric community. In C. R. Kneisl and H. S. Wilson (Eds.), *Current perspectives in psychiatric nursing: Issues and trends.* St. Louis: C.V. Mosby.

Wortis, J. (1984). Introduction: Quality of life. *Mental Retardation and Development, 13,* 17–20.

13. Health Care Beliefs and the Use of Medical and Social Services by the Elderly

ALEXANDER SEGALL
NEENA L. CHAPPELL

THE USE OF HEALTH AND SOCIAL SERVICES BY THE ELDERLY

The relationship between age and health services utilization behavior has been the subject of considerable research (e.g., Snider, 1980; Haug, 1981; Wolinsky et al., 1983; Wolinsky, Mosely, & Coe, 1986; Chappell & Blandford, 1987). To a certain extent, this research is based on the assumption that the elderly are disproportionately heavy users of services. Furthermore, it is assumed that as the number and proportion of the elderly in the population increases, their disproportionate consumption of health services will also increase.

Is this an accurate portrayal of the effect an aging population will have on the health care system? According to Barer et al. (1987), our present understanding of health services utilization by the elderly is characterized more by fallacy than by fact. They argue that the expected growth in the number of potential elder users does not necessarily translate into an inevitable disproportionate increase in the use of health services. In fact, the equivocal nature of the relation between age and the use of services is illustrated by the findings of several studies. For example, Haug (1981) concluded that her study did not provide clear evidence that the elderly consistently utilize physicians more frequently than younger persons. Similarly, Wolinsky et al. (1983) report that age is not a strong or significant predictor of health services utilization. In addition, some evidence suggests that the elderly, as a

Aging and Health: Linking Research and Public Policy, © 1989 Lewis Publishers, Inc., Chelsea, Michigan 48118. Printed in U.S.A.

whole, do not make excessive demands on the health care system (Roos & Shapiro, 1981). Instead, a small proportion of those over the age of 65 use a disproportionately large share of the services.

Future research initiatives should attempt to identify the characteristics of this group of elderly users and to assess the factors which shape their utilization behavior. Furthermore, the focus of this research should be expanded to include not only the use of health services, but also the use of a range of alternative community-based services. It is important to determine if the same factors influence the use of health and social services. A more comprehensive understanding of the current utilization behavior of the elderly is vital if we are to plan the types of services necessary to meet the future needs of an aging population.

IDENTIFYING THE CORRELATES OF SERVICE UTILIZATION BEHAVIOR

The objectives of the present study were: (1) to identify the characteristics of the elderly attending day hospitals and senior centers; and (2) to evaluate the predictive utility of these characteristics in explaining utilization behavior among the elderly (i.e., the use of both medical and social services). Studies of service utilization behavior among the elderly are typically guided by the conceptual model developed by Andersen and Newman (1973). These authors outlined the three main determinants of utilization behavior as needs, enabling, and predisposing factors. According to this framework, need is the basic and direct stimulus for the use of health services and is usually measured by self-reported symptoms, perceived health status, functional limitations, or the number of conditions diagnosed by a physician.

Enabling factors are conceptualized as those individual characteristics and family/community circumstances which can either facilitate or hinder the use of services once a need has been recognized. These include, for example, income, health insurance, place of residence, and knowledge of services (Ward, 1977). The final component of the model, predisposing factors, reflects the fact that individuals with certain personal characteristics have a greater propensity to use services. According to Andersen and Newman, predisposing factors exist prior to the incidence of illness and may influence the individual's propensity to use health services. These factors may be classified as either: sociodemographic (age, sex, marital status); social structural (education, occupation, ethnicity); or beliefs and attitudes (locus of control).

The factors that comprise this model have been tested as predictors of medical care utilization in the general adult population and among the elderly. Research evidence suggests that both groups are essentially similar in terms of the factors that affect their behavior. In addition, the model has been used in a limited number of studies (e.g., Wan & Odell, 1981; Coulton & Frost, 1982) to determine whether the same dimensions can be used to explain the utilization of both medical and social services. Coulton and Frost (1982) report that the use of medical care and social services is largely explained by need factors and that enabling and predisposing factors account for little additional variance. It seems that "most factors that are known to be important in explaining medical care utilization are also important in predicting the use of selected social services" (Coulton & Frost, 1982, p. 336).

However, findings based on this model are not conclusive. Despite the popularity of the framework as a guide for research, there are a number of unresolved conceptual and methodological problems. For example, the three categories of determinants are rather broad and have been operationally defined and measured in different ways. Chappell and Blandford (1987) provide a detailed summary of the lack of uniformity in the literature. Studies also do not use comprehensive sets of indicators of the three dimensions of the model. In particular, Wolinsky et al. (1983, p. 326) contend that research seldom includes measures of health beliefs and attitudes as predisposing factors. Thus, the Andersen and Newman model has not been tested in its entirety, and the relative importance of health beliefs as a part of the model and potential determinants of service utilization are still typically neglected.

HEALTH BELIEFS AS DETERMINANTS OF UTILIZATION BEHAVIOR

Despite the volume of research in this field, Wolinsky et al. (1986) argue that little is actually known about the reasons for utilization. Most studies emphasize either the importance of need factors or the demographic characteristics of service users. In order to move from description to explanation, more attention must be paid to health beliefs as predisposing factors. The Wolinsky et al. (1983) survey of the noninstitutionalized elderly is one of the few studies to date to incorporate a measure of health beliefs as a determinant of utilization (i.e., internal locus of control). Obviously, this component of the model warrants much fuller attention.

The primary goal of the present study was to identify health beliefs prevalent among the elderly and to evaluate their relative importance as determinants of the use of both medical and social services. A review of the literature suggests several beliefs which may be salient for the elderly. Service utilization behavior is presumably based upon an underlying conception of what constitutes health and illness. These lay conceptions are quite complex and fundamentally shape the interpretation of the meaning of symptoms and the way sickness is experienced. Unfortunately, very little is actually known about the nature of lay conceptions of health and illness and the influence of these beliefs upon help-seeking behavior.

Despite its methodological limitations, one of the few empirical studies (Apple, 1960) found that interference with usual activities may be the most important condition associated in the layperson's mind with illness. In other words, social functioning plays an important part in shaping lay conceptions of illness. According to Baumann (1961), lay conceptions encompass three different orientations to health: (1) a symptom orientation—health is interpreted as the absence of symptoms (physical level); (2) a feeling state orientation—health is interpreted as a feeling of well-being (psychological level); and (3) a performance orientation—health is interpreted as the ability to perform one's usual social roles (social level). While age does not appear to have a consistent effect on these health orientations, Baumann reports that there is some evidence that a symptom-oriented conception of health is found less frequently at successive age levels. For the purposes of the present study, lay conceptions were categorized in terms of Baumann's typology, and the relation between health orientation and service utilization by the elderly was investigated. It was hypothesized that a symptom orientation to health would be associated with the use of medical services, and a performance orientation would be associated with the use of social services.

In addition, it has been suggested that there is a "tendency for the younger adults to be somewhat more 'scientific,' whereas those over 60 years of age tend to be more 'old fashioned' in their explanations" of health and illness (Mabry, 1964, p. 381). While it is assumed that traditional folk beliefs and practices are likely to be found among older persons, there is little supporting empirical evidence. The present study investigated adherence by the elderly to traditional "popular" beliefs about health. These beliefs were characterized as popular because they are part of the collective wisdom of the lay community, and the cultural context which provides the individual with an explanatory framework for making sense out of sickness and deciding on a course of action (Helman, 1978; Blumhagen, 1980). Thus these beliefs may influence help-seeking behavior. It was hypothesized that adherence to popular health beliefs would be associated with the use of social (rather than) medical services.

Finally, service utilization behavior among the elderly may be influenced by beliefs about physicians, such as medical skepticism and antiprofessionalism (Kleiman & Clemente, 1976; Nuttbrock & Kosberg, 1980), or by beliefs about the individual, such as independence and self-confidence (Kleiman & Clemente, 1976; Leventhal, 1984). In the first case, it is argued that doubts and uncertainties resulting from past experiences with physicians may encourage the elderly to rely on their own resources and self-care practices. This argument presumes that the elderly are more skeptical of professional medical care than younger age groups. This lack of confidence in technical medical expertise and a negative image of the physician may, in turn, shape utilization behavior. "Many reasons have been advanced for medical skepticism among the elderly including: an image of physicians and medicine as ineffective in the treatment of chronic ailments; and a perceived lack of competence on the part of medical professionals to promote health in later life" (Segall, 1987, p. 49).

Alternatively, it has also been argued that early life experiences of the elderly may have resulted in the internalization of a strong belief in independence and individualism and a general reluctance to accept help (Moen, 1978). This argument is based on the assumption that a belief in self-reliance will have a bearing on the utilization of all formal health and social services. It was hypothesized that medical skepticism and a belief in personal responsibility for health and illness would be associated with the use of social (rather than medical) services.

RESEARCH DESIGN AND METHODOLOGY

Sample Selection

Information about the health beliefs of the elderly and their use of medical and social services was collected using face-to-face interviews with respondents attending day hospitals and senior centers in Winnipeg, Manitoba. Data collection involved a two-stage process. First, all five day hospitals in the city provided a list of their members. Interviewers contacted all participants (n = 218), except those considered ineligible by staff due to physical deterioration or mental confusion (n = 94). Only 18 refused to be interviewed, 8% of the population considered eligible. Thus a total of 200 day hospital participants (aged 50 and over) were interviewed.

In the second stage, a matched sample was drawn from the population of elderly persons attending senior centers in Winnipeg. All seven operational senior centers in the city provided membership lists from which a random sample was drawn. Participants were matched on age, sex, and ethnic background with the day hospital respondents and then randomly selected within categories until a total of 200 interviews were obtained. The refusal rate in the senior center sample was 26%. Each interview lasted one hour on average, and all of the interviewing was completed between January and October 1986.

Data Collection and Analysis

Utilization of services was examined in terms of the total number of health and social services used in the six-month period prior to the interview. Formal health services use included general practitioners, medical specialists, dentists, public health nurses, chiropractors, occupational and physical therapists, podiatrists, pharmacists, optometrists, nutritionists, audiologists, hospitals, emergency clinics, community health, and walk-in clinics. These formal health care utilization behaviors scaled quite well for both day hospital and senior center participants ($\alpha = 0.61$). Social services use included social workers, home care, and clergy. These utilization behaviors did not form as clear an additive scale ($\alpha = 0.45$).

The independent variables were categorized as need, enabling, or predisposing factors as suggested by the Andersen and Newman model. Measurement of need included functional disability, number of chronic conditions, health satisfaction, and perceived health status. Functional disability was measured by the number of activities of daily living (such as use of the telephone, shopping, dressing, and bathing) that the individual is unable to do alone ($\alpha = 0.86$). Health satisfaction was measured by a single indicator. Respondents were asked to indicate how satisfied they were with the present state of their general health on a scale ranging from terrible (1) to delightful (7). Finally, to measure perceived health status respondents were asked to rate their own health (for someone their age) as excellent, good, fair, poor, or bad.

Enabling factors included average monthly personal income, including old age security payment, and (for those not living alone) average monthly total household income. Two types of predisposing factors were measured, i.e., sociodemographic characteristics of the individual and health beliefs. Sociodemographics included age, sex, marital status, and education. The health beliefs investigated included (1) lay conceptions of health (e.g., a symptom, feeling-state, or performance orientation); (2) adherence to traditional popular health beliefs; (3) belief in the efficacy of professional medical care (e.g., medical skepticism); and (4) belief in personal responsibility for the onset of illness.

Lay conceptions of health were measured by the open-ended question, What do you think most people around your age mean when they say they are in good health? Baumann's (1961) typology was used to guide the coding of responses. Health is clearly a multidimensional concept, and individual responses sometimes contained evidence of more than one orientation. Consequently, health orientation was recoded for the purposes of analysis as physical (1), psychophysical (2), psychological (3), psychosocial (4), and social (5). In other words, higher scores indicated a more performance-oriented conception of health/illness.

To measure adherence to traditional health beliefs, respondents were given a list of nine popular beliefs about health and were asked to indicate which ones they thought were correct. This list was derived from previous research on age differences in lay health care beliefs and practices (Segall, 1987). These items form a reliable additive scale ($\alpha = 0.76$).

Finally, respondents were presented a list of 10 general statements about illness and medical care. They were asked to indicate whether they strongly agree (5), agree (4), are uncertain (3), disagree (2), or strongly disagree (1) with these Likert-type items. Responses were subjected to a varimax rotation factor analysis and two factors emerged: medical skepticism (6 items, eigenvalue = 2.58); and personal responsibility for illness (2 items, eigenvalue = 1.38). These belief subscales had overall alphas of 0.72 (medical skepticism) and 0.69 (personal responsibility).

Correlational analysis was used to evaluate the relationships between the four health beliefs investigated and to determine whether the elderly possess an integrated system of beliefs. For example, do those older adults, who have a physical (symptom) orientation to health, also reject popular health beliefs as incorrect and place their faith in professional medical expertise?

Finally, hierarchical multiple regression was used to assess the relative explanatory power of health beliefs in accounting for differences in the number of medical and social services used. Health beliefs were compared with other predisposing characteristics (sociodemographics) as well as enabling and need factors in explaining the variance in utilization behavior among the elderly.

THE HEALTH BELIEFS OF THE ELDERLY

The sociodemographic characteristics of the elderly who attend day hospitals and senior centers were quite similar. Respondents were matched by sex and age during the sample selection process. Forty-six percent of all those surveyed were male and 54% were female. Respondents ranged in age from 50 to 96 and the mean age was 76 years. No significant differences were found between the two groups in marital status, education, or total personal income. The proportion of day hospital and senior center participants who are married (36%/42%) or widowed (41%/45%) is about the same. The mean number of years of schooling completed was nine. Most respondents (54%) had an average personal monthly income between $250 and $750.

In contrast, significant differences were found between the two groups on the health measures. Those attending senior centers are apparently in better health. For example, they are more likely to report no functional disability, fewer than four chronic conditions, and perceive their health to be good or excellent. Not surprisingly, the senior center elderly were also much more satisfied with their health status.

Respondents most frequently displayed a social orientation to health. In other words, to the elderly interviewed in this study, good health typically means being able to perform one's usual roles and tasks. This was followed, in order, by a psychological (feeling state) orientation and a physical (symptom) orientation, and thus supports prior research on lay conceptions of health and illness. However, there were significant differences in the health orientation of the day hospital and senior center participants. Those attending day hospitals were more symptom-oriented, while the elderly attending senior centers were more performance-oriented. In view of the differences in the type of service being used and self-rated health status, this finding was not unexpected.

The findings of this study also suggest that the level of adherence among the elderly to traditional popular health beliefs is very low. Overall, 20% of those interviewed rejected all of these beliefs as incorrect. The mean number accepted as correct was only 2.14. The specific beliefs most frequently accepted were: Bowels should move every day without fail (43%); and If your feet get wet, you will get a cold (33%). Day hospital participants accepted significantly more of these beliefs than the elderly attending senior centers.

The two groups of respondents did not differ in their beliefs about the nature of personal responsibility for illness and the efficacy of professional medical care. The mean scores for both groups were identical. Respondents displayed a moderate level of skepticism about doctors and accepted some responsibility for the onset of illness.

The evidence suggests that these four health beliefs are not highly interrelated. Health orientation did not correlate with any of the other belief measures. The correlations among popular beliefs, medical skepticism, and personal responsibility were highly significant ($p = 0.0001$), but were not very strong ($r = 0.25$). In other words, there was a moderate association between these particular beliefs.

Correlations among need, enabling and predisposing sociodemographic characteristics, and the four health belief measures were examined next. It is important to note that age is a significant correlate of health beliefs in only one case (i.e., popular beliefs, $r = -0.10$) and the relationship is negative. This indicates that older respondents accept *fewer* traditional beliefs about health as correct!

THE RELATIVE IMPORTANCE OF HEALTH BELIEFS IN EXPLAINING UTILIZATION BEHAVIOR

In the final stage of the analysis, hierarchical multiple regression was used to assess the relative explanatory power of all of the factors in the model in accounting for variance in the utilization behavior of the elderly. Health beliefs were included as predisposing factors along with other individual characteristics (sociodemographics) and received special attention as potential predictors of the number of health and social services used. The results of the regression analysis are presented separately for the two measures of service utilization (see Table 1 and Table 2).

Table 1 indicates that together these factors are good predictors of the use of health services by both the elderly attending day hospitals and senior centers (i.e., $R^2 = 0.34$ and 0.36, respectively). This compares favorably with previous research on health service use by the elderly. Also, as is

Table 1. Standardized Regression and Hierarchical R^2 Coefficients for the Need, Enabling, and Predisposing Factors Used in Predicting Health Services Utilization Among Elderly Day Hospital and Senior Center Participants

	Day Hospital Sample (n = 200)	Senior Center Sample (n = 200)
Need factors (N)		
Functional disability	−0.079	0.139
Number of chronic conditions	0.395***	0.303***
Health satisfaction	0.042	−0.117
Perceived health	−0.217*	−0.059
Enabling factors (E)		
Personal income	−0.080	−0.121
Predisposing factors		
Sociodemographics (PS)		
Age	−0.103	−0.065
Sex	−0.141	−0.143
Married	0.215*	−0.075
Widowed	0.284*	0.189
Education	−0.068	0.063
Health beliefs (PB)		
Health orientation	0.129	0.012
Popular beliefs	−0.102	0.237**
Personal responsibility	−0.093	−0.046
Medical skepticism	0.021	−0.190*
R^2 (N)	0.245***	0.239***
R^2 (N + E)	0.249***	0.240***
R^2 (N + E + PS)	0.297***	0.290***
R^2 (N + E + PS + PB)	0.336***	0.365***

*$p < 0.05$.
**$p < 0.01$.
***$p < 0.001$.

typically the case, need factors (particularly the number of chronic conditions) emerged as the best predictors of the use of health services. Enabling factors accounted for little additional variance. Both categories of predisposing factors contributed, to a limited extent, to the explanatory power of the model (i.e., 9% to 12%). Overall, health belief measures ranked a distant second to need factors in terms of predictive utility. It should be noted that health beliefs accounted for more of the variance in the use of health services among the senior center sample (r^2 change = 0.08) than the day hospital sample (r^2 change = 0.04).

Table 2 indicates that these factors are not quite as good at predicting the use of social services by the elderly. While the model explains 34% of the variance for the senior center sample, it accounts for only 14% of the variance in utilization among the elderly attending day hospitals. Need factors are once again relatively important predictors of this type of service utilization. Health beliefs seem to play a more important part in shaping the service utilization behavior of senior center participants (r^2 change = 0.10) than the elderly attending day hospitals (r^2 change = 0.04).

Table 2.   Standardized Regression and Hierarchical R^2 Coefficients for the Need, Enabling, and Predisposing Factors Used in Predicting Social Services Utilization Among Elderly Day Hospital and Senior Center Participants

	Day Hospital Sample (n = 200)	Senior Center Sample (n = 200)
Need factors (N)		
Functional disability	0.106	0.297**
Number of chronic conditions	0.181	0.258**
Health satisfaction	0.039	0.004
Perceived health	−0.105	0.068
Enabling factors (E)		
Personal income	0.056	−0.223*
Predisposing factors		
Sociodemographics (PS)		
Age	−0.060	−0.138
Sex	0.014	0.038
Married	−0.168	−0.016
Widowed	−0.006	0.151
Education	−0.084	0.058
Health beliefs (PB)		
Health orientation	0.184	−0.189*
Popular beliefs	0.074	0.145
Personal responsibility	−0.006	−0.077
Medical skepticism	−0.045	−0.224*
R^2 (N)	0.070	0.157***
R^2 (N+E)	0.071	0.179***
R^2 (N+E+PS)	0.103	0.237***
R^2 (N+E+PS+PB)	0.140	0.336***

*$p < 0.05$.
**$p < 0.01$.
***$p < 0.001$.

As a final step in the data analysis, stepwise multiple regression was used to assess the importance of each of the specific health beliefs held by senior center participants. As anticipated, lower levels of skepticism are associated with more extensive utilization. Adherence to traditional health beliefs does not apparently discourage the use of formal medical services. Health orientation and belief in personal responsibility for illness do not explain much of the variance in this type of utilization behavior. Medical skepticism was identified as the best predictor of the use of social services and accounted for half of the variance explained by all of the health belief measures. Low levels of skepticism are associated with the use of both formal health and social services. The remaining health belief measures accounted for approximately 1% of the variance in social service use.

SUMMARY AND CONCLUSIONS

Day hospital participants use significantly more social *and* health services than the elderly who attend senior centers. However, the Andersen and Newman model was more effective at predicting the service utilization behavior of senior center participants. Also, health beliefs emerged as significant predictors only for respondents in this sample. Thus, it seems that health beliefs are important, but only among the elderly who are in better health. Additional research is required to determine whether beliefs held by the well elderly in the general community are also related to utilization behavior. It is possible that this relationship may be unique to the well elderly already participating in particular networks, such as senior centers.

Certain findings regarding the health beliefs of the elderly should be highlighted. It is notable that a social orientation to health was most prevalent among the respondents in this study. That is, the elderly, especially the well elderly, tend to view health primarily in terms of their ability to perform various day-to-day functions. This finding has implications for the nature of the interaction between elderly patients and formal health care workers. From a medical perspective, physical improvement may be the main criterion; however, from the elderly patients' point of view, side effects of treatment that interfere with social functioning may be more important.

It is equally vital that health care workers recognize that stereotypical notions about the health beliefs of the elderly were not empirically supported by the findings of this study. For example, few of the elderly accepted popular health beliefs as correct. Furthermore, age alone was not a significant factor in explaining the use of either health or social services. When this finding is combined with the relative importance of chronic illness and functional disability (need factors) as predictors of service utilization behavior, and the differences between the well and ill elderly, it is obvious that the major challenge facing society today is to find an effective means of maintaining the health of the population rather than simply focusing upon the rate at which we are aging.

ACKNOWLEDGMENT

This research was conducted while both authors were National Health Research Scholars (#6607–1376–48 and #6607–1340–48 respectively), funded by Health and Welfare Canada. Data reported are from a study funded by NHRDP, Health and Welfare Canada (#6607–1390–42).

REFERENCES

Andersen, R., & Newman, J. R. (1973). Societal and individual determinants of medical care utilization in the United States. *Milbank Memorial Fund Quarterly/Health and Society, 51,* 95–124.

Apple, D. A. (1960). How laymen define illness. *Journal of Health and Human Behavior, 1,* 219–225.

Barer, M. L., Evans, R. G., Hertzman, C., and Lomas, J. (1987). Aging and health care utilization: New evidence on old fallacies. *Social Science and Medicine, 24,* 851–862.

Baumann, B. (1961). Diversities in conceptions of health and physical fitness. *Journal of Health and Human Behavior, 2,* 39–46.

Blumhagen, D. (1980). Hyper-tension: A folk illness with a medical name. *Culture, Medicine and Psychiatry, 1,* 197–227.

Chappell, N. L., & Blandford, A. A. (1987). Health services utilization by elderly persons. *Canadian Journal of Sociology, 12,* 195–215.

Coulton, C., & Frost, A. K. (1982). Use of social and health services by the elderly. *Journal of Health and Social Behavior, 23,* 330–339.

Haug, M. (1981). Age and medical care utilization patterns. *Journal of Gerontology, 36,* 103–111.

Helman, C. G. (1978). Feed a cold, starve a fever—folk models of infection in an English suburban community, and their relation to medical treatment. *Culture, Medicine and Psychiatry, 2,* 107–137.

Kleiman, M. B., & Clement, F. (1976). Support for the medical profession among the aged. *International Journal of Health Services, 6,* 295–299.

Leventhal, E. A. (1984). Aging and the perception of illness. *Research on Aging, 6,* 119–135.

Mabry, J. H. (1964). Lay concepts of etiology. *Journal of Chronic Diseases, 17,* 371–386.

Moen, E. (1978). The reluctance of the elderly to accept help. *Social Problems, 25,* 293–303.

Nuttbrock, L., & Kosberg, J. I. (1980). Images of the physician and help-seeking behavior of the elderly: A multivariate assessment. *Journal of Gerontology, 35,* 241–248.

Roos, N. P., & Shapiro, E. (1981). The Manitoba longitudinal study on aging: Preliminary findings on health care utilization by the elderly. *Medical Care, 19,* 644–657.

Segall, A. (1987). Age differences in lay conceptions of health and self-care responses to illness. *Canadian Journal on Aging, 6,* 47–65.

Snider, E. L. (1980). Awareness and use of health services by the elderly: A Canadian study. *Medical Care, 18,* 1172–1182.

Wan, T. , & Odell, B. G. (1981). Factors affecting the use of social and health services among the elderly. *Ageing and Society, 1,* 195–115.

Ward, R. A. (1977). Services for older people: An integrated framework for research. *Journal of Health and Social Behavior, 18,* 61–70.

Wolinsky, F. D., et al. (1983). Health services utilization among the noninstitutionalized elderly. *Journal of Health and Social Behavior, 24,* 325–337.

Wolinsky, F. D., Mosely, R. R., & Coe, R. M. (1986). A cohort analysis of the use of health services by elderly Americans. *Journal of Health and Social Behavior, 27,* 209–219.

PART II

Money, Politics, and Public and Private Choices

14. Reading the Menu with Better Glasses: Aging and Health Policy Research

ROBERT G. EVANS

HOBSON'S CHOICE

"Every man desires to live long; but no man would be old." Indeed not. "The cold friction of expiring sense . . . "; on the whole, I'd rather be in Philadelphia. But Swift puts the dilemma rather well, both our individual condition and our public, collective problem. If aging troubles you, consider the alternative.

In this respect there is a significant parallel between the aging process and the use of health care. We undergo each, not by choice, but in the belief that the alternative is worse. Few people actually look forward to either for its own sake. Anyone who wants to use health care services when s/he is not sick, is sick. And the strenuous effort and expense that people undertake to avoid the symptoms of age suggest that it is not widely regarded as a thing of beauty either. Cicero was faking it. Furthermore, these two dubious benefits, aging and health care, tend to be quite closely correlated with each other, since both are associated with declining health.

AGING: THE FISCAL FOCUS

At this point the individual experience becomes the collective concern. The provision, or at least the regulation and finance, of health care is in every civilized country a public responsibility (Culyer, 1988; OECD, 1987; Scheiber & Poullier, 1987). This collective concern, however, can lead to a serious narrowing of focus and a loss of perspective. In those countries

Aging and Health: Linking Research and Public Policy, © 1989 Lewis Publishers, Inc., Chelsea, Michigan 48118. Printed in U.S.A.

which, like Canada, are passing through a major demographic transition and shifting to a much older, slow-growing or static population, the individual experience with aging is too easily projected as a "crisis" in the collective funding of health care, to the virtual exclusion of other dimensions (Evans, 1985).

In this process, fiscal issues and concerns tend to crowd out other substantial questions. As a counterweight to the immediacy of health budgets, one must try to keep in mind that the process of aging involves much more than changes in health status and risks, important though these may be. Moreover, the most appropriate responses to the health problems that do arrive, or worsen, with age are not always health *care* interventions. Health and function, at any age, depend on many other factors in the public and private environment, which may be more significant in the long run. Too often, the most that health care can offer is salvage and partial repair, in response to illnesses whose real origins lie elsewhere.

Accordingly, the health policy questions connected with aging must be defined more broadly than the health care system itself and *a fortiori* much more broadly than simply questions of health care finance. Useful research can still be done in the narrower framework, but those who do it, and particularly those who rely on its findings, must be clear that they are looking only at one piece of a much larger, interlocked puzzle.

CLEARING THE FOG: CHOICES, NOT CONSTRAINTS

Older people need, or at least use, more health care (on average—many are actually quite healthy, but some are very sick indeed). As the average age of the population increases, the demands on the health care system will inevitably rise—are rising—with consequent massive requirements for additional personnel, capital equipment, buildings, and finance to pay for it all. How can we afford all this, and who will pay?

Furthermore, in addressing this puzzle, it is well to keep in mind both parts of Swift's aphorism. Policy questions have a way of becoming policy problems, in the sense of a burden rather than a challenge, and the "aging of the Canadian population" is no exception. From a broader perspective, however, a *failure* of the population to age should be a good deal more disturbing. The mathematics of demography tell us that this would imply either static or falling individual life expectancies, or high birth rates and rapid population growth—the latter being unsustainable, and the former, to say the least, unattractive. We may find it comforting, and possibly even helpful, to remember that we are trying to cope with the problems of success.

Like any major policy issue, this one has attracted or generated a considerable amount of rhetorical fog, which has to be cleared away before anything sensible can be said (Evans, 1986). It is particularly unhelpful to talk about aging and health as a question of whether we, as a community, can "afford" the financial burdens of caring for our aging population. Although you could rarely tell from our public rhetoric, we are a remarkably rich and privileged population. We do not, of course, share equally in that wealth, and for some of us questions of what can be "afforded" are stark reality.[1] Similarly, there *are* communities in the world in which questions of what can and cannot be "afforded" are real and binding constraints on policy—for many things, the resources simply are not there. But as a group, as a community, Canadians have ample resources to support a major expansion in health spending.

We may not wish to. We perhaps should not wish to. The principal advocates of the argument that health care is "underfunded" and deserves a higher priority have up to now been the providers of health care, who by elementary arithmetic logic would receive any such increased spending as increases in their incomes. But the real issue is one of setting priorities, of deciding how we, as a group, want to use our really rather substantial resources.

Further confusion is sown by those who claim that the "inevitable" increase in health care costs to care for an aging population will bring about a collapse, or at least a major change, in the present Canadian arrangements for funding hospital and medical care (Evans, 1987). As a community, we may be able to afford greater outlays, but some would have us believe that we cannot afford to pay for them all through the public system as we do at present. Private sources of finance, user-pay and private insurance, must be tapped to supplement inadequate public funds.

This of course is a simple accounting confusion. Canadians must pay the total bill for their care, through whatever administrative channel. That total does not become more or less "affordable" by virtue of going through one set of budgets rather than another. If we can afford increased private expenditure, then we can also afford increased public expenditure. If it were really true that we could not afford more public expenditure, then we could not afford it privately either.

Different systems of finance *do* shift the burden of paying for health care. Generally speaking, shifting from public to private funding sources tends to shift the distribution of the cost burden from the healthy and wealthy to the poor and sick, and conversely. Each society makes a political choice as to how this burden will be distributed; the critical point is that in a developed society at least it *is* a choice. The specious plea of "insufficient funds" in the public sector in particular is simply a strategy to promote a particular pattern of choice by the assertion of a pseudoconstraint.

The channel of payment does, however, affect the overall amount which must be paid, as well as who must pay it. The comparative international evidence seems very clear that systems of mixed public and private finance cost a great deal more, both for care and particularly for administration, than universal public ones (Culyer, 1988; Evans, 1986; Evans, Lomas et al., forthcoming).[2] Thus a greater reliance on private funding sources not only does not increase the overall capacity of the community to pay for care, but tends to increase the economic burden of that care, and move it to weaker shoulders.

It is perhaps not surprising, therefore, that the confusion between questions of aging and health, and those of public versus private finance, tends to be generated by spokesmen for the insurance industry and for physicians, who never liked the universal programs in the first place. (And their arguments find greater acceptance among those who are relatively both healthy and wealthy.) These groups expected, quite rightly it seems from the U.S. experience, to do better financially in a mixed public/private system; and they have apparently not yet given up hope of reestablishing direct contact with patients' wallets (Weller & Manga, 1983; Stoddart & Labelle, 1985). As for the logical connection between this agenda and the aging of the Canadian population, well, any stick will do to beat a dog.

WE AND THEY, OR NOW AND LATER?

Once we clear away this sort of fog, however, the central question remains. Not, Can we (all) afford to grow old? but, How much do we want to spend in the process? What share of our resources do we want to give up, in our youth and middle age, to support *ourselves* in an increasingly extended old age, and how would we like these resources to be spent?

This formulation of the problem, however, represents a choice of perspective or time frame which is by no means value-free. The ethical content of the policy choice appears in a very different light depending on whether we view the issue at a single point in time or as unfolding through time. Nor is it clear that there is any analytic way of reconciling these two perspectives, or choosing between them.

The dilemma arises naturally from the simple demographic fact that a combination of falling birth rates and rising life expectancies must eventually raise the aged dependency ratio, the number of elderly persons *per* each member of the working population. Since, apart from changes in inventories and external debt, current consumption can only come from current production, it follows that whatever resources are made available to the elderly must be provided by the rest of the population. What they get, we lose. The truth of this proposition is not seriously challenged by changing retirement patterns. In addition, that the elderly may have contributed to health plans during their working lives does not refute the fact that when they draw on these "entitlements" they are *at that point in time* drawing on the product of others, just as when they were building up the entitlements, others were drawing on them. In other words, the elderly are not about to be self-sufficient at the time they use health services, in the strict sense of contributing present wealth sufficient to cover current utilization.

Intergenerational conflict, the "we/they" confrontation, is, however, a result of the choice of time perspective. If we view aging as a process, unfolding over time, rather than seeing youth and age as a snapshot, frozen in time, it becomes obvious that each of us (with a few unfortunate exceptions) passes through the same stages of life. The choices we face can be thought of as decisions about how we ourselves want to be treated, or rather to allocate our own resources. In this rather Kantian perspective, our decisions about aging policy are in fact our choices as to how we want to allocate our own resources over our own life cycles.[3]

In the process, of course, we will also be addressing issues of interpersonal distribution—presumably (but by no means only) from the more to the less economically well off. But in the longitudinal or life-cycle perspective, these interpersonal redistributional issues are logically separate from the intertemporal questions.

From this perspective, the balance between health care and other forms of activity looks very different. Each of us might very rationally (and quite ethically) decide—looking forward over the life cycle—that some forms of life prolongation were not at all worth their current cost. After all, impoverishing one's working life to provide for ever more expensive "heroic measures" at death, which merely prolong the agony, is not the obviously rational way for an individual to manage the long retreat.

By extension, it seems inappropriate for a society as well. We can certainly "afford" to provide ever more elaborate health care for an ever older population—ourselves, when old. But we will equally certainly have to give up some other sources of satisfaction in return. "Staying alive," in whatever condition and at whatever cost, is not the only good in life.[4]

One way or another, however, in ignorant fog or clear-eyed acceptance of fate, we as a community will eventually make, indeed are currently making, these choices. But these are political and ethical issues, problems of discovering and giving effect to what it is that we want to do. What role does research have in all this?

RESEARCH AND THE RANGE OF CHOICE

As always, truth in advertising should compel us to emphasize that more knowledge will *not* by itself make these choices for us. The fundamental questions we face do not have objective "right" and "wrong" answers, discoverable by sufficiently clever and energetic application of technical expertise. There is a common temptation, often encouraged by researchers, to try to recast inherently political choices into the form of technical problems which can be passed over to the "expert"—at least as a delaying mechanism.

The maneuver never works; in the end the political choice has to be made, even if it is only not to act. But the veneer of expertise can buffer the consequences to the decisionmaker.

What research *can* do, of course, is to clarify the nature of the real choices, and help to avoid diversion of effort and attention over nonissues (like, What can we afford? and Must we abandon universality?, noted above). Sound research can "refine the class of allowable hypotheses," clarifying the policy menu by eliminating the things which really are not available, identifying the real choices, and getting the prices right. Certain apparent options or threats can be shown to be illogical, inconsistent, or simply unsustainable from the existing data.[5]

DEMOGRAPHIC TRENDS AND THE COSTS OF HEALTH CARE

The first point, which emerges from a series of analyses by different researchers over the last decade, is that we should not be too worried about the demographic transition *per se*. The increased proportion of elderly people in our population, combined with the well-documented tendency for elderly people to use more health care than younger ones, will indeed tend to push up average per capita utilization and costs; but the key question is, How much? The answer is, Not much, or at least not as much as you think.

The general approach of such studies has been to measure the age-specific utilization rates at a point in time, and then to assume that these age-specific rates are held constant while the population ages according to various alternative population projections (Boulet & Grenier, 1978; Denton & Spencer, 1983; Woods Gordon, 1984). This procedure isolates the pure demographic effect of the changing mix of age groups in the overall population; the average utilization/cost per capita rises as the proportion of elderly people increases, even though the utilization/cost per capita at each age remains constant.

Results vary, depending on base year and fineness of the age breakdown. In general, however, such studies show rates of increase in per capita use for all health services in the neighborhood of 1% per capita per year. This is below the long run trend rate of economic growth, implying (assuming past trends continue) that a constant share of national income devoted to health care could fund the increase in utilization arising from demographic factors alone, and still leave some room for service expansion—if that is wanted.

The research results are clear and remarkably consistent. Yet the policy debates, particularly at the political level and in the media (but not only there), continue to refer to the demographic trends as if they were the source of major utilization and cost trends, both now and in the future. Obviously, the quite straightforward answer that current research gives to the demographic question is either unheard, or misunderstood, or found unacceptable for other reasons.

The first two possibilities suggest that the research community has a greater responsibility to communicate its results (and people who make and carry out health policy, as always, ought to be listening better). But the third, that the results are unacceptable for other reasons, is a more interesting avenue for further exploration. The findings could be unacceptable because the assumptions underlying these projections are wrong, or because the projections are incomplete and inappropriate, or simply because they yield conclusions which are unpalatable.

Taking the last point first, all such projections of the impact of aging on health care utilization indicate not only relatively slow *per capita* growth, but growth at very different rates for different sectors. Utilization of long term care or home care services may grow at rates closer to 2% or more per year per capita (over the whole population), but for physicians' services the rates are much smaller, about 0.33% per year. The implication is that population aging may not require massive new infusions of resources to the whole health care field, but it *will* require a redeployment of resources from the high-prestige sectors of acute care hospitals and physicians' services to what the British call the "Cinderella services"—home help, psychiatric services, and long term care.

Require, however, is too strong a word, tending to lead us across the boundary between *is* and *ought*. These studies do *not* tell us how patterns of health care provision *should* respond to the aging of the Canadian population. Rather, they measure what the impact *would* be, if we chose to hold constant the current levels of provision of each type of service, per person in each age group.

Whether present patterns of provision of, say, home care or physicians' services are appropriate is a very different kind of question. It leads back to the central issue of the relation between particular types of health care, and health or, more generally, well-being. What is it that we really want to buy, or do, or have done?

Some argue that we should expand the home care system dramatically, suggesting that this may reduce the proportion of the elderly population in long term care institutions. Others note that our present rate of utilization of physicians' services appears to be a historical accident, rather than the result of any systematic assessment of "need," or even any conscious political choice (Lomas, Barer, & Stoddart, 1985). The demographic impact studies show only that *if* the objective is simply to maintain the health care *status quo,* in the face of an aging population, then the principal problem is one of redeploying resources, not funding a massive increase.

The problem with "redeployment" is that as noted above, expenditures are always identically equal to incomes. Thus the utilization projections provide little comfort for, e.g., medical school deans, trying to justify perpetuation of the current levels of production of physicians, when the growth of physician supply in Canada currently outstrips population by 1.5–2% per year.[6] The physician supply is thus expanding considerably faster than any reasonable projection of population needs, at least based on current demographic factors.

If finance does not expand in proportion, i.e., if the rest of the Canadian population cannot be persuaded, one way or another, to increase its outlays for physicians' services, then their average incomes must, by simple arithmetic, fall. The findings are no more comforting for those trying to promote the expansion of "high-tech" services in acute care hospitals—such expensive facilities may or may not be justified on the basis of explicit clinical evaluations, but they are not simply a response to increasing needs which arise from the aging process *per se*.

In these circumstances, it makes eminently good political sense to ignore the research findings and rely on loose generalizations. Hence the continued claim that the aging population will require large increases in all sorts of health services, and particularly large amounts of new money—from whatever source. The present pressure for growth of expenditures in the medical and acute care hospital sectors is not consistent with "redeployment" away from those areas, and the current research findings threaten to undermine what might otherwise be a powerful political lever for extracting additional public (or private) support.

But there are grounds for questioning the relevance of these findings, other than economic interest. Are they a safe basis for health policy; is the impact of aging likely to be as innocuous—in total—as they suggest? (Redeployment of resources away from the high-visibility and high-tech areas of health care is of course by no means *politically* innocuous!) Again, truth in advertising reminds us that all projections, like all generalizations, are false.

In particular, these projections depend on assumptions about future birth and death rates, which imply that the future will be more or less like the past. The birth rate assumptions are not too dangerous; patterns have been rather stable in Canada since the end of the baby boom in 1965, and even an immediate new boom would not have much impact on the overall projections. (It would cause *per capita* utilization projections to fall.) But the assumptions about mortality rates, particularly among the oldest-old (85 and up) are much more important, because unexpected changes at this end of the age distribution have immediate effects on utilization and costs.

Furthermore, the increases in life expectancies, which were decelerating into the early 1970s, have now apparently begun to accelerate again (Wilkins & Adams, 1987). If one projects the rate of *acceleration* of life expectancies observed over the last decade, which no study quoted has done, the impact of projected demographic changes on the health care system becomes greater, and/or sooner. Health policy has to be based on *some* projection, implicit or explicit, and the current research is still the best we have, but whatever projections we use, we need to keep a very close eye on trends in mortality rates at the upper end of the age distribution.

CHANGING TREATMENT PATTERNS: WHO DOES WHAT TO WHOM?

These potential errors, however, are matters for the future. The major current source of concern with projections of the impact of demography on health care use is the assumption that age-use patterns, the per capita rate of utilization at each age, will remain constant over time. This has obviously not been true in the past, and there is no reason to expect it to hold in the future.

As a criticism of the demographic projections themselves, this point is misplaced. The purpose of the assumption of constant age-specific use rates, which could also be called constant technology, is *not* to yield a "best-guess" projection of what overall utilization rates are going to be. Rather, it is used to isolate the *component* of any increase in such rates which is attributable to demographic factors alone.

The changes which have occurred in age-specific use rates in the past, and which presumably will occur in future, are changes in the pattern of delivery of health care, responding to pressures from within the health care system (e.g., the increased supply of physicians), or outside it (e.g., AIDS), or some combination (e.g., advances in diagnostic imaging technology).

Such changes may have a much more profound impact on the health care system than demographic trends; it has certainly been true in past decades that changes in how patients were treated have been much more significant than changes in how many patients, of what ages, were available for treatment. But that observation merely reemphasizes the importance of focusing on how choices are made within the health care system as to who to treat and how, rather than on external demographic changes which, while real, are likely to be quantitatively much less important (Roos, Montgomery, & Roos, 1987).

THE MOVING TARGETS: MORTALITY, MORBIDITY, AND HEALTH CARE

These two forces, demographic trends and treatment patterns within the health care system, do not, however, exhaust the set of factors influencing health care utilization. The "technology" of health care, in the broadest sense, could conceivably remain constant (although it never has), yet age-specific use rates could shift because of changes in the age-specific rates of morbidity in the population. People could be getting healthier, or sicker, at different ages, a possibility which brings us into the fascinating and important set of issues surrounding the controversy over the "compression of morbidity," "natural death," and the possible convergence of life expectancies to the preprogrammed and ineluctable natural life span of the human organism (Fries, 1980, 1983; Schneider & Brody, 1983).

This field of discussion is large, and once again projections play at least as large a role in the discussion as hard research data (and are themselves less well linked to that data). Nevertheless, a bit of logical analysis may provide a framework within which to view the research information which *is* available.

The general line of argument is well known, and is discussed in more detail in other chapters in this volume. It is observed that, over time, the plot of survival probability against age for human populations has become increasingly "rectangularized"—early death is less and less common. Further, the biological limits on the number of times a given type of cell can divide (the "Hayflick limit") suggest that there are corresponding impassable upper limits to human life expectancy. There must, somewhere, be a (probabilistic) right-hand wall bounding the survival curve. But the implications of these observations for aging and health policy turn out to be profoundly ambiguous.

The optimistic scenario places "The Wall" of life span relatively close to current (female) life expectancies—85 years plus or minus 15. Furthermore, it posits that approaching the wall will be associated with improved health and progressive deferral of onset of the common chronic diseases of old age—heart disease, cancer, osteoarthritis. Thus morbidity will be "compressed" into a narrower and narrower span of years just before death, and healthy life free of chronic ailments will make up a larger and larger share of the total life span. Finally, when the allotted span is reached, the individual will undergo "natural death"—general failure of a number of systems at once—rather like the wonderful one-hoss shay.

All of this is very good news for the average individual, and economic disaster for the health care industry. Age-specific use curves will *fall* throughout most of the life span, as the major sources of illness, disability, and health care use will be deferred to later and later in life, and perhaps missed entirely. Finally, when "natural death" is reached, it will be obvious that there is no point in prolonging the imminent inevitable by the famous or infamous "heroic measures," and the terminal process can be conducted with dignity and economy.

And it may all be true—the time-scale of the progression to this future state is not clearly identified. Both "compression" and "natural death" may be another generation away. But this scenario is by no means the logical and inevitable consequence of the observed "rectangularization of mortality," whether or not we are in fact presently close to the biologically determined life span. The rectangularization of *mortality* is a measurable, and measured, fact, but that of *morbidity* is a hypothesis which does not follow from the former, and the compression (and thereby reduction) of health care utilization and cost requires still further questionable assumptions (Barer et al., 1987).

The progressive deferral of death is consistent with either increased or decreased morbidity, either of which is consistent with increased or decreased health care utilization, depending on one's causal scenario. A health care system which provided more and more "successful" salvage services could yield a population which lived longer, but was on average sicker, and in consequence used more health care. Patients who would otherwise have died would be kept alive, but not "cured," so that sicker and sicker survivors would be included in the total population.

Alternatively, the "compression of morbidity" could be a consequence of substantially expanded, and successful, preventive and truly curative interventions by the health care system—better health outcomes and reduced morbidity over most of the life span. But the price of this achievement might be a substantially increased utilization of, and expenditure for, new and more effective health care services.

Finally, "natural death" is as much a behavioral as a physiological hypothesis. All systems may be failing and the end may be inevitable, but will clinicians recognize that fact and act on the recognition? There seems no reason, in principle, why any amount of resources might not be devoted to the terminal care of the dying; death may indeed be "natural," but so, it seems, is intervention. *Nunc dimittis* is not explicitly part of the Hippocratic oath. It is certainly included as one of the components of *primum non nocere,* but the specific applications are problematic, and may not be so clear to patients (or their families).

WHEN ALL ELSE FAILS, LOOK AT THE EVIDENCE

There are thus no *a priori* grounds on which to predict the direction of future shifts in the age-specific health care use curves. Past and present trends in morbidity and use patterns, however, may give one some clues as to how the (near-term) future is likely to unfold. And current research is revealing some rather startling changes in utilization patterns. (I focus on some of my colleagues' and my own work, not because it is the only or even the most important in the field—it is not—but because I know it better.)

As noted above, the age-specific use rates in Canada have definitely not been constant in recent years. A convenient device for displaying their changes is the age-use curve, by which per capita utilization (or expenditure) rates for some particular service are measured on the vertical axis of a graph, with ages or age groups on the horizontal axis. The resulting curve shows how utilization rates vary with age at a particular point in time; a plot of such curves for two or more years (or regions) shows differences specific to each age group.

A number of such curves have now been generated, displaying changes in use rates for physicians' and hospitals' services (e.g., Barer et al., 1987). In general, age-use curves for physicians' services are being displaced vertically over time. But those for hospital utilization—either separations or patient days—are twisting, falling under some age ranges and rising over others. (The Canadian hospital data system does not permit one to compile age-expenditure curves directly; these would be very useful to show whether there are offsetting changes in the intensity of servicing per patient day or episode of care.)

Hospital use is rising among the very old and the very young, and falling in between. In British Columbia, hospital days per capita among children aged 28 days to 14 years has fallen by two thirds since 1966, while rising for those under 28 days at admission (Evans, Robinson, & Barer, 1988). Among the adult population, the fall in utilization (since 1969) is almost as pronounced up to the age of 50. The intertemporal displacement in the curves then begins to narrow, until for the age group 70–74 utilization is virtually unchanged between 1969 and 1985–1986. The curves then cross again, and for the older age groups use has increased over time (Evans, Barer et al., forthcoming). (As noted above, for physicians' services the whole curve is displaced upward over time, but it rises fastest at the upper age groups.)

The impact of this shift in use patterns is most remarkable when one examines all hospital use, including that of extended care beds in acute and extended care hospitals. Between 1969 and 1985–1986, the unadjusted rate of hospital days per capita rose by just over 5% in total. But within this total, acute care use dropped by about one third, while the rate for long-stay patients nearly tripled. By the latter year, patients whose hospital stays were 60 days or longer accounted for just under *half* of all patient days, although only 2% of all separations.

PROLONGING LIFE, OR PROLONGING DYING?

Even more striking, one fourth of those long-stay patients, or 0.5% of the total of all separations, died in hospital. This subgroup accounted for a quarter of all hospital patient days in the province. In 1969, long-stay patients who died in hospital made up only 0.25% of all separations, and about 6% of patient days.

Almost all of these patients were 75 years of age or older, and most were over 85. These data therefore reflect a massive reallocation of hospital space to the institutional care of the very elderly, in large part during their increasingly prolonged terminal episodes (see also Stout & Crawford, 1988). Since the total rate of utilization is very little changed—in age-adjusted terms it actually fell—the transfer has been away from the hospitalization of people between the ages of 28 days and 70 years. More generally, the "ordinary" hospital patient, who stays for two weeks or less and comes home alive, accounted for about 85% of all separations in both 1969 and 1985–1986, but his/her share of patient days fell from 46% to 31%—less than one third.

The number of patient days thus reallocated is enormous, about 1.33 million, or between one fifth and one fourth of all the days in the province. This is the equivalent of ten 400-bed hospitals, operated at 90% occupancy, among a population of just under 3 million.

Of course, the corresponding transfer of *resources* may be much less. Extended care patients presumably receive primarily custodial care with a much lower procedural intensity. But it seems clear that either by design or by accident, British Columbia has developed a "policy" of greatly increased institutionalization of the elderly population—recall that all the above measures are *per capita* and already adjusted for the increased numbers of elderly—matched by a substantial reduction for the rest of the population. Similar changes in utilization patterns have been observed in other provinces.

There are a number of reasons why this might have come about. Much has been written about the declining ability and/or willingness of children, particularly daughters, to support aging parents (Walker, 1987). More advanced medical and nursing technology, and/or more aggressive styles of intervention, may be extending the terminal episode—prolonging death, not life (Fuchs, 1984; Scitovsky, 1984; Roos et al., 1987). Ironically, a healthier population of seniors may at the end simply take longer to die. There is obviously room for considerable further research to pin down in more detail the factors which account for this dramatic change.

MORE MEDICAL CARE, OR JUST MORE DOCTORS?

As noted above, the elderly are also increasing their use of physicians' services, both in absolute terms and relative to the rest of the population. Here, however, there is another interesting factor. Analysis of the Manitoba experience shows that the increase in use per capita is associated with an increased average number of physicians contacted per patient (Roch, Evans, & Pascoe, 1985; Evans et al., 1987). Moreover, the increase in average number of physicians seen is greatest among the oldest age groups.

Nor does this reflect only increased numbers of consultations. There has also been a marked increase in the average number of general practitioners seen, per patient, in the period since 1971. Nor does this reflect simply increased patient sharing through physicians covering each others' on-call time, because the average annual number of services per patient seen has not declined. Thus there has been an overall expansion in servicing.

The physician-to-population ratio in Manitoba has risen rapidly over this period, while average physician incomes and workloads have nevertheless remained stable. But this stability has not been achieved through each physician's servicing a shrinking pool of patients more intensively. Rather, the same person is turning up in the practice population of a larger number of different physicians, so that the size of each physician's practice, the apparent patient count, is in fact rising, not falling. Thus although the average number of both persons and discrete patients (persons who contact one or more physicians) per physician is falling, the average number of apparent patients is not.

The reasons for this pattern are obscure. A cynic might identify it as "pinball medicine"—physicians, and especially GPs, referring patients (informally; these are not billed as consultations) among themselves to keep busy. A spokesman for a medical association would be more likely to criticize "shopping" by patients who take the same complaint to a number of physicians until they get a diagnosis or a treatment they like—or just to pass the time. The observed data are consistent with either.

But they are not consistent with the hypothesis of compression of morbidity and declining utilization. Of course, we know very little about morbidity compared to what we know about utilization. But what we do know seems more consistent with the view that morbidity is increasing, not decreasing. The optimistic scenario, of compression of morbidity followed by natural death, with declining need for health care, has not been demonstrated to be invalid for the much longer run, but we are certainly not approaching it at the moment (see also Verbrugge, 1984, forthcoming).

TO WHOSE PROBLEM IS MORE HEALTH CARE A SOLUTION?

On the other hand, precisely because we *do* know so little about morbidity independent of utilization statistics, we have no basis for assuming that the large increases in health care servicing rates for the elderly population are an appropriate way to respond to their needs. Is there really much benefit from having the average elderly person see a larger number of different general practitioners in any one year, or spend twice as long in an extended care bed before dying? What does all this activity have to do with health?

This is both an evaluative and a conceptual issue. At the evaluative level, it represents an application of clinical epidemiology and program evaluation—what is the balance of positive and negative consequences associated with the increasing array of interventions to which the elderly in particular are exposed? To what extent do these enable the blind to see and the lame to walk, as against simply prolonging the dying process. And what other benefits could be provided to the elderly population—or to the rest of us—with the same resources?

But it is also a conceptual issue, as we have to think harder about what our objectives are—what do we mean by health? The patient with late effects of CVA, who appears no longer sentient—would we want to support prolongation of life, if that were ourselves? And if the answer, as honestly as we can give it, is no, then are we ethically justified in doing so for others? It is doubtful if we are prepared to contemplate euthanasia, at least not in this generation, but the patient's right to place limits, in advance, on the extent of intervention, is receiving increasing attention.

Both the conceptual and the evaluative questions surrounding the relation between the health of the elderly and the expansion of their health care are eminently researchable. The problem of deciding what we want to do as well as how is, however, compounded by the unfortunate fact that while, from most perspectives, the health care of the elderly is a problem, to some it is a solution.

We have already noted that the supply of physicians is increasing in Canada at a rate substantially faster than the general population. Again as simple arithmetic, and without implying any malfeasance by physicians, this implies that either utilization per capita must rise, or physician workloads must fall. In the latter case, either fee increases that are more rapid than the general inflation rate must be bargained for or physician incomes must fall. What has in fact happened is that utilization per capita *has* risen to match the increased numbers of physicians so that workloads have not fallen (Barer & Evans, 1986). But these increases have been most rapid among the elderly (Barer et al., 1987; Roch et al., 1985). If the "compression of morbidity" had led to *falling* utilization rates in the elderly population over the last two decades, the economic position of physicians would have deteriorated significantly.

Nor are physicians the only ones with an economic stake in the servicing of the elderly. By transferring hospital capacity from acute care to extended care, British Columbia hospitals (and behind them the provincial government) have effectively "downsized" the hospital industry over the last 20 years, without the political backlash that might have accompanied actually closing beds. Extended care patients are much cheaper to look after, precisely because they *are* the "bed blockers" that physicians complain of. If they could be transferred elsewhere and the beds freed up for acute care patients, overall service intensity, costs, and medical billings would rise. Bed blockers are a medical problem but an administrative solution.

It is, however, both impolite and impolitic to present the changing patterns of utilization by the elderly in this way. Far better to focus on external forces—major demographic trends, for example, or the uncontrollable advance of technology. And of course these external factors do matter; but they are not the *only* forces at work.

RESEARCH TO KNOW AND RESEARCH TO DO: WINNERS AND LOSERS

The conflict of motivations and interests at stake in the care of the elderly has important implications for the conduct and climate of research in this field. The objectives and the process of research in the field of policy generally differ in a fundamental way from those in the "hard sciences." The latter is in a sense a "game against nature," the former is to a considerable extent a game against ourselves.

The game against nature is not by any means easy—subtle is the Lord. But we have no reason to believe that nature plays actively against us and changes its behavior when it appears that we are winning a point—malicious He is not. The natural world is assumed to be a stable structure, subject to uniformitarian laws, even if our understanding of it may change radically over time. At each point in time our knowledge gained through research is cumulative. As a society, as a species, we are continually adding to a total corpus of understanding, and the processes whereby we do so are independent of the objectives we seek in doing so.

The motivations for doing or supporting research are various—individual fame, national pride, commercial advantage, morbid curiosity, keeping gainfully employed, and passing the time. But the connection to subsequent action is not an essential part of the process; knowledge is of value for its own sake. (The publication is its own reward.) This is particularly clear in such fields as cosmology; a better understanding of the origins of the universe may profoundly affect our sense of who we are and where we fit in to the larger picture, but has no direct policy implications.

Research on public policy, however, addresses a target that is constantly moving, in essence a historical process. The knowledge gained is not cumulative and permanent, but constantly decaying as the objects of knowledge are transformed by time. The descriptions and the causal structures which such research generates are at best temporary; as Heracleitus pointed out, you cannot step into the same river twice. Laplace's Demon has been exorcised and, anyway, Laplace is dead.

The purpose, then, of describing and analyzing ephemera is to guide decisions and actions. The research process cannot be separated from the conclusions in the form of "what is to be done"; the justification of the research *is* the consequent action (or inaction—to do nothing is also a decision).

An enormous amount of hopeful policy research goes on which is never completed in action—it is in consequence completely useless, a trivial pursuit. But the process can be justified on two grounds. First, when policy decisions *are* influenced, and improved, by research, the payoffs can be enormous. And second, the effects of policy research may often be indirect in both time and space—good analysis can influence the way people see the world around them, and lead to subtle changes in behavior impossible to predict in advance. So, of course, can bad.

The intimate connection between policy research and action, however, means that intelligent observers can identify the implications of research findings, and particularly the economic implications. Winners and losers can be identified in advance. The policy game is not simply zero-sum, a process in which every winner is matched by a loser. "Good" policies presumably yield results that, on balance, do more good than harm, when aggregated in some way over the whole society. But it is very unusual to find policies that do not make *somebody* worse off. The secret of implementation, and progress, is to identify portfolios of policies which assemble constituencies of support—political entrepreneurship.

THE BUGS WON'T STAY ON THE SLIDE ... THEY WANT TO BE COAUTHORS

In this process, research can contribute by making much clearer what the relevant payoffs and costs are, and what the alternatives may be. But insofar as research influences the probability of adoption of particular policies, the gainers and losers can be expected to enter the research process itself. The distribution of consequences is identifiable, and subject to contention, so the "objects" of research take a hand in it as well, and research becomes very difficult to separate from advocacy.

The advocacy of alternative theoretical interpretations and conflict over the validity of particular observations are, of course, found in the "true sciences" as well. But such advocacy is usually separable from the advocacy of policies based on those interpretations. Nuclear physicists may disagree over the morality of developing and using weapons based on their research, but these disagreements are logically separable from any disagreements they may have over the body of knowledge in subatomic physics.

In the policy fields, the *ought* penetrates the *is*, and disputes over policy become translated into disputes over the research on which advocacy of those policies is based. The result is equivalent to "Ban-the-Bomb-ers" and "Nuke-the-Reds-ists" each taking an active part in debates over the physics of fission and fusion as well as the proper applications (or bugs advancing alternative theories of pathology). In this environment, the development of consensus over the conclusions to be drawn from research comes rather more slowly. Policy debates are thus extraordinarily difficult to settle decisively, even though in real time actions are or are not taken. Old arguments come back over the years, like bad dinners.

Research in health care spans both the "hard" and the policy fields. Biomedical research, with all its subdivisions, fits the former description. Its focus and funding may be politically contentious, but its findings are not. In this area, we are all on the same team, engaging in or cheering on the game against nature. But health policy research is inherently divisive, in that its conduct and its findings are under constant dispute by the winners and losers from the policies which they support or oppose.

This raises the possibility that policy research which is *not* challenged by some threatened interest may have no implications, or none of importance. Accordingly, a body like the Saskatchewan Health Research Board, or any other agency conducting or supporting health policy research, is inevitably launched into a politically contentious field—unless it chooses to be impotent. The other alternative, of course, is to slide sideways into biomedical research—getting out of the kitchen—in the alleged pursuit of "science" or "rigor."

Unfortunately, there is no reason to believe that progress in biomedical research, now or soon, is going to resolve any of the major problems in health policy, or for that matter to make a major contribution to the health of the elderly or anyone else. That is not to say that biomedical research does not matter—clearly it does—but its contributions tend to be slow and small, while the costs of its application are rapid and large. Decisive "breakthroughs" are very rare. The virtual elimination of polio probably qualifies, but that of smallpox was a triumph of organization, not research.

Indeed, a recent survey of eminent biomedical researchers revealed a general consensus: the greatest improvements in human health in the near term will come not from their work, but from changes to healthier lifestyles and environments—smoking cessation, dietary improvement, exercise, stress management (Taylor & Voivodas, 1987). These are problems for policy.

In recent years, the progress of biomedical research appears to have exacerbated the problems of caring for the aged population, insofar as it has tended to extend the range of "salvage" capability more rapidly than that of "cure" (or rehabilitation), or prevention. The dilemma of the named individual—how can we let *this person* die?—has made it extraordinarily difficult for us to address the broader question of how we want to allocate our resources over our own lives—how much do we want to sacrifice now, to be salvaged later? Alternatively, how should the resources the presently working population is prepared to devote to the dependent aged be used? When the choice boils down to bread or bypass grafts, the latter win out because of their perceived greater immediacy and the degree of organization of their advocates, who *may* in fact be advocates for named individuals.

There is no *a priori* reason why progress in biomedical research should always take this direction. In Lewis Thomas' terms, we may hope with enough knowledge to escape from "halfway technologies" and eventually discover the decisive interventions that effectively (and perhaps cheaply) resolve current sources of morbidity. This may be one road to the eventual "compression of morbidity." But it is not happening yet, and experts in the field do not hold out much hope of "magic bullets" in the near term.

Accordingly, we shall have to continue to address the difficult questions of choice, the problems of discovering our collective wishes and intentions and giving them effect through health policy. As emphasized above, more and better research can never substitute for these political decisions. But it can certainly improve our understanding of our current situation, our perception of the range of choices available to us, and their probable consequences. As an act of faith (and in the absence of clear supporting evidence), those of us in the research field are required to believe that this process will lead to better policy choices.

The realities of politics, however, dictate that a necessary (though not sufficient) condition for such a result is the dissemination of research findings well beyond the research community itself. To justify our activities, if not our existence, we need connections to the wider society.

ACKNOWLEDGMENT

Comments from Steven Lewis and Morris Barer are gratefully acknowledged. The author's research is supported by a Research Scientist Award from the National Health Research and Development Program, Health and Welfare Canada.

NOTES

1. What medical care we could "afford" would become stark reality for a good many more of us, if we did not have a collective system for funding health care. The wonders of modern medicine are rarely cheap, and the costs of care for a severe illness could easily be beyond the resources of most low and middle income families in a "user-pay" system. Questions which present themselves as choices for the community as a whole would be absolute constraints for the individual. Thus *every* developed society—even the United States—funds the bulk of its health care through collective institutions, and makes explicit or implicit collective choices in the process.
2. These observations contradict a line of argument which arises from the naive application of elementary economic models. A number of economic commentators, particularly those without much experience of health care, believe that when care is "free" (at point of service), "consumers" will "overuse" it, leading to increased costs. "Deterrent" charges are advocated to control costs by reducing this "frivolous" use. This argument fails, because it misspecifies the processes determining the utilization of health care services, and abstracts from the central role of the providers of care in interpreting and responding to the "needs" of the patient (Stoddart & Barer, 1981; Evans, 1983, 1984).

On the other hand, Canadian physicians have consistently argued for the re-imposition of direct charges on the ground that this would *increase* overall outlays for health care, which they believe to be currently "underfunded" (e.g., Canadian Medical Association, 1981). On the international evidence, the doctors would appear to have the direction of effect right.

The question has been confused by findings from studies of individual patients, carefully isolated by experimental design from the normal interaction of patient and provider behavior, which show that under these circumstances direct charges will reduce utilization by such selected groups (Newhouse, 1981; Manning et al., 1987). But it is an elementary "fallacy of composition" to generalize those findings to the system-wide level; and the reasons for the failure of this generalization are well documented (Barer, Evans, & Stoddart, 1979).

3. Steven Lewis (personal communication) has pointed out, however, that this "life-cycle contract" perspective implicitly assumes that the potential interventions which the health care system can deploy will remain constant over time. In reality, the individual "contractor" at age 20, or 30, can be sure only that the technological possibilities will be very different, when s/he reaches 90. Thus to agree (not) to pay for particular interventions now, on the understanding that they will (not) be made available to oneself 50 or 60 years hence, is nonsense—the needs and interventions may then be totally different.

   He suggests an alternative perspective, a "Rawlsian" principle. What would one choose to undergo, and pay for, and through what institutional channels, if one were behind the veil of ignorance and did not know how old, ill, or wealthy one was? This seems to me to be even more difficult to operationalize than the life-cycle contract viewpoint, and yet his point about the unpredictability of future intervention possibilities—and needs—seems to me to be entirely correct and important. Another paper, perhaps.

4. We do not think it ethically reprehensible for individuals to engage in risky activities such as mountain-climbing, which apparently yield current satisfactions at a cost of current risk to (their own) life and limb. The life-cycle allocation process merely spreads this trade-off over a longer period—current satisfactions versus future morbid or mortal consequences.

5. On the other hand, some choices may become substantially more difficult, as they are clarified. Fundamental conflicts of values, which may be between individuals or within each of us, pose dilemmas that the political process may be able to blur and bypass—if no one looks too closely.

6. Not all of this is domestic production. Net immigration of physicians continues to add several hundred per year to the Canadian stock even after the sharp cut-back of 1975. But even if net immigration went to zero, which there is little likelihood that it will, domestic production would still exceed current population growth rates (Barer, Gafni, & Lomas, 1989).

REFERENCES

Barer, M. L., & Evans, R. G. (1986). Riding north on a south-bound horse? Expenditures, prices, utilization and incomes in the Canadian health care system.

In R. G. Evans & G. L. Stoddart (Eds.), *Medicare at maturity: Achievements, lessons & challenges.* (pp. 53–183). Calgary: University of Calgary Press.

Barer, M. L., Evans, R. G., Hertzman, C., & Lomas, J. (1987). Aging and health care utilization: New evidence on old fallacies. *Social Science and Medicine, 24*(10), 851–62.

Barer, M. L., Evans, R. G., & Stoddart, G. L. (1979). *Controlling health care costs by direct charges to patients: Snare or delusion?* (Ontario Economic Council Occasional Paper No. 10). Toronto: Ontario Economic Council.

Barer, M. L., Gafni, A., & Lomas, J. (1989). Accommodating rapid growth in physician supply: Lessons from Israel, warnings for Canada. *International Journal of Health Services, 19*(1), 95–115.

Boulet, J. A., & Grenier, G. (1978). *Health expenditures in Canada and the impact of demographic changes on future government health insurance program expenditures* (Economic Council of Canada Discussion Paper No. 123). Ottawa: ECC.

Canadian Medical Association. (1981). Evidence presented to the Special Committee on The Federal-Provincial Fiscal Arrangements, House of Commons, Canada, *Minutes of Proceedings and Evidence* (Issue No. 10, pp. 10–3 to 10–54, and 10A-1 to 10A-44), Tuesday, May 12, 1981, First Session, Thirty-Second Parliament, 1980–81.

Culyer, A. J. (1988). *Health expenditures in Canada: Myth and reality, past and future.* Toronto: Canadian Tax Foundation.

Denton, F. T., & Spencer, B. G. (1983). Population aging and future health costs in Canada. *Canadian Public Policy, 9*(2), 155–63.

Evans, R. G. (1983). The welfare economics of public health insurance: Theory and Canadian practice. In L. Soderstrom (Ed.), *Social insurance.* Amsterdam: North-Holland.

Evans, R. G. (1984). *Strained mercy: The economics of Canadian health care.* Toronto: Butterworths.

Evans, R. G. (1985). Illusions of necessity: Evading responsibility for choice in health care. *Journal of Health Policy, Politics and Law, 10*(3), 439–67.

Evans, R. G. (1986). Finding the levers, finding the courage: Lessons from cost containment in North America. *Journal of Health Politics, Policy and Law* (Tenth Anniversary Issue), *11*(4), 585–616.

Evans, R. G. (1987). Hang together or hang separately: The viability of a universal health care system in an aging society. *Canadian Public Policy, 13*(2), 165–80.

Evans, R. G., Barer, M. L., Hertzman, C., et al. (forthcoming). *The long good-bye: The great transformation of the British Columbia hospital system. Health Services Research.*

Evans, R. G., Lomas J., Barer, M. L., et al. (forthcoming). Controlling health expenditures: The Canadian reality. *New England Journal of Medicine.*

Evans, R. G., Robinson, G. C., & Barer, M. L. (1988). Where have all the children gone? Accounting for the paediatric hospital implosion. In R. S. Tonkin & J. R. Wright (Eds.), *Redesigning relationships in child health care* (pp. 63–76). Vancouver: BC Children's Hospital.

Evans, R. G., Roch, D. J., & Pascoe, D. W. (1987). Defensive reticulation: Physician supply increases and practice pattern changes in Manitoba, 1971 to 1981. In J. M. Horne (Ed.), *Proceedings of the Third Canadian Conference on Health Economics, 1986* (pp. 91–126). Winnipeg: University of Manitoba, Dept. of Social and Preventive Medicine.

Fries, J. F. (1980, July 17). Aging, natural death, and the compression of morbidity. *New England Journal of Medicine, 303*(3), 130–35.

Fries, J. F. (1983). The compression of morbidity. *Milbank Memorial Fund Quarterly/Health and Society, 61*(3), 397–419.

Fuchs, V. R. (1984). Though much is taken: Reflections on aging, health and medical care. *Milbank Memorial Fund Quarterly/Health and Society, 62*(2), 143–166.

Lomas, J., Barer, M. L., & Stoddart, G. L. (1985). *Physician manpower planning: Lessons from the Macdonald report.* Toronto: Ontario Economic Council.

Manning, W. G., Newhouse, J. P., Duan, N., Keeler, E. B., Leibowitz, A., & Marquis, M. S. (1987). Health insurance and the demand for medical care: Evidence from a randomized experiment. *American Economic Review, 77*(3), 251–77.

Newhouse, J. P. (1981). The demand for medical care services: A retrospect and prospect. In J. Van der Gaag & M. Perlman (Eds.), *Health, economics, and health economics* (pp. 85–102). Proceedings of the World Congress on Health Economics, Leiden, The Netherlands, September 1980. Amsterdam: North-Holland.

Organization for Economic Co-operation and Development. (1987). *Financing and delivering health care* (OECD Social Policy Studies No. 4). Paris: OECD.

Roch, D. J., Evans, R. G., & Pascoe, D. W. (1985). *Manitoba and medicare, 1971 to the present.* Winnipeg: Manitoba Health.

Roos, N. P., Montgomery, P., & Roos, L. L. (1987). Health care utilization in the years prior to death. *Milbank Quarterly, 65*(2), 231–254.

Scheiber, G. J., & Poullier, J. P. (1987). Trends in international health care spending. *Health Affairs, 6*(3), 105–12.

Schneider, E. L., & Brody, J. A. (1983, October 6). Aging, natural death, and the compression of morbidity: Another view. *New England Journal of Medicine, 309*(14), 854–6.

Scitovsky, A. A. (1984). The high cost of dying: What do the data show? *Milbank Memorial Fund Quarterly/Health and Society, 62*(4, 591–608.

Stoddart, G. L., & Barer, M. L. (1981). Analysis of demand and utilization through episodes of medical service. In J. Van der Gaag & M. Perlman (Eds.), *Health, economics, and health economics* (p. 149). Proceedings of the World Congress on Health Economics, Leiden, The Netherlands, September 1980. Amsterdam: North-Holland.

Stoddart, G. L., & Labelle, R. J. (1985). *Privatization in the Canadian health care system: Assertions, evidence, ideology and options.* Ottawa: Health and Welfare Canada.

Stout, R. W., & Crawford, V. (1988, February 6). Active-life expectancy and terminal dependency: Trends in long term geriatric care over 33 years. *Lancet,* 281–283.

Taylor, H., & Voivodas, G. (1987). *The Bristol-Myers report: Medicine in the next century*. New York: Louis Harris for the Bristol-Myers Company.

Verbrugge, L. M. (1984). Longer life but worsening health? Trends in health and mortality of middle-aged and older persons. *Milbank Memorial Fund Quarterly/Health and Society, 62*(3), 475–519.

Verbrugge, L. M. (forthcoming). Recent, present, and future health of American adults. In L. Breslow, J. E. Fielding, & L. B. Lave (Eds.), *Annual Review of Public Health* (Vol. 10). Palo Alto, CA: Annual Reviews Inc.

Walker, A. (1987). Meeting the needs of Canada's elderly with limited health resources: Some observations based on British experience. In *Aging with limited resources: Proceedings of a colloquium on health care* (pp. 27–39). Ottawa: Economic Council of Canada.

Weller, G. R., & Manga, P. (1983). The push for reprivatization of health care services in Canada, Britain, and the United States. *Journal of Health Politics, Policy and Law, 8*(3), 495–518.

Wilkins, R., & Adams, O. B. (1987). Changes in the healthfulness of life of the elderly population: An empirical approach. *Revue D'epidémiologie et de Santé Publique, 35*(3–4), 225–35.

Woods Gordon Management Consultants. (1984). *Investigation of the impact of demographic change on the health care system in Canada—final report.* Prepared for the Task Force on the Allocation of Health Care Resources— Joan Watson, Chairman. Toronto: Woods Gordon.

15. Death, Ethics, and Choice

ANDREW MALCOLM

I am not a health professional—I am a storyteller, professional storyteller, a journalist, although in the course of my research in recent years I have spent many, many long and fascinating hours with those dedicated people who provide the health care in North America. I come to the issues as a consumer on one level, and as a professional journalist on another with a fascination for human stories, the human condition, and I have come to have a fascination with the human spirit as well.

With that in mind, I would like to share with you some thoughts about what I believe to be quite possibly the most serious issue facing our society today. And at the same time, it is quite possibly the least discussed, the least understood, and no doubt the most feared. That issue of course is death—our own mortality, that of our loved ones, our friends, strangers. Probably most of us have at one time or another been at a family dinner table—perhaps Thanksgiving—when an elderly family member starts to speak. "Some day when I am not here," she begins, comfortable in the acceptance that real life is thinning, it does come to an end at some point. But she is cut off by a unanimous chorus of everyone speaking instinctively: "Oh, Grams," they say, "you are going to be here long after we are gone." The subject is changed, some laugh uncomfortably, but everyone smiles and gets on with the business of eating and living and forgetting the subject and the momentary discomfort at the thought of all of us being united by our mortality. And of course, the children, sitting there so silently and attentively, have all been passed the unspoken message about the unspoken subject with five letters which in French, of course, is a four-letter word.

We don't have trouble on TV or in the movies or books showing people getting blown to bits in the most imaginative and colorful ways possible. But when it comes to a natural demise it is a different story. The advertising industry struggles with death—how can they sell life insurance for the day you die without talking about death?—so we see a fatherless family still absolutely happy and delighted thanks to the thoughtfulness and foresight of

Aging and Health: Linking Research and Public Policy, © 1989 Lewis Publishers, Inc., Chelsea, Michigan 48118. Printed in U.S.A.

the missing dad. My favorite is the commercial with an apparent angel escorting an unsuspecting father onto an escalator into the big sky. "You mean," says the man, "it is that time?" The angel does not reply, so of course we all know. But that one dread day does come with the solemn phone call and the reality no longer can be ignored and we all feel sick with that kind of hollow empty feeling in the gut.

I remember talking with my father about five years ago. He had some serious chronic medical problems—painful, debilitating—and he had chosen to have some surgery. It had not gone well. Over the course of several months in those wonderful warning words of George Burns, my father had fallen in love with his bed. I was urging him as only an only son of 37 might to get up and out and about and find something to engage his mind other than the next round of pills or what the doctor had said at the last appointment. There seemed to be so little to engage his mind anymore other than the latest twinge of pain or annoyance at a world that seemed too easily baffled by his simple demands. "You know," he said to me, "quite honestly, I would just like to go to sleep and not wake up."

Well, that is one way to shut up a nervously chattering son, I can assure you. Here I was naively stuck in the useful belief that everyone outside of a war zone would want everyone else to stay alive as long as humanly and, in these days of medical miracles, mechanically possible. Now my father said he didn't want to anymore. He wasn't planning suicide, but the quality of his life as only he could define it was no longer worth it. Five days later he got up about 4:00 A.M., showered and shaved, wrote me a note, and also wrote detailed instructions to my mother on what to do in case of an emergency. Then he went back to bed, lay down and went to sleep quite naturally and did not wake up. Now, that was too bad for me and my mom and my children, but fortunately for him no one found him until it was too late. And later that morning I got the dreaded phone call with the finite news that produced the awful ache in the gut.

My father was lucky in a way. There is nothing I would rather have back again than my vibrant father full of ideas and talk and questions and his energy for me and his grandchildren. But I say he was lucky because he never spent any of that awful time in between life and death, when no one knows what he wants because we never thought or talked about it.

Now, a lot of the time when that phone call comes, it brings the news not of life or death, but of a kind of foggy middle ground where feelings are faint, where questions are many and where the rules are unwritten. And in this murky, new realm where medicine, law, and emotion merge into a volatile mix, lies both a threat and a challenge for our society as we approach the 21st century. For mankind has developed a most amazing array of medicines and machines. They can bring sight to sightless eyes, they can restart hearts. They can and do keep failed bodies operating to save perishable parts for transfer into other troubled bodies. I wrote a long story for the *Times* not long ago following the death of two women and the 10 other people who received parts of them—how their 10 lives were changed and how the lives of those of the donors' families were affected as well. Experts are now experimenting with transplanted limbs, and on moving parts of monkeys' brains back and forth. This progress is not going to stop. Without a doubt, these advances have given precious extra hours, days, weeks, even years of meaningful life to thousands, if not millions, of people.

I spent some time in a neonatal ward not long ago in California and saw babies no heavier than a couple dozen business letters being fed and aspirated and kept alive until that hoped-for day when their own tiny organs could take over for themselves. "Would you like to see this little guy's heart?" one doctor said to me. He took an instrument the size of an electrical shaver, stuck it in the incubator, put it gently on the baby's chest, and there up on the screen, in living black and white, was the tiny throbbing muscle working away so hard. That machine cost $150,000.00. He has to buy a new one every three, four, or five months.

I also spent time in an intensive care unit where several of the 10,000 U.S. bodies in permanent vegetative states were being maintained in various stages of being, hooked to machines that fed them, monitored them, drained them, breathed for them with mechanical sighs programmed in every 32 seconds. No one could ask for more devoted care by health professionals or machines. When we do think about death, we would all like to think that sometime after our eightieth or ninetieth or hundredth birthday perhaps we will be walking along the street when a huge truck will come from out of nowhere and snuff us out with no suffering, no pain, no lingering, no financial drain on us, our family, or our society—no messy decisions that trouble the living who never anticipated that middle ground. But the fact of the matter is that, thanks to the medical advances of recent decades, we can now live through so many diseases and conditions once considered inevitably terminal, so that we can die from the next layer of diseases and conditions presently considered inevitably terminal.

As a result, over 80% of us will die in institutions where the technology is gathered—not at home where the family was gathered. Most of us will die after a long period of suffering from a chronic, painful condition. What about the people for whom that extra period of life is a commitment to a living hell? What about the ultimate civil right of a patient to control the medical treatment of his or her own body?

But what about the parents of those 24-ounce babies who told the doctors they wanted their sons' precious lives in God's hands, not the doctors'. The doctors had the lawyers get the court order at 4:00 A.M.; while the doctors and the lawyers and the judge could go home to their healthy families every evening, the new parents got to spend many months of long visiting hours in that neonatal intensive care unit watching their long dreamed-of child wilt away. He died, and the hospital and the doctors which had placed their set of ethics and rules above the rights of that family and child presented them with the medical bill for $1 million.

More important, what about the baby whose mouth only knew a sterile plastic tube, whose total nutrition was pumped in through the nose, whose arms were bruised from necessary needle punctures—was that a life? Was that a fair decision by the powerful medical establishment? And who is to say? Did the doctors and the nurses really have a choice? Did the patient? What kind of freedoms do we as free society, do we as health care providers grant to the ill or take from them because they are ill, or because we decide they may just be depressed for awhile, or because they refuse to be what patients are supposed to be, namely, patient. Do we as a society have a choice about what kinds of freedom we will allow to individuals because they happen to be sick in an age of medical marvel?

These are obviously very difficult decisions—decisions where there is no right and wrong, just difficulty. They are the flip side of our medical miracles. But I think our society is so accustomed to wealth and abundance that we assume all things are fixable if only enough money and technology are thrown at them. I think our societies must begin considering new rules to guide us all in these painful new times—decisions about life and death, and what they are and when we should use the awesome powers we have created. One woman told me that it was much easier when God made all the decisions.

I don't believe any doctors actively seek the power to decide whether to unplug someone this afternoon, but the onus has fallen to them because so few of us want to think about any of this in advance. Democratic societies, by and large, get the kind of politicians (and press) they deserve or demand, and we are heading for the kind of medical decisionmaking that we deserve by our default: colored by the fears and demands of others (say, doctors afraid of malpractice or criminal charges) and too often too little shaped by the desires of the patient and the family. We have seen some painful controversy in Oregon, where they are reallocating money from transplants to neonatal care—there is only so much to go around. Who, for instance, is going to get the limited number of organs available for transplant—the one most in need or the one who gets on the evening news with the saddest story? Should we be spending so much of our increasingly limited money on medical care in the waning weeks of life, or might we better invest these funds in improving the health care at the other end of life, on those little folks who can't vote yet? What politician would be crazy enough to make such a suggestion and take on the motivated legions of the elderly who have the time, the vote, and the self-interest and who, not coincidentally, are the fastest growing sectors of our societies in North America.

A few months after my father's death I read a short item in the *New York Times* about an elderly Texan who had gone into the hospital to visit his wife of 52 years. The woman had long suffered from Alzheimer's disease. She no longer recognized anyone and thought her dutiful husband was the devil. Her husband, alone with her that day, had purchased a small pistol; he shot her in the heart and then he shot himself in the heart. A few weeks later I called the hospital spokesman to talk about the man who had come into the hospital and killed his sick wife. The hospital spokesman said to me, "Which one?" I remember that chilling sense that I had that day, the realization that what I had thought was such an isolated incident really had become frighteningly ordinary. One freak happening in Dallas, Texas, another in Chicago, one in San Francisco, Toronto, Montreal, and pretty soon you have a pretty disturbing pattern of people who, desperately wanting out but finding no exit, create their own. In January 1988, an ill man in New York City, rather than go back to the hospital, threw himself off the upper balcony of the Metropolitan Opera House, nearly killing a couple of other people on the way down. The former head of the New York Bar Association, ridden with cancer, called his doctor and, in the course of the telephone conversation, shot himself. In California, an ailing couple, one of whom faced long term care on a machine, rented an apartment, wrote a lot of notes, left them around, put poison in their wine and died in each other's arms.

Now no one had really ever explored these kinds of issues in the newspapers. I wrote two long stories for the *Times;* and that was supposed to be it. But the flood of mail and the pleas from both public and private organizations alike indicated a desperate hunger for more information. Basically, they were saying, "Thank God somebody is writing about it," but where are the institutions facing this question rather than dodging it? The basic problem is, I think, we have created a marvelous medical technology without creating an accompanying marvelous set of rules and guidelines. Doctors in hospitals can with impunity do everything technologically possible without creating a counterbalance to consider the desires of the patient should they be contrary. When should we not do everything we can? Whose life is it anyway?

How many of us have ever remembered to discuss with our doctor what kind of treatment we want should something go wrong with the minor surgery tomorrow. We plan for fires in the home, we plan for life insurance, we even plan for automobile accidents, wearing seat belts in the unlikely event that we get smashed by somebody, but we don't prepare for what certainly will come to everyone of us: only a third have a will when we die. This sometimes seems to be an age where there are no more acts of God. Anything that goes wrong must have been caused by someone, someone to blame, someone to sue. In this litigious age, what doctor, trained to believe that death is a defeat, is going to say, "Of course I am certain the surgery will go well tomorrow, Mrs. Jones, but just in case it doesn't and you fall into a permanent vegetative state, what kind of care or withholding of care would you like and do you think your family might sue me?" It is something we have to think about in advance, not the day before.

So we have out of our collective inattention created a continental open secret—a kind of negotiated death. Someone gets sick, we try treatments, something else goes wrong, the patient deteriorates, the doctor meets with the family. The caring doctors never crush all family hope, so they use euphemisms. My personal favorite: the gambling odds—there is a 1 in 5 chance. Of course, for the patient it is 100% or zero. There is also the sports euphemism—he has two strikes against him. The doctors may try to educate the family to give them time to adjust to the reality, or even plant the seed of choice to see if the family responds. Maybe the daughter has been caring for the old man these many years, and agrees he would not want to be on these machines—he was terrified of them. "Just let my father be comfortable." But then the son arrives from the East, feeling awfully guilty, not having come home the last two Christmases because of all the disease and unhappiness in the house. He has left the care to his sister and now has to strut a little bit about caring about his dad. So he says, "By God, Doc, I want you to do everything you can for my pa." Now what do you, as the doctor, do?

You probably do everything you possibly can for his father—hope and costs be damned and perhaps the patient's wishes, too. But even if over the next few days or weeks the family comes around to the realization that the end really is near, a decision is made in secret. No one in the family is ever going to mention at next week's cocktail party that they just negotiated their father's death. The doctors who don't need any prosecutors nosing around and labeling them Dr. Death in the tabloids aren't going to make that announcement or admit that they unplug people every day. So when you or I or anyone else faces the same set of circumstances with our loved ones, we think we are the first poor souls in the world ever to face this awful dilemma unprepared.

Sad to say, the financial burden keeps growing. Today about 40% of all money spent by Medicare in the United States is spent on the last few weeks of life, in those last vain efforts to fight the inevitabilities of death for reasons, I suspect, that have more to do with making the living feel good about all that they did than for the brief benefit to the dying. As Dr. Christian Barnard has said, "Sometimes death can do what doctors can't—it can relieve suffering."

But how do we permit reasoned exits for some members of our society while protecting the rights of the larger majority who may want to try everything for awhile? There are obviously no easy answers here, but a variety of attempted solutions have just begun to emerge, some of them almost in a clandestine manner. Many hospitals have formed ethics committees under one name or another, which try to educate, to guide actual decisions, or to arbitrate when disagreements emerge in this emotional area.

There are about 5700 deaths on the average day in the United States. Experts I have talked with estimate that at least several hundred of these deaths are, in effect, negotiated. That is, the doctor and the family, maybe an ethicist, maybe a specially trained nurse, maybe even a lawyer or two, and maybe even the patient, if he or she is still conscious, meet and over the course of sometimes prolonged discussions they will reach an agreement to provide less aggressive care—they will make the patient comfortable and allow nature to take its course. The cause is not listed as unplugging, of course; it is cardiopulmonary failure or some such term, and so long as no one runs screaming to some local prosecutor crying foul, everyone goes on about his business of living without legal complication and seemingly without memory. There is also in North America a developing array of legal precedents based on a growing number of cases settled in courts. We are all probably familiar with the Karen Ann Quinlan case of 1975, when the New Jersey Supreme Court ruled that an artificial breathing machine could be removed from a permanently comatose patient. But in recent years the courts have approved removal of other means, most recently the artificial feeding tube. A majority of American states have also approved living wills and durable powers of attorney signed by the patient naming a proxy decision-maker in the event the patient becomes incompetent. Millions of people have signed these wills, which may only indicate a general wish to avoid any extraordinary treatment, but today's extraordinary treatment is tomorrow's routine treatment. There is also the issue of whether last year's signatory still feels the same today. Many of the 38 states have slightly different wording requirements in living wills and, as a result, you may have one in Arizona and get sick in California, and you still have problems.

Just as important in this whole process is frank discussion within the family and certainly with the doctor. We are certainly getting away from the old days where the doctor was God. In almost all North American political jurisdictions, suicide is perfectly legal, but assisting an act of suicide is illegal. That means that someone can be prosecuted for helping someone do something that is legal. We have also a patchwork of prosecution depending, in many cases, on the personality of the prosecutor and the juries. In Florida, one elderly man shoots and kills his wife, a long-suffering victim of Alzheimer's; they find him standing next to the wheelchair sobbing with a smoking gun in his hand and the grand jury refuses even to lay charges. In the same county two years later, another man does the same thing, and he is now at the age of 73 serving a life sentence in prison. More typical is the true story that I detailed in *This Far and No More*, which NBC happened to call *A Right to Die* because it probably got more people to watch. It is the story of a young mother stricken with amyotrophic lateral sclerosis. At first she determines to fight it—she is going to be the first person ever to beat the disease. I have her diary, and you can see her attitudes change as she becomes increasingly confined by the paralysis. But then she comes to feel that her increasingly restricted life—its emotional and financial weight on her and all of her family members—is not the kind of life she wants to live. And so she sets out with her husband's reluctant help to let her body die despite the hospital's many objections and obstacles. In one scene, the little girl comes to play show-and-tell. At one point the little girl of about three goes over to her mother and takes the skin on her bony arm and pinches it as tightly as she possibly can trying to get a reaction, but of course she gets none, because there can be none. She then leans up and looks in her mother's eyes deeply for a couple of minutes, goes back to her father and says, "Is mommy really in there?" And before the tears came, her father was able to say, "Yes, of course she is," and then warn her that her mother can hear everything that she is saying. This shows up in the diary and feeds the desire of this woman to get out of the life she has found completely unacceptable. She or her husband find sympathetic doctors and arrange a pattern of home visits. One Saturday a doctor gives her a sedative, the respirator is turned off, she dies, another comes, certifies on the death certificate that so far as he can tell it is a natural death. She is cremated, and the hospital, knowing full well the complete plan, looks the other way, relieved. This is happening every day.

And so it seems we are all being left to work out our own answers in emergency conversations with our families and doctors—Emily's was an example of that. How could her husband, who said he was in this fight to the end with her, ask, "In case there is a breathing problem along the way, do you want to go on a respirator or not?" This was seen as defeatist by his wife, so there was no decision until her eyes started rolling and she couldn't breathe, and to play it safe, he put her on the respirator and then it was three years down the road. We need to talk about this in advance and then also pray that the doctor is not out on the golf course when our day comes. The polls indicate a growing awareness of the problem, and over 70% know that patients do indeed have the right to ask the doctor to turn off a life-sustaining machine.

I suppose it should not be surprising that societies that cannot yet agree on when life officially begins cannot also agree on when it can end. But I think that if any of us here thought that the debate over abortion or other social issues was emotional, we have not seen anything yet until the debate really gets going over euthanasia and the right to die. I hope that my reporting and the book and, perhaps in some small way, the words in this chapter may have contributed something to the thinking side of that debate.

16. *The Politics of Change in the Health Arena*

DAVID BARRETT

INTRODUCTION

As Ray Jackson (1985) noted a couple of years ago in a Science Council of Canada discussion paper entitled *Issues in Preventive Health Care,* in the past century, there have been two health revolutions. The first was the result of general improvement in public health measures: water supplies, hygiene, vaccines, and better food and living conditions. The second followed the introduction of sulfa drugs, penicillin, and other antibiotics. The greatest strides in increasing life spans and health followed the first revolution. As the emphasis switched from public health measures to the powerful drug and surgery techniques practiced in a doctor's office and hospital, life expectancy increased, but much more slowly in the past 30 years. In Canada and the United States, only about 1% of persons die of infectious diseases before they live the biblical span, whereas the proportion of people being treated for chronic or degenerative diseases such as mental illness, cancer, stroke, cardiovascular, arthritis, injuries, and so on continues to rise steadily. We are entering a third revolution in health care as we grapple with chronic and degenerative diseases of the elderly, because such diseases are clearly not as susceptible to treatment as they are to prevention.

CAUSES OF DEBILITATING DISEASE

Although they can be genetic, more often than not debilitating diseases develop from long-term social, environmental, nutritional, and lifestyle situations. Affluent lifestyles can influence the rate of chronic and degenerative illnesses, but poverty breeds these illnesses as well. Men at the bottom of the income scale live six fewer years than men at the top income scale. On

Aging and Health: Linking Research and Public Policy, © 1989 Lewis Publishers, Inc., Chelsea, Michigan 48118. Printed in U.S.A.

average, men at the top income scale can expect 14 more disability-free years than men at men at the bottom. Canadians who are poor are more likely to die as a result of accidental falls, chronic respiratory diseases, pneumonia, tuberculosis, and sclerosis, and they have more mental illness, high blood pressure, and disorders of the joints and limbs. But the diseases of the elderly do not suddenly spring up as a result of some birthday. Chronic and degenerative conditions take years to develop and may have had their origin in nutritional or other deficiencies going back to early years. Poverty ages people far more quickly.

Meanwhile, millions of dollars are funneled to a commercial bank in financial trouble, but food banks are allowed to go broke. Prevention of illness is too often ignored in favor of the cheapest cures after the fact. Expenditures on health care have increased dramatically, but more and more hospitals have become impersonal industrial plants where patients endure "the managed maintenance of life on high levels of sublethal illness" (Jackson, 1985). We do not necessarily have just a sick population, however—we have a sick society.

Degrading the environment for the sake of profit, laying off millions for the sake of profit, skimping on education taxes for the sake of profit, cutting back worker protection or compensation for the injured for the sake of profit will result in an unhealthy and unhappy population. These degenerative processes eventually produce a society that can be kept alive only by expensive, heroic procedures and only for a very short time—in other words, a society that is brain-dead.

SOLUTIONS

The prescription for better and more affordable health is not an exponential increase of drugs and surgical procedures for the diseases of civilization, but a more enlightened society that realizes by tolerating, or even inducing, poverty by economic and social policy, it lights the fuse of an expensive treatment time bomb. It is not in the operating theater but in the political arena that the massive reductions in chronic and degenerative illnesses are more likely to be produced. Medicine's severest critic, Ivan Illich (1975), offers this prognosis: "The level of public health corresponds to the degree to which the means and responsibility for coping with illnesses are distributed amongst the total population."

The remedy lies in the political process, but it will not be found in those philosophies obsessed with the bottom line, which focus only on one aspect of life—the financial payoff—to the exclusion of all else. Political parties that take a holistic approach to society and all its problems are the only ones that can lead us back to rationality.

The approach to a healthy population must be holistic in both the socioeconomic and the medical sense. The elderly know that social programs have an enormous impact on their health and well-being. But this is not being done. (A significant number of elderly—particularly women—do not have enough money. Women aged 55 and over, when compared to men, have been relegated to a level of poverty that is startling, yet no Canadian national or provincial programs for women have been designed.) They also know it is *cheaper* to provide them with a homemaker's service at home than with bedpans in a hospital.

To carry through the new revolution, we will need the active involvement not only of the health professions and the politicians, but of the people. (To their credit, doctors have been at the forefront of campaigns against nuclear weapons, smoking, and unsafe cars, but inevitably are caught up in such government programs as ParticipAction [Canada's national fitness program], healthy cities, and the like.) One such mechanism that proved successful and very economical in my own political experience was a combination of human resource boards in community health and service clinics. The resource boards and service clinics were among the recommendations of a royal commission to the government of British Columbia in 1974, headed by Dr. Richard Ffoulkes, which advocated a holistic approach to the problems of health delivery. Several self-governing human resource boards, a mixture of local citizens directly elected by the communities, were established, and they appointed professionals to oversee the allocation of health and social welfare department expenditures in their communities. In British Columbia in the mid '70s, the government established pilot programs in five communities, from metropolitan settings to the isolated wilderness. They operated successfully for several years, and both government and British Columbia Medical Association audits verified notable efficiencies in delivering a vigorous health maintenance program. I am convinced that, over a generation, those projects would have had an enormous impact on improving general health as well as reducing cost, but one by one they were closed, despite vociferous protest, essentially for ideological reasons.

Do partisan considerations impede optimal development of health systems for the elderly? Can policymakers reconcile necessary but politically difficult decisions such as reallocation of resources? Should policies and programs be planned with a coherent philosophy rather than an ad hoc set of objectives? The answer to all of these is yes, and the solution is more democracy at the grass roots. People must be involved in making basic decisions—it can't just be left to the professionals—excluding, of course, social workers. Nor can it be left to the those politicians who regard citizens as mere producers or consumers rather than as whole human beings.

Politicians should be sensitive to the right to privacy and the right to choose among options, such as a range of social and housing options, including programs identifying with minorities and religious groups. We have to encourage decentralization of programs rather than trying to fit all people into the same particular service—a false efficiency.

The times are changing quite rapidly in the health care field. The population is aging, and the shift from infectious diseases to chronic and degenerative conditions is accelerating. The very nature of these changes inevitably involves the political process. Are we who work in the health care industry really ready to say to people: "Hey, you may know more than us"?

REFERENCES

Illich, I. (1975). *Medical nemesis*. Toronto: McClelland and Stewart.
Jackson, R. (1985). *Issues in preventive health care*. Science Council of Canada. Ottawa: Minister of Supply and Services.

17. Politics and the Limits of "Rationality"

FRANK S. MILLER

INTRODUCTION

An oxymoron, so the dictionary says, is a group of words that do not mean what they say literally. A favorite example is *postal service*. One can quickly conjure up others. But to me, even while I was Minister of Health in Ontario (1974–77), an obvious contender had to be "health system." Indeed, our health system in Ontario often struck me as being about as sensitive to central control as China's warlords were under Sun Yat-sen. Each component went its merry way, expecting little more than continuous, unlimited central funding! And woe betide the minister who tried to coordinate, inventory, rationalize, restructure, or—heaven forbid—close part, or all, of any component.

Perhaps, 14 years after I took on the duties at Bill Davis' behest, one could say "Plus ça change plus c'est la même chose." The aging of a population has inexorably crept along as predicted. Our fixations are focused in acute care still.

LOOKING BACK TO THE EARLY 1970s

I remember vividly being told I, as a chemical engineer, was to head the Ministry of Health. I asked my premier, "Why me, why not a physician?" His answer was "I've had a physician. I need someone to control costs—that's your job."

Remember that state medical care was maturing after a rocky start in the late '60s. Hospital care was still cost-shared by the federal government only in acute care facilities. Not only was the bookkeeping heroic, the emphasis on cost-shared (hospital/medical) elements caused planners to opt for dollars,

Aging and Health: Linking Research and Public Policy, © 1989 Lewis Publishers, Inc., Chelsea, Michigan 48118. Printed in U.S.A.

not needs. The elderly were especially hard hit. So much of the care they needed lay outside the "insured" (cost-shared) definitions, that health facilities growth virtually ignored them.

Ontario in 1972, under Dr. Richard Potter, made nursing home care an insured benefit for those who needed something less than chronic care and something more than families would provide at home. It was sold to the Finance Minister as a cost-saving device. People would occupy $12.50 beds and we could close $75 beds. And the first law of health care was discovered: all beds in all levels of care will be full all the time. The alternative had become a necessary add-on. Still, the hospitals were jammed with geriatric patients.

We then had a study of our health care system by none other than my fellow panelist, Dr. Fraser Mustard, and a top-quality committee which included my soon-to-be cabinet colleague Dr. Bette Stephenson. Its recommendations read well even now. The report undoubtedly shaped Ontario's health system's configuration and form. And from it flowed our District Health Councils—seen as a tool to move decisionmaking to the regional level and to sensitize its members to the horrendous costs of health care. I suspect that some ministers would be honest enough to admit that its most useful function seemed to be its ability to lose individual demands for more services in an extremely lengthy process without end. But I could be too cynical!

In 1974, Ontario spent about $2 billion on health care—almost half for hospitals, one fourth for physicians—or 7% of the Gross Provincial Product. Today, almost $10.5 billion is spent, with the proration remarkably similar. At first glance, one could say not much has changed. But I believe it has.

Influence of Partisan Considerations

Indeed, the first suggested question—To what extent do political and partisan considerations impede the optimal development of the health system (for the elderly)—begets a bit of a defensive reaction in me. It seems to imply that "political" or "partisan" considerations are petty, mean, and not reflective of public need. Just the opposite seems true to me. I can hardly remember a year as Treasurer when I was not required to vote extra money for health and geriatric-related social services.

These votes stemmed directly from a grass roots system in which constituents let their elected members of all political persuasions know in no uncertain terms that *their* community needed new or better services, and better get them, or *else*.

If the question should be taken to mean how does this impede the rationalization and elimination of surplus, outdated, redundant, and sometimes professionally unsafe facilities—to allow for more effective use of existing budgets—then I'd say yes. The democratic process does, and will continue to, prevent effective use of health dollars. We can all see the waste and duplication. We all know it exists (in someone else's facility or town).

The elderly, while a potent voting force, do not profit from the health spending generated by political pressure as much as they should. Modern science creates amazing technology. This creates demand for more and more sophisticated and costly equipment. We all support—nay, *demand*—it. Thus, it is much easier to obtain monies for laser beam equipment than it is for chronic care beds.

The professionals can't escape blame either. The glamour for them, too, is in the acute side of health care. Their whole professional beings are trained to equate success (and job satisfaction) with the discharge of healthy (or healthier) people. Chronic care by too many individuals and the institutions they represent is seen as second-class health care. In my opinion, institutions that provide acute treatment seldom deliver good chronic care.

Resource Reallocation

The second question asks how senior policymakers react to politically difficult conclusions (e.g., the closing of small hospitals and resource reallocation to the community sector). This is one I have had considerable personal experience with. To carry out my mandate—i.e., cost savings in health—I instructed senior health ministry staff to prepare a detailed plan of action (political considerations aside) to cut waste, eliminate competition, and to identify areas of need, with proposals to meet them. The request was made late in 1974 or early 1975 on the premise that a likely 1975 election would return the Progressive Conservatives with a majority. It was also my assumption that any politically sensitive actions would have to be effected in the first two years following the election.

The staff reacted with great enthusiasm. They were as keenly aware of the misuse of resources as any, and were anxious to bring order to the far-flung health care facilities—which had grown like Topsy—and which, in many parts of the province, were closer together than modern travel times required. My recollection is that some five large books of analysis and proposed actions were presented to me by mid-1975, awaiting political approval for a postelection campaign.

Targets were set for acute beds (3.5/1000), nursing home beds, chronic beds, psychiatric care, children's mental health, and much more. We planned to close quite a few redundant general hospitals, a few private hospitals, effect amalgamations of obstetrics, pediatrics, food and laundry services—to limit certain highly specialized equipment to teaching facilities, to convert a number of general hospitals (especially in two-hospital towns) to chronic care, close wards where total closures were deemed to be impossible, and to cut budgets of hospitals where costs per bed exceeded their peers. And that was only the beginning. It was ambitious and, I believe, exciting to all of us involved. I can firmly say that the senior staff were anxious to make the system more effective—subject to political will. They were not as anxious to let the money decisions be made at the local level.

Of course, the 1975 election resulted in a perilously thin Conservative win—and a minority government. I remember saying to staff, "We can shelve the reports for good." How wrong I was. Three months later by cabinet decree, "constraint" became policy. The books came off the shelf and, only slightly amended, became the blueprint for action.

As a footnote, I would say that years later we can conclude the constraint action of 1976 improved the delivery efficiency of health care in Ontario in ways we did not expect, failed in ways we expected would succeed, and probably taught every politician who observed it from a safe distance not to close hospitals—ever! As for me, I observed its closing chapters from the comfort of the Coronary Care Unit at Wellesley Hospital in Toronto.

COORDINATION OF HEALTH CARE FOR THE AGED

Health policy for the aged has been fragmented and, despite attempts to centralize planning, probably always will be. I believe Ontario, at least, is seriously trying to bring the many providers together under some semblance of coordination. To respond to the third question, the constituencies most influential have been, in my mind, the providers of care, in very disparate ways. Planners would like one neat, coordinated package. But senior people—their needs, frailties, ills—do not fall into nice neat organizational pigeon holes. Nor should they.

Thus, governments at all levels provide services to meet seniors' needs—from home care, housekeeping, senior citizen apartments, homes for the aged, nursing homes to chronic care. These cross municipal-provincial-federal financing and jurisdictional boundaries, and within provincial ministries, often caused turf wars. It always seemed to me to be a bit ridiculous to have one ministry run a home for the aged, which quickly graduated into a nursing home as well, while a second ministry built nursing home beds, but wouldn't allow the less infirm in. We tended to set a series of standards converted into mathematical points, which rather unintentionally determined where the human should end up. Thus, the most powerful constituency to me has been bureaucracy—protecting their own special, narrow niches in a senior's spectrum of need. Indeed, at times it seemed like a macabre game of musical chairs. Imagine if you were acutely ill, and moved from nursing home to hospital to be cured—only to find that, in your absence, your nursing home bed had been taken.

A second constituency is very strong—the families of the elderly, who often equate anything but hospital care with inadequate care.

But, I am an optimist. I believe the whole area of geriatric care is improving—perhaps of necessity—and will be designed more with the comfort, needs, and quality of life of the patients in mind. Outstanding examples like Baycrest in Toronto are there to guide us.

EVALUATION OF CURRENT RESEARCH

It is hard for me to assess the current quality of policy research as posed in our fourth general question. Because of the daily firefighting nature of a Minister of Health's life, I fear that much research goes unnoticed. I believe that papers like Dr. Mustard's are the most effective route to political awareness and action. They allow acknowledged experts to review and summarize much that politicians have neither the time nor inclination to pursue, permit public input, and create a certain awareness (and expectation of action) in the press and therefore the public.

In a large Ministry of Health like Ontario's, a coherent philosophy and set of objectives have generally existed. The actions and reactions forced on the system by external pressures create ad hoc decisions that may not conform to policy.

THE POWER OF POLITICIANS

The last of the general questions—Do politicians sense that they have real control over how the health system develops, or are they constrained by the system's own momentum and/or by the desires of powerful constituencies— causes me to look into the mirror of reality. I guess I'd have to say that if a politician answers, "Yes, I have control," I would worry about him or her a lot. I'm not sure the control should be so complete, and I am sure that in a democracy it will not be. The constituencies are powerful. How quickly a hospital can have beds in the halls. How fast we can learn about a death that could have been prevented if only more funds were available. How often rival hospitals duplicate each other's underutilized, highly specialized equipment—then use it heavily to prove they were right, and on and on.

But we are limited by the parameters of the human being's gifts of intelligence and determination. Given those, I think Canada can be proud of having as good, as efficient, and as responsible a health system as the world has been fortunate enough to produce.

18. Aging and Health: Research, Policy, and Resource Allocation

J. FRASER MUSTARD

INTRODUCTION

Any approach to this subject will be strongly conditioned by the values, beliefs, and knowledge that a society has about health and aging. Over the centuries, the broad philosophical concepts of health have ranged between an emphasis on the important role of social and economic factors and individual choices in determining health status (the ecology of health), and a focus on the cause of disease and specific therapeutic measures for the treatment of the sick. In the seventh century B.C., the concept of health in Greece was personified by the goddess Hygeia. She was not involved in the treatment of the sick, but was the guardian of health who symbolized the belief that people could remain in good health if they lived according to reason. In the fifth century B.C., the philosophy of the healing god Aesculapius gained ascendancy. This god, in contrast to Hygeia, was concerned with the identification of the cause of disease and the treatment of the sick.

Most human action is inevitably driven by current belief. We act as we do because we have a belief about the consequences of our actions. Thus at any time, the dominant theory or belief about health affects how we approach health problems.

At the beginning of this century, the ecology of health, as manifested in public health policies, was a dominant force. With the emergence of scientific medicine as the major thrust during the middle part of the century, the dominant philosophy became the concept of a unitary cause of disease that could be treated (e.g., antibiotics for infectious disease, insulin for diabetes, vitamin B_{12} for pernicious anemia—the concept of a "magic bullet"). Today the theories about health are confused. The recent report from National

Aging and Health: Linking Research and Public Policy, © 1989 Lewis Publishers, Inc., Chelsea, Michigan 48118. Printed in U.S.A.

Health and Welfare of Canada, *Achieving Health for All: A Framework for Health Promotion* (Epp, 1986), is much more in the ecology of health framework than in the "magic bullet" framework.

Our understanding of infectious diseases illustrates how belief influences our views about health. René Dubos (1959), writing about the ecology of health, made the point that although the tubercle bacillus can be demonstrated in all people with tuberculosis, the opposite does not hold true; all the individuals who have been exposed to or harbor the tubercle bacillus do not develop tuberculosis. The concept of each disease having a specific treatable cause excludes consideration of conditioning factors such as behavior and the environment, which influence the susceptibility of individuals to disease. The importance of these other factors in the decline of mortality from infectious disease that occurred long before we had antibiotics has been well described by McKeown (1976) and Trowell and Burkitt (1981). The public is becoming increasingly aware of the limits of medicine in terms of the unique cause, "magic bullet" theory, because of the multiplicity of factors that appear to influence the development of chronic disorders such as cancer, cardiovascular disease, and mental illnesses. The major thrust of our therapeutic intervention for most chronic disorders is the treatment of symptoms, not of the underlying causes.

Over the last 10 years, there has developed a better understanding of the factors that determine or influence the health status of individuals and their ability to function. This trend could mean that the dominant theory about health will again become the ecology of health. If so, this perception about health will influence how we view the aging process and diseases associated with elderly people and will strongly influence our policies and resource allocation for older citizens.

AGING AND HEALTH CARE

Our knowledge of the aging process and the supporting role of individuals for the elderly is still limited. It is clear, however, that as we age there is a progressive decline in the function of our organ systems which is not due to disease, although disease can influence the rate of decline (Fries, 1984; Brody, 1985). Also, the decline in the function of organ systems can make individuals susceptible to some diseases.

Since man has a finite span estimated to be about 85 years (Fries, 1984), but possibly longer (Brody, 1985), we can anticipate the care that will be required by an aging population as individuals gradually lose the function of their organ systems and suffer from a variety of chronic illnesses. Some have proposed that morbidity due to illness may be compressed into the later years of life, with intermittent or continuous care primarily required during the final months before natural death. It is at this point that medical intervention may actually extend the dying process, adding a substantial burden to the health care system, but often only a few additional months of poor quality life for the individual. A difficult philosophical and ethical question is, How much medical technology should be applied to the terminal stages of life? It is important to point out that although one might believe that morbidity can be compressed into the last years of life, on the basis of present evidence this does not appear to be likely (Brody, 1985; Roos, Shapiro, & Havens, 1987). Those between 65 and 84 years of age use hospitals about three times as much as those between 25 and 64, whereas those over 85 use hospitals about five times as much. However, the majority of older individuals are infrequently hospitalized. A small group of the elderly (less than 5%) use the most hospital days; this group is a concern for health care planners. Most of these individuals are at the terminal stages of their lives.

CARING FOR THE ELDERLY

There are three important elements of research policy and resource allocation for care of an older population. These are: (1) the social, economic, and cultural factors that determine the health status and function of older people; (2) the informal supportive care structure that is available to older people; and (3) the professional services in medicine and social work that are provided for older people.

SOCIAL, ECONOMIC, AND CULTURAL FACTORS

Individuals who have adequate income and control over their own housing and transportation, as long as they are of sound mind and body, have a better quality of life and live longer than individuals who have fewer economic resources and control over their lives. A society's policies on pensions, housing, and other forms of economic support are all significant for the quality of life, health status, and function of older individuals. There has been relatively little population-based research that integrates all the factors in this complex area. This is partly because of the complexity of the problems, the limited data base, and the difficulty of analysis. Without an adequate data base and appropriate research priorities and policy, the development of such research will be impaired. The need for research in this area is apparent because of the changes in family structures, the changing role of women in society, the changing nature of jobs, and the changes in the concepts of retirement. Knowledge of how social, economic, and cultural factors influence the health status and function of older individuals is important if we are to develop sound policies and sensible resource allocation. This kind of research has as its focus the ecology of health.

INFORMAL CARE

Traditionally, close relatives have been the primary providers of informal care for the elderly. Tomorrow's senior citizens will have fewer sons, daughters, siblings, and cousins because families have grown smaller. Sibling relationships may become more important than they once were, because it is common for families to experience one or more divorces or separations, and siblings offer an anchor of continuity in families. It is also becoming increasingly difficult for several generations of a family to be in close proximity to each other, in part as a result of the mobility of the work force.

In our society, it is not unusual for older women to become isolated because, in general, they live longer than their spouses, but either women or men who are left on their own tend to have a higher rate of morbidity, including severe mental symptoms, than those who remain in contact with other individuals. Mechanisms to keep individuals in touch with other members of society must be given serious consideration.

Another aspect of informal care is the concept of developing "tools for living" adapted to the mental and physical needs and abilities of older people. One simple example is the walkers to help children learn how to walk, which can serve a similar function for older people. Glasses are another "tool" developed to compensate for changes in our visual capacity as we age. Living facilities need special consideration, and tools for simple chores in the kitchen and around the house can also be specifically developed for older people. The special devices older people need should not be thought of as medical devices, however. One of my friends advocates setting up a retail chain focused on "tools for living" that serve the needs of all ages.

Informal or nonprofessional care for the aged is obviously of crucial importance. As indicated above, family structures are different than in the past because so many women are now in the work force. Many women, however, are still providing informal, unpaid care for the aged. In the United Kingdom, it has been estimated (Qureshi & Walker, 1986) that if informal care decreased by 5%, the medical and social services would be swamped. Countries that have researched the changes in their social and economic structure have been developing new policy approaches. Among the subjects that need to be addressed in informal care are:

1. a clear understanding of the meaning and purpose of informal and community care (this has usually meant care by females) and its differentiation from care provided by social and medical services.
2. the limits to community care and informal care that may be influenced by professional and political interests (doctors with a tendency to hospitalize patients could have a greater impact on hospital use than change in population demography)

3. the limits of what the existing informal care sector can do as a result of the social and economic changes
4. the political pressures to reduce government support for health and social services by dumping problems into an informal care sector that cannot cope because of insufficient resources
5. the further development of informal networks of care based on kinship, religion, and ethnic groups (with our diverse cultural and ethnic backgrounds, this would involve a diversity of arrangements rather than a single solution)
6. the development of interrelated community care services (social and medical) to ensure the success of a policy for more informal care
7. recognition of the cost of informal care and the benefits to society

Groups who have thought deeply about the social and economic changes occurring in most societies have begun to think of new arrangements for informal care. In Sweden, it is estimated that the application of advanced technology will cause unemployment for as much as 10% of the work force in the next decade (Lagergren, Lundh, Orkan, & Sanne, 1984). However, employment could be maintained by reducing the hours of work, and the Swedes have suggested that, in the free time thus created, everyone should have to make some commitment to community-based programs such as informal care for the elderly. In addition, it may be economically feasible to have informal care provided by a relative or friend, who will be given time off from the activity at which she or he earns a living with no loss of income, benefits, or seniority. Obviously, this approach would only be feasible if the caregiver occupied a position in the work force which could easily be filled by another individual. This type of arrangement removes the economic penalty faced by most women who provide informal care at the present time. An experiment in Nova Scotia in which relatives are paid up to $4800 per annum to care for elderly people is a small step toward recognizing the cost of informal care to individuals.

HEALTH CARE

The health care side of caring for the elderly is of secondary importance to economic issues and informal care, but it has significant economic and ethical considerations. It is important that the limits of medicine be kept in mind when policies are being established for health care services for the elderly. Although there is a common belief that as individuals live longer they become sicker, this is not true for the majority of the elderly. Only 5% of the elderly account for the high utilization of hospital days. The evidence indicates that if we supply effective health care services efficiently, we can easily meet the health care needs of our older population over the next 40 years (Evans, 1986). It is essential, however, that health care services not assume functions that properly belong in the informal care sector. The excess number of physicians now being produced in Canada creates risk that the nonmedical care of the elderly will be taken over by the medical profession. This could have a negative effect on the quality of life for older people and could add an additional financial burden to society.

We have a much less sophisticated understanding of the biological and psychological aspects of aging than we do of child development. This is partly because only recently have we shifted our attention to a more in-depth understanding of the aging process and associated conditions such as osteoporosis, dementia, depression, and musculoskeletal problems. Understanding the normal process of aging, the associated disease processes, the psychological changes, and such things as sensitivity to drugs is of importance for our care of the elderly and how we allocate resources.

Finally, society must face the fundamental question of whether to use intensive and expensive medical therapy to extend the life of individuals for a few months at the end of their lives. This question is of major importance when the intervention will not improve the quality of life for an individual with a terminal illness.

SUMMARY

The following issues are among those that are important for research and policy development in order to maintain a high quality of life for the elderly as the demography of the population changes:

1. the financial and other resources available to the elderly to help maintain their independence and social interaction
2. the policies for informal care and community care that take into account the social and economic changes that are taking place in our society
3. the arrangements and effectiveness of community-based health care services that relate to the consumer and informal care sector (the health care services should operate under incentives that promote the efficient provision of effective care)
4. the establishment of community-based health services, with minimal central government involvement, that enhance the consumer-provider interaction and reduce the provider-government focus of the present arrangements
5. increased research on the important questions concerning the aging process and associated disorders

Research on these topics could help in developing policies and resource applications that take into account the influence of social, economic, cultural, and health care factors on the elderly. Without a strong research program, it will be difficult to design sensible policies in relation to our older population that are based on an understanding of aging and the changes that are taking place in our society.

REFERENCES

Brody, J. A. (1985). Prospects for an aging population. *Nature* (London), 315, 463.

Dubos, R. (1959). *The mirage of health.* New York: Harper-Row.

Epp, J. (1986). *Achieving health for all: A framework for health promotion.* Ottawa: Ministry of Supply and Services.

Evans, R. G. (1986, November). Hang together or hang separately: Universal health care in the year 2000. In *Health care for the elderly in the year 2000* (pp. 63–94). Proceedings of a symposium conducted at Victoria, BC, by Ministry of Health, BC, and Faculty of Human and Social Development, University of Victoria.

Fries, J. (1984). The compression of morbidity. In P. K. Robinson et al. (Eds.). *Aging and technological advance.* New York: Plenum Press.

Lagergren, M., Lundh, L., Orkan, M., & Sanne, C. (1984). *Time to care.* A report prepared for the Swedish Secretariat for Future Studies. New York: Pergamon Press.

McKeown, T. (1976). *The modern rise of population.* London: Edward Arnold.

Qureshi, H., & Walker, A. (1986). *The caring relationship: The family care of elderly people.* London: Macmillan.

Roos, N. P., Shapiro, E., & Havens, B. (1987). Aging with limited resources: What should we really be worried about? In *Aging with limited health resources, proceedings of a colloquium on health care, May 1986* (pp. 50–56). Ottawa: Canadian Government Publishing Centre, Supply and Services Canada.

Trowell, H. C., & Burkitt, D. P. (1981). *Western diseases: Their emergence and prevention.* Harvard University Press.

19. Informal Social Support Systems in China

WILLIAM T. LIU
ELENA YU
MINGYUAN ZHANG
SHIN-CHENG YANG

INTRODUCTION

This chapter describes the informal social support system of the elderly in China, using data collected from a probability sample survey conducted in Shanghai, China. Gerontological research of the social and health needs of older people in China has been largely based on verbal descriptions of needs through analyses of official policies and interviews with informants (Davis-Friedmann, 1983, 1985; Liu, 1982; Yuan, 1981; Zeng, 1983). Systematic sample surveys have not yet appeared in print, although several such studies have been conducted in Tianjin (Pang & Lin, 1987; Gui et al., 1987). This chapter is based on 5050 interviews of older persons, aged 55 and over, residing in one of the 10 administrative districts in metropolitan Shanghai. The random probability sample was drawn specifically to oversample the older age groups (65–74 and 75 and older) to produce near-equal numbers of elderly in three age cohorts: 55–64, 65–74, and 75 years and older. Sample design has been described elsewhere (Levy, 1987) and will not be repeated here.

THE FAMILY AS AN INFORMAL SOCIAL SUPPORT SYSTEM

To begin a study of the informal social support systems in China, it is impossible not to touch upon the role of the family, which in a sense differs from our normal usage of the word in the West. The generic term *chia*, or

---

Aging and Health: Linking Research and Public Policy, © 1989 Lewis Publishers, Inc., Chelsea, Michigan 48118. Printed in U.S.A.

"the family," includes anyone who is a member of the *domestic group*. There have been some drastic changes of the concept of the domestic group during the three decades of repeated political campaigns. As a collective movement, there is a certain fundamental incompatibility between commitment to a radical revolutionary ideology and intense collective identification, on the one hand, and family solidarity on the other. Kinship is based on the maintenance of intergenerational ties and a certain basic continuity of transmitted tradition. Between the nonselective and nonideological kinship obligations and universalistic criteria of ideologically based comradeship, boundaries of the domestic group shift on both the national and the individual levels as social change continues to take place in mainland China.

The Party and state leadership have been ambivalent about the role of the family. On one hand, family identity promotes the maintenance of a particularistic relationship that could run counter to the interest of the state and the revolutionary goals. On the other hand, many of the issues with respect to welfare, housing, old age pensions, health care, and social problems, which normally would require huge state investment, have been relegated to the family. To the Party leaders, old age and child care, for example, could be only domestic problems unless one does not have close kin. The assignment of familial obligations can be taken as strengthening the mutual identity of family members and, at the same time, reaffirming a culturally accepted perspective that such problems really did not exist for the state.

There are additional historical and demographic reasons for the absence of the problems of the elderly until the beginning of the '80s. A relatively small proportion of the huge population was 65 and over, the result of a high fertility pattern, encouraged by Mao Zedong in the beginning of the Socialist regime. Furthermore, China has had a national pension program since the beginning of 1951 (Davis-Friedmann, 1983, 1985). Even though eligibility criteria for state retirement pensions had excluded about 80% of the labor force, the vast majority of the people resided in rural communities where the aged, as compared with their urban counterparts, do not experience discontinuity of either employment or cash income. Finally, besides being supported by their adult children, old people often depended on marginal employment in the neighborhood. Thus despite the limited access to old age pensions, few elderly become destitute. China is probably one of the few countries in which nursing homes and elderly residential facilities are scarce in comparison with the number of people aged 65 and over.

In short, informal support systems for the elderly must be viewed within the larger context of their familial and kinship structure, social networks, demographic patterns, housing, and welfare patterns of the society.

GOVERNMENT POLICY ON RETIREMENT

Government policies on retirement are closely associated with, and explained by, the modernization policy, which takes precedence over other issues germane to the elderly. These modernization programs, more directly related to economic reforms, have important and profound implications for the retirement of older workers, the pension incentive system to counter lower bureaucratic resistance, and continuation of a favorable wage system to keep pace with the life cycle of individual workers. Modernization policy should be viewed as the context for the assessment of the informal support system for the elderly.

On Economic Reforms

The dramatic change of population policy announced in the '70s—from a pronatal to a one child per couple—will have a direct impact on the population structure for decades to come. Though exceptions were allowed for ethnic minority populations and for remote rural areas, the Chinese government has generally been rather uniform in enforcing the one-child policy.

Along with the explicit population growth control policy is state investment in housing construction in older cities, which had been badly needed for years. The abolition of the rural commune, the opening of free markets for goods and services, the institutionalization of work incentive policy, and implementation of a mixed centrally controlled and market economy have resulted in remarkable short-term economic growth throughout the system, along with the sharp rise of consumer prices and, in some sectors, increased standard of living in both the rural and the urban sectors.

Modernization of the economy inevitably calls for the retirement of older, ideologically promoted cadres who were in key economic and political positions at the end of the Gang of Four era. To this end, the Party leaders announced in the early '80s the abolition of life tenure for old cadres and the promotion of younger cadres to leading posts. In spite of increased pension incentives for the newly retired cadres, there remain many elderly without the protection of a pension system.

On Retirement Pensions

Government policy on retirement, pensions, and other benefits for the elderly have been periodically reported in official media publications. A summary of the Chinese policy on pensions is available in both Chinese and English language publications (Parish & Whyte, 1978; Liu, 1982; Ascher, 1976; Davis-Friedmann, 1985). A thorough treatment of the issue by Davis-Friedmann reported that pension remains a privilege for a minority of state workers, and not as a universal entitlement program. Thus the number of

pensioners has not kept pace with the rate of increase in the elderly population (Davis-Friedmann, 1985, p. 296).

Davis-Friedmann reports that before 1978 there was no compulsory retirement policy for state employees. In fact, during several political struggle
periods, retirement of healthy older workers was considered antisocialist.
The 1978 revision of the Labour Insurance Regulations specified that ages
60 and 50 were retirement ages for male and female workers, respectively,
though enforcement might not have been universal (Davis-Friedmann,
1983). Retirement became a more prominent issue when, in 1982, senior
government officials were asked to retire. The age set for officials at the
ministerial level was 65, and 60 for those at the subcabinet level. To compensate for the loss of bureaucratic privileges and political power, the Party
increased significantly the retirement pensions to those who served the Party
before 1949. Here again, mandatory retirement was not implemented across-
the-board; many highly skilled state employees were asked to stay. Juvena-
tion of the huge bureaucracy had initially met formidable political opposi-
tions even when adopted as a part of modernization programs. In a socialist
totalitarian state, such resistance has been described in part as a form of
bureaucratic politics in that the significant interest groups are those persons
and units within the bureaus of government, rather than those out in the
public arena (Olson, 1987a; 1987b, p. 245). The increased pension and other
benefits (better and larger housing quarters, for example) provided incentives
for aged bureaucrats to lower their collective resistance.

On Postretirement Employment

A substantial proportion of retirees continue to work in marginal jobs or
in jobs not connected with their previous employment units. With their
pensions and the supplemental income, the total incomes for the retired
persons may be much higher than their incomes prior to retirement. Thus
among men and women between 55 and 65, it is not unusual to find the
highest income in the five years after retirement.

Our survey data in Shanghai, based on more than 5000 interviews with
persons 55 years or older, showed that a little less than 10% of current
retirees are working on a full-time basis and another 1.2% on a part-time
basis. Only 1.6% of respondents said that they could not find jobs. On the
other hand, about 88% said that they did not wish to continue work after
retirement.

The unwillingness to continue working is probably best explained in economic terms. The income structure favors senior workers and old age cadres,
especially those who receive retirement pensions. Taken as a whole, our data
show that the reported aggregate income of persons in preretirement status
is significantly lower than that reported by the postretired elderly.

The important factor, however, was the way family members pool their income in one way or another. Preliminary analysis indicates that retirees are economically, or at least psychologically, more secure when compared with the preretirement elderly. In addition, most of the urban elderly in China share their residence with their married adult children, who often pool their resources and hand over at least a part of their income to the elder parents. Thus the government, through its low-wage structure and a generous retirement pension policy, has in effect provided both economic security and social prestige for the elderly population. In general, older people have a higher income and a wider network of connections than younger people. Such a network of connections, known as *quanxi*, is in fact an asset of potential personal influence.

INFORMAL SUPPORT SYSTEMS FOR THE ELDERLY IN SHANGHAI

The formal support system for the elderly in China appears to be rather weak compared to the West because of the philosophical and cultural emphasis on filial piety, which defines the child's duty to care for the aged. The pension system favors those who contributed to the earlier stages of the Revolution and to the Party and the State. Retirement programs are implemented through bureaucratic political processes at present, and probably will be universally administered in the future when the current cohort of older cadres retires and a new generation of young old leave their posts to allow younger leadership to take charge of the country's ambitious modernization programs.

These changes notwithstanding, the family is the chief care unit for the elderly in spite of the fact that the Chinese family structure has shifted dramatically since the Revolution of 1949. State work assignment, mass internal migration during the mid- and late '50s, various political movements and the Great Cultural Revolution all have contributed to the changes of the domestic group. Crises, the utilitarian requirements of the Party with respect to the desired place of residence and work, and the one-child policy have added to the strengthening of the family as a domestic group. The demands of work and change of residence have segmented the kin group. It is therefore impossible to describe the Chinese family system in static terms.

What remains true, however, is that generation extension and cohesion are still considered an ideal form of familial relations. Due primarily to the improvement of public health and the standard of living for the poorer and rural populations since 1949, there has been a noticeable increase in persons surviving into old age. There has also been a concomitant decrease in fertility rates: the average household in the early 1970s had an average of about three children, compared with the one child per couple widely practiced in the 1980s. The extension of longevity is supported by the fact that close to 8% of those selected for interview (aged 55 and over) have living parents over the age of 70. Eleven percent of those who reported both parents still alive at the time of interview were people over 75 years of age. Fifty percent of those interviewed have four or more living children.

Such being the case, there is statistical evidence of an informal support system for the elderly at the end of the 1980s in China. Future studies will periodically monitor the changes in the de facto informal support system in the context of an ever-increasing number of older people.

Nuclear Family as an Informal Support System

The spouse is considered the most important source of emotional and social support for the elderly (Shanas, 1979a). In the Shanghai data, 62% of the elderly are married and living with their spouse, whereas 31% are widowed. This figure is comparable with the U.S. data in the 1980s, though in both countries the percentage of married males over 65 is about twice as high as females of the same age cohort.

Siblings provide support as well. In the United States, more than 70% over the age of 70 have living siblings (Shanas, 1979b). In the Shanghai survey, 68% of those 55 and over reported having living siblings. Figures for those over 75 and over 65 are not available at this time.

Coresidence with adult children is infrequent in the United States. However, it is common that adult children live close by. In the same study, Shanas (1979b) reported that 75% of her respondents have children living within 30 minutes by car. The Shanghai data show that more than 73% of the elderly actually live with their children; 63.7% also reported that there are other relatives sharing residence with them. Of those who do not live with their own children or other relatives, only 6% (N = 314) of the more than 5000 cases reported living alone. The affective component between generations appears on the average to be strong, though measures of affectivity are difficult to define. Eighty-four and six-tenths percent said they see their children on a daily basis, although another 8% see them on a weekly basis.

Interaction with children often goes beyond just providing companionship for each other. For the majority there is mutual help, most frequently with household chores. Children render more health care to their parents, but the latter provide material things for their children. Living in the same household, however, makes such specific functional contributions to one another somewhat ambiguous. There have been studies, for example in the United States, which show that although the elderly report higher levels of affection in their relationships with children, they tend to minimize the amount of assistance or exchange of services. The Shanghai data pose similar questions as to how such data can be interpreted. Singling out services and assistance between cohabitants may not be applicable in the Chinese family, because it is expected that people who live in the same household share common tasks.

In short, the overwhelming majority of our respondents reported strong and cohesive nuclear family ties.

Contacts with Kin-Relatives

Contacts with more distant kin, including grandchildren, are equally intensive. More than 50% said that they have their grandchildren live in, and close to 68% said that they helped with the caring of their grandchildren.

Living with other relatives, such as in-laws, siblings, and cousins, ranged from more than 33% for daughters-in-law, to less than 1% for siblings. More than 6% reported living with other female relatives, and 2.4% with other male relatives. Our tentative conclusion is that the intergenerational cohesion exceeded cohesion with distant relatives. Siblings are among relatives with whom there are the least contacts, judging from the patterns of coresidence.

On the other hand, close to 15% of the respondents said that they have get-togethers with their kin-relatives at least once a month. Another 60% said that they have kin gatherings at least once a year, probably during the Chinese New Year's holidays.

Types of relations make a great deal of difference with respect to emotional intimacy and trust. Spouses are mentioned by one half of the respondents as their confidants; another 20% named one or more of their children. Sixteen percent, however, named their coworkers as their confidants; about 6% are siblings. Only about 3.5% named their neighbors as their close confidants to whom self-disclosures were reported. Similarly, nonspecific confidants, or "friends," constituted only 5% of the total responses. It raises serious conceptual questions about the concept of "friend" and "friendship" in Socialist China (see Liu, 1986 for a discussion).

CONCLUSION

In an earlier paper based on a separate sample survey on stress and psychological illness conducted in 1983, the senior author argued that in spite of the revolutionary commitment, the Community Party leaders did not minimize the importance of the family in the new society. Social welfare policies, particularly those pertaining to the care of the elderly, made paramount a closer interdependency among members of the family, which goes beyond the nuclear family. Intergenerational cohesion takes priority over all other types of relations. Like other countries in the West, spousal and adult-children support constituted the core of the informal support system.

The continuous political movements, attempts to flush out ideologically deviant elements in the socialist society, have failed to establish comradeship based on friendship. Informal support with respect to life crises may have to depend on neighbors and friends, such as the organizational monitoring system established in urban China. Emotional intimacy, however, is found mainly among closest relatives, within the nuclear family, and to a much lesser extent among other relatives.

Finally, because of the organizational imperative within the huge bureaucracy in China, one's work unit has become a total institution in Goffman's sense. The supervisory cadre serves not only as superior at the workplace, but also in the role of "confessor," teacher, and one who can really help in time of needs and crises. It is therefore not surprising that more than 16% named coworkers as their intimate confidants.

REFERENCES

Ascher, I. (1976). *China's social policy*. London: Anglo-Chinese Education Institute.

Davis-Friedmann, D. (1983). *Long lives*. Cambridge, MA: Harvard University Press.

Davis-Friedmann, D. (1985). Chinese retirement: Policy and practice. *Current Perspectives on Aging and the Life Cycle, 1,* 295–313.

Gui, S., Li, L., Shen, Z., Di, J., Gu, Q., Chen, Y. & Qian, F. (1987). Status and needs of the elderly in urban Shanghai: Analysis of some preliminary results. *Journal of Cross Cultural Gerontology, 2*(2), 171–186.

Levy, P. (1987). *Statistical sample design of the Shanghai elderly survey by P/ AAMHRC*. Unpublished working paper. Chicago: Pacific Asian American Mental Health Research Center.

Liu, L. (1982). Mandatory retirement and other reforms pose new challenges for China's government. *Aging and Work, 5,* 119–130.

Liu, W. T. (1986). *Friendship and kinship in contemporary China*. Paper given at the East Asian Research Center Symposium.

Olson, P. (1987a). A model of eldercare in the People's Republic of China. *International Aging and Human Development, 24*(4), 279–300.

Olson, P. (1987b). Modernization in the People's Republic of China: The politization of the elderly. *Sociological Quarterly, 29*(2), 241–262.

Pang, Y. K. & Lin, N. (1987). *Family structure in China: Changes, life course, and networks*. Paper read at the Annual Meeting of the American Sociological Association, Chicago.

Parish, W., & Whyte, M. (1978). *Village and family in contemporary China*. Chicago: University of Chicago Press.

Shanas, E. (1979a). The family as a social support system in old age. *Gerontologist, 19*(3).

Shanas, E. (1979b). Social myth as hypothesis: The case of the family relations of old people. *Gerontologist, 19*(3).

Yuan, J. (1981). *Living conditions of elderly retirees in Shanghai*. Paper presented at Conference on Retirement in Cross-Cultural Perspective, Bellagio, Italy.

Zeng, S. (1983, January). China's senior citizens. *China Reconstructs, 31,* 5–8.

20. Australian Services for the Elderly—Some Structural Difficulties

ANNE CRICHTON

In order to understand the present provision of services in Australia, it is necessary to provide some historical background. This will emphasize policy rather than research issues.

THE CONTEXT

Australia has many similarities to Canada and many differences. It was founded after the American War of Independence, is a federation of states that developed independently until confederation in 1900, and its patterns of settlement have been fairly similar to Canada's—much of the population arriving after World War II came from a wide variety of countries other than Britain. So the demographic "pyramid" is much the same as ours—the peak numbers of elderly, as a proportion of total population, are still to come as the baby boom ages—in a population somewhat more than half the size of Canada's.

Other similarities are cultural and political. The heritage is British, and both nations follow the Westminster Parliamentary system, adapted to local conditions. Australian television reveals the continuing strength of the British ties in Australia, but the British influence in Canada began to lessen after World War II. The differences between the two nations probably began to widen when the British Empire began to fold up after the war, though some major ones did preexist.

Australia has always been a country of cities, despite the rural image of "Waltzing Matilda" and other bush songs and legends. These cities were linked to Britain (rather than one another) by ships, and their hinterlands

Aging and Health: Linking Research and Public Policy, © 1989 Lewis Publishers, Inc., Chelsea, Michigan 48118. Printed in U.S.A.

were sparsely populated. There is still very little interstate movement. In the 19th century, Australia developed urban cultures modeled on British city life rather than following the Canadian pattern of rural settlement. Thus we find that hospitals were established on the same lines as English charity hospitals; workers formed friendly societies for insurance against life's crises, particularly sickness care for themselves and their families; and the medical profession had a sliding scale of charges according to the assessment of the patients' ability to pay. It was a philanthropic/entrepreneurial system of care. Although this may sound rather like Canada's own structures, in fact there were considerable differences in the approach. Australia is a much more class-conscious society, and the doctors are much more concerned about maintaining their elite position than in most Canadian provinces.

BACKGROUND AND SOCIAL LEGISLATION

As in most of Canada, there had been from the start a rejection of the English Poor Law, but where the Canadian provinces came to rely on charities and the municipalities to help those in need, Australia had chosen to subsidize the charities alone as its agents for relieving the poor. Where the states did not have sufficient charities (e.g., Queensland), they gave care of a kind, but they believed in "Out of sight, out of mind" and put the institutions in inaccessible places. Evans (1976) has explained the ideology as the classical liberal approach. Australians were expected to work hard to succeed in their enterprises. Failure had no place. Working men were expected to be thrifty, to prepare for bad times.

Roe (1976) has identified three groups who used professional and social services—the well enough off, who could command resources as and when they were needed; the "respectable working class"; and the poor, about 20% of the population, who relied on charity in times of need.

There grew up strong mutual aid organizations in this largely working class society. The respectable working class helped one another informally through "mateships" and formally through friendly societies, which provided support in crises and usually contracted with doctors to look after workers and their families. But the doctors resented these mutual aid contracts and curtailed them by the mid-1920s. They wanted to be in control of an entrepreneurial/philanthropic system of providing medical services.

Labour Party Governments

In the 1890s, Australian workers began to form labour clubs and a Labour Party similar to their contemporary British counterparts. They wanted to establish better social security policies, not so much to deal with existing indigency as to prevent the respectable working class from falling into indigency.

Although the labour clubs discussed universal and comprehensive social security, in the 1890s they were ahead of their time. The first Acts of Labour governments did not follow through on these principles, but imposed means tests and other conditions on age pensioners and invalids (following German models). Not until the government decided to assist war veterans after World War I was a universal and comprehensive pension and rehabilitation "Repatriation" program introduced, and it is still for only this group that such a total care package exists.

The early social security schemes were cash transfer programs, not service-providing programs. At that time, there was no intention to intervene in service provision, though soon after the logic led the Labour governments of New South Wales and Queensland toward the concept of state provision of services. (This idea did not make much progress except in Queensland, which like Saskatchewan introduced state-controlled medicine in 1944. Private medicine was reintroduced there in 1958 and now coexists with state-controlled medicine.)

Liberal Party Governments

At the federal level, a second wave of interest in establishing a welfare state emerged in the late '30s and lasted until the early '50s—a period of conflict between Labour and Liberals (right wing in Australia). When Labour was in power during the war years, the conflict between those who believed in maintaining the traditional entrepreneurial/philanthropic system and others who supported state control of health and social services came to a head. Labour was prevented from introducing socialist programs, partly because it had not thought them through until the late '40s, but mainly by constitutional challenges largely orchestrated by the medical profession. The Liberals then took power for 23 years and determined that any new programs should reward the deserving rather than the needy. (Though they said they would meet need, it was "expressed need" rather than "assessed need" that they meant [McLeay, 1982].) Thus their programs profited the more articulate respectable working class rather than the poor.

SERVICES IN KIND FOR THE ELDERLY

There was a housing shortage at the end of the war, and the Liberals were persuaded to help with subsidies to the elderly under the Aged Persons Homes Act, 1954. Grants were given to volunteering organizations (profit and nonprofit), which agreed to build accommodation for those who wished to lead normal lives as married couples (or singly). More often than not, the organizations wanted contributions from prospective clients (founder-donor arrangements). Only a few took in the poor.

HEALTH SERVICES

The evolution of health services is a long and complex story, but by the 1950s:

1. A range of public and private prepaid hospitals existed. Those who could pay were expected to pay. Private hospital insurance schemes began to be provided for all who wished to contribute about 1950, but the elderly often found it difficult to get insurance.

2. Medical care insurance had existed under contract doctor schemes since the mid-19th century, but doctors resented them. A breakthrough occurred about 1950, with doctor-sponsored schemes opening up insurance to a much wider range of Australians. Again, the elderly might have had problems in getting insurance.

3. In 1953, the Liberal government agreed to subsidize the insurance companies. In 1952, this government had introduced a Pensioner Medical Service, which was means tested and restrictive, for some of the poor. The next 20 years saw conflict between government and doctors resistant to this scheme. Doctors wanted to continue giving their own charity, to remain in control.

4. Mental hospital care was provided by the states. It had followed moral treatment objectives in the late 19th century, but by the mid-20th century was outdated. Federal review in 1955 revealed deficiencies in institutional care and predated reforms and a shift toward community care in the '60s.

5. A Pharmaceutical Benefits Program that had been introduced by Labour had produced a constitutional crisis in 1945, but had been revised to meet the doctors' objections to "civil conscription."

6. A home nursing program had begun to be subsidized in 1957 to relieve hospital shortages.

7. Public health services tended to concentrate on sanitary problems. There were some public health nursing services in New South Wales, but these were not closely linked to medical services.

A CHANGE IN DIRECTION

The decision of federal government to move into the provision of Aged Persons Homes, 1954, led to the development of that program in the '60s. As the population in the homes grew older there arose pressures to provide continuity of care and the federal government began subsidizing nursing homes. In the '60s, this became a more comprehensive program of institutional care:

1. Private hospitals giving long term care were taken out of the hospital subsidy scheme and became separately subsidized nursing homes. The number of nursing home beds grew immediately by 48%, especially in the profit-making sector.
2. Mental hospital patients were moved into big boarding homes (shared cost rather than state cost only).
3. Residents of sick bays or infirmaries in Aged Persons Homes became eligible for subsidies (1963). The program was extended later (1966, 1969).
4. Subsidies for hostel accommodation (i.e., personal care) were introduced in 1969 "to keep people functioning." The population in institutions grew rapidly from 25,535 in 1963 to 67,912 in 1981 (Commonwealth Department of Health), or from 26.6 to 46.9 beds per 1000 people aged 65 and over.

INSTITUTIONALIZING COMMUNITY CARE

The states were offered some help to develop community care services in 1969. The following cost-sharing programs were included in the offer: (1) home care, housekeepers, senior citizens' centers, welfare officers; (2) paramedical care; chiropody, OT, PT, speech therapy; (3) delivered meals and senior citizens' center meals; and (4) single persons' dwellings. The states did not take up the offer with much enthusiasm.

DISCONTENTS ARISE 1965–72

Health insurance was costly for all and not always accessible to the elderly. Concerns arose about geographic maldistribution of health services and lack of community care services. Doctors' conservative attitudes were revealed by quarrels following the Nimmo Report in 1969 about fee payments. Concerns about the poor, ethnics, disabled and the elderly were growing. Some thought there was failure of the philanthropic/entrepreneurial system of organization and wanted more planning by governments.

REFORMS 1972–75

Labour was reelected in 1972 with an aggressive program of reform. How much was to be socialist reform (concerned with assessed needs) and how much was to be concerned about better management? Reformers were concerned with both.

1. The federal government requires states to intervene directly in private nursing home planning and to review admissions, growth, and fee policies. An *Australian Medical Journal* editorial (November 1972) argued that 25% of institutionalization was unnecessary.

2. A Domiciliary Nursing Care Benefit for relatives was introduced.

3. More hostel support was provided "to keep people functioning."

4. There was new emphasis on home care and outpatient services by nursing homes.

5. Medical Care Reforms:
   a. Medibank 1975: An Act introduced government-administered universal health insurance, generating great hostility among Liberals and doctors. The scheme was operated for only one year before it was replaced by prepayment schemes to private insurance companies. (In 1983, a Medicare Act reinstated government-administered universal health insurance.)
   b. Under the Hospital and Health Services Commission, community health programs were set up by special grants to states to strengthen primary care, support services, rehabilitation and geriatric medicine, rural services, hospital development, manpower, and facility planning.

6. Royal commissions and public inquiries continued throughout the '70s, addressing poverty, disability, access, and involvement in policy development. These all had implications for the elderly.

FISCAL RESTRAINT 1976–82

By now, governments were committed to providing a wide range of services. The entrepreneurial/philanthropic model was superseded. Both parties recognized the need to take control, particularly over institutional services, and to increase community care services. The main difference in their policies was the extent to which private services should be controlled/encouraged.

New management techniques and improved accountability began to develop. From 1976–82 the governing Liberal/Country Party wanted (1) to increase the private sector; (2) to delegate fiscal control to states; (3) to rationalize existing services; and (4) to improve services to the elderly and disabled. The last two objectives were shared by Labour. Task forces began to sort out federal/state/voluntary organization responsibilities (Bailey, 1977–78; Jamison, 1981). The Bailey Committee recommended simplification of granting mechanisms. A three-year budget cycle for Aged and Disabled Persons Homes was implemented in 1976. Efforts to increase home nursing and the Community Health Program were hindered by cost restraints and a shift to general revenue financing. Institutions continued to be maintained. Continuing reviews of service structures for the elderly culminated in a comprehensive review by the House of Representatives Subcommittee on Expenditures (McLeay, 1982). The McLeay Committee described some of the problems as follows:

> It appears, therefore, that what started out as a housing scheme for the fit aged, based firmly on welfare criteria, has, in effect, become a program providing capital subsidies predominantly for nursing home care. This outcome sits uneasily with the government objectives to limit the growth of nursing homes and work towards improving the balance between institutional and community care in accordance with patients' needs and requirements. (Paragraph 2.71)
>
> The policy objective of restraint applied to the domiciliary care sector may have been self defeating. (Paragraph 2.73)
>
> In general terms . . . the emergence over the years of policies and programs for accommodation and care of the aged points to a lack of concern with evaluation in relation to the stated purposes of schemes and programs. There is evidence of a lack of attention to considerations of cost effectiveness and program effectiveness, particularly in relation to the development of strategies for alternative means of providing accommodation and care. (Paragraph 2.73)

RECOMMENDATIONS OF THE COMMITTEE

1. Need to clarify philosophy and purposes to go beyond seeing care for the elderly as "a health matter."

2. Need to move toward three programs (for simplification): (1) Extended Care; (2) Nursing Home Care; and (3) Subsidized Housing (to be developed).
   Extended Care Programs—senior citizens' centers, home support services, more money for assessment teams, more staff training, planning by states down to local levels, monitoring of expenditures.

Nursing Home Care—within five years, states (not federal government) should take responsibility for: standard setting, whether to have contract care, respite care, open ownership, and complaints machinery.

The Committee took its preliminary report around the country for discussion in order to involve consumers and providers of services in the final recommendations.

SUBSEQUENT DEVELOPMENTS

In 1981, a National Survey on Disablement showed the considerable extent of disability in the elderly (Australian Bureau of Statistics, 1981).

In 1983, a further survey asked the disabled themselves what they would like. This coincided with plans for opening doors of institutions for the handicapped and a shift to community care in small homes.

From 1983 onward, Hawke's Labour government set up the Department of Community Services to develop programs, and offices of age care services at federal and state levels for consumer inputs.

In 1987, the Ministry of Health merged with the Department of Community Services to improve communication. The new Department had the following subsections:

- Community Programs
- Health Benefits
- Hospital and Residential Programs
- Housing Services
- Health Advancement
- Disability Programs
- Health Research and Services
- Therapeutics
- Corporate and Information Services

SUMMARY AND CONCLUSION

1. The statistical indices show that Australia is demographically similar to Canada, as is the epidemiology. Long term care institutional rates are high, particularly compared to Western Europe. In 1982–83, community services accounted for 12.5% of the budget for accommodation and home services for the elderly.

2. Key factors impeding development of optimal policies for health of the elderly are mainly structural. For historical reasons funding of institu-

tional and community care services is divided between federal and state authorities. Incentives encourage institutionalization, often for profit of private owners.

3. Another key factor is ideology. There are political party differences relating to the concept of deservingness. Labour defends universality. Liberals believe in rewarding the thrifty.

4. The McLeay Report (1982) identified lack of concern about outputs/evaluation/resources. There has been more concern regarding processes (particularly political processes). Attempts are being made to introduce more evaluation.

5. Major policy and research trends relate to streamlining—improving management of services. Much research effort has arisen from Royal Commissions and Committees of Inquiry. Whether or not this is research per se, the main efforts have come here. Evaluation and planning departments are being set up. Academic research is being conducted on demography, retirement issues, family, home life, social justice, and service organization. As indicated, the main emphasis on research with policy implications is on framework or structural research. Improving program evaluation and considering how to improve financial incentives toward community rather than institutional care are current priorities.

NOTE

Research published up to 1982 is listed in the McLeay Report. For further information, follow through on researchers listed in that bibliography.

REFERENCES

Australian Bureau of Statistics. (1981). *Survey of handicapped persons.* Canberra: Australian Government Publishing Service.

Bailey. (1977–78). *Australia. Task Force on Coordination in Welfare and Health: Proposals for change in the administration and delivery of programs and services.* Canberra: Australian Government Publishing Service.

Evans, R. L. (1976). The hidden colonists: Deviance and social control in Colonial Queensland. In J. Roe (Ed.), *Social policy in Australia: Some perspectives 1901–75* (pp. 74–100). Sydney: Cassell.

Jamison. (1981). *Australia. Commission of Inquiry into the Efficiency and Administration of Hospitals: Report.* Canberra: Australian Government Publishing Service.

McLeay. (1982). *Australia. House of Representatives Standing Committee on Expenditure. In a home or at home.* Canberra: Australian Government Publishing Service.

Roe, J. (1976). *Social policy in Australia: Some perspectives 1901–75.* Sydney: Cassell.

21. Institutionalization of Elderly Canadians: Future Allocations to Non–Health Sectors

COPE W. SCHWENGER

INTRODUCTION

This chapter reviews some of the more important non–health care factors impinging on present and future health care costs for elderly Canadians. The focus here will be on the utilization of long term institutional care. Emphasis will be placed on housing as an alternative to long term institutional care, and briefer mention will be made of family, income, and social services as examples of other non–health care factors influencing levels of institutionalization.

Health as a concept can be very broad indeed; the European office of the World Health Organization (1984) describes health as a resource and a matter of realizing aspirations, satisfying needs, and changing or coping with the environment. This concept is the basis for a recent report by the Canadian Federal Government (Epp, 1986) and three Ontario reports sponsored by the Ministry of Health (Evans, 1987; Spasoff, 1987; Podgorski, 1987). In these reports it is hard to imagine what is not included under the rubric of health (e.g., peace, income, housing, food, family, work, community).

The definition used here is closer to that used by Bob Evans (1984). Health status is based on a rather narrower definition of health (absence of disease or infirmity). He describes health care as "goods and services which consumer/patients use solely or primarily because of their anticipated (positive) impact on health status." Included are such things as health personnel institutional and formal community care. The non–health (care) sectors are everything other than this.

Aging and Health: Linking Research and Public Policy, © 1989 Lewis Publishers, Inc., Chelsea, Michigan 48118. Printed in U.S.A.

A GERIATRIC CRISIS?

There has been much "crisis rhetoric" regarding future health care costs for elderly Canadians. The major villains are said to be demography, technology, and utilization.

Demography

The familiar projections of the growth of the elderly population do not, in themselves, indicate an impending geriatric crisis. Other developed nations already sustain a much higher proportion of elderly people (e.g., 15% in the United Kingdom). Of more concern is the aging of the aged population. The oldest old (85 and older) are projected to rise at 3 times the rate of the youngest old over the next 25 years. Although much smaller in numbers, they represent a much higher proportion of high-risk older people living on their own, with lower incomes, more fragile health, and in greater danger of needing institutional care. There appears to be a growing consensus, however, that the oldest old, although they certainly have cost implications, are not the major factor in driving the system (Barer et al., 1987).

Technology

More important than demographics is the ever-greater use of sophisticated and expensive technology by increasing numbers of elderly patients, especially in hospitals and particularly at the time of death (Roos, Shapiro, & Havens, 1987). Three fifths of all men and three fourths of all women in Ontario die after 65 years of age. One fourth of all these deaths occur in long term care institutions and one half die in general hospitals (Gross & Schwenger, 1981).

In his book *Setting Limits* (1987), Daniel Callahan, Director of the prestigious Hastings Institute, has a good deal to say about care of the dying elderly. He implores physicians to "forsake their goal of averting death at all costs and focus their tremendous powers on improving the quality of peoples' lives." He wants to set limits on expensive technology and confine its use to those with a "natural" life span and a high quality of life. He agrees with the British system of rationing life-extending acute care medicine to the elderly. Callahan's critics argue that his proposed alternatives of better medical services, rehabilitation (to improve quality of life), and adequate long term institutional and community care services, although perhaps more humane and compassionate, would not necessarily be less costly.

Allocation by age rather than need is highly suspect among North American gerontologists, who have stressed the differences in individual needs and heterogeneity of the elderly (Neugarten, 1982). Rationing expensive high technology by whatever means and the development of cheaper, cost-effective low technology will in any case become matters of increasing concern.

Utilization

By far the greatest factor driving the whole system is the ever-increasing utilization of health care resources by the elderly, more particularly utilization of physicians and institutions (both acute and long term care).

The ratios of population to physician in 1979–1981 were 538:1, 522:1, and 617:1 in the United States, Canada, and United Kingdom, respectively. In a study for Health and Welfare (Schwenger, 1985), key informants in all parts of the country were asked what they regarded as priority health care needs of the elderly in Canada. Contacts included senior provincial health and social service officials, voluntary and professional organizations, and gerontologists and clinicians in geriatrics and geriatric psychiatry. There was a consensus about the dangers to the long term care system resulting from too much power in the hands of too many physicians. Exceptions were the matter of maldistribution and the lack in some areas of certain categories of physicians to care for the elderly, especially geriatricians. Disquieting were the number of reports indicating lack of expertise (or even interest) in elderly patients and the lack of recognition by all medical schools in Canada of the demographic imperative of an aging population.

Canada's rate of long term care institutionalization of the elderly is significantly higher than in the United States and United Kingdom. It is not, however, as high as the 9.5% (65 and older) which the Canadian Medical Association (1984) has proclaimed in the so-called Joan Watson Report in which short term hospital care was mistakenly included in the category of long term care institutions. It is much closer in this country to 7% (65 and older), compared with some 5% in the United Kingdom. Keep in mind that the difference of 2% of elderly Canadians occupy some 60,000 beds (approximately 3 million Canadians 65 and older in 1988).

In Ontario in 1982–83, over two thirds (69%) of all health care costs for the elderly in the Ministry of Health were devoted to institutional care, compared to less than 3% spent on home care and a similar small amount available for other public and community health programs.

DEINSTITUTIONALIZATION

The term *deinstitutionalization* is increasingly being used in the discussion of future policy regarding elderly Canadians. Cost implications of long term institutional care are important, and it is predicted that there will be increasing pressure to keep older people at home or move them out of such institutions back into the community, as is the case in the United Kingdom. Even more important is that home is where the elderly and their relatives wish to be.

There are at least four non–health care factors that must be kept in mind in preventing premature institutionalization: family, income, social services, and housing.

Family

Estimates suggest that some 80% of all care provided to the elderly comes from family and friends (Chappell, Strain, & Blandford, 1986). By far the commonest support is provided by the spouse, followed by children. Walker (1987) states that family support is much more important than demography in the potential future demand for health and social services. "If only 5% of families refused to provide care then formal services would be swamped." He warns of the importance of preventing the exploitation of female caregivers and avoiding unbearable financial, physical, social, and psychological costs that may be incurred.

There are some ominous portents concerning future demographics of the family. With higher rates of divorce and separation, one wonders whether the person who has been married for five years will have the same sense of responsibility to give long term care as the spouse of 50 years.

There will be decreasing numbers of children available as caregivers, together with increasing numbers of elderly relatives needing care. Furthermore, with the impending boom of the oldest old (85 and older), their children (65 and older) do not have the same energy or physical resources and may not be able to supply the same level of care as when younger. In addition, what is the commitment of children of second and third marriages toward their stepparents and stepgrandparents? It is said that maturing post-war baby boomers should in the future look to their siblings as potential caregivers as an alternative to the production of an insufficient number of available children.

An increasing emphasis is being placed everywhere on the needs of caregivers, whether they be family, relatives, friends, neighbors, or volunteers. Many express concern that professionals will encroach into areas where the elderly and their caregivers could be doing things for themselves. The question is whether a larger share of funds should be used to support the relatives rather than more services for the elderly.

Various methods of family support have been developed such as day care, day hospitals, respite (relief) care, and intermittent (periodic) admissions. All of these, in addition to helping the patient, make looking after difficult cases at home more bearable.

The cost savings of using family support are recognized everywhere as significant, especially at the time of death. Governments, partly because of the mounting costs of the last few days in hospital, are considering the possibility of looking after the dying elderly at home. In this case, one must provide not only comfort for the suffering and dying patient, but a great deal of additional support for the caregiver. Older people themselves don't necessarily want to go to hospital; they have been persuaded by societal attitudes that hospital care must be included as a last resort, even though all hope of recovery is lost. Hospitals have become the place to die. An attempt to counteract this attitude has been launched by the New Brunswick Extramural Hospital Program and elsewhere.

Income

It is a lot healthier to be rich in old age. Mortality and morbidity rates of the more affluent are lower and life expectancy is higher. Richer old people have fewer admissions and reduced lengths of stay in institutions. This raises the question of whether it would be better and more cost-effective to give low income elderly more money instead of ever more health services.

Many have conceded (Schwenger, 1985) that income is extremely important in keeping older people out of institutions, but it was considered simplistic to just hand them more money and expect them necessarily to know how to spend it wisely on health maintenance. An intriguing experiment is going on in Nova Scotia, where caregivers are being paid up to $4800 annually to look after elderly relatives who would otherwise be going into institutions.

One of the persistent myths about elderly Canadians is that they are the poorest segment of society. Between 1979 and 1984 both in families and individuals, the prevalence of low income (a reasonable proxy for poverty) went up in all groups except the elderly, where it went down substantially. Elder-headed families (mostly couples) were much below the average. Within five years, elder-headed families (mostly couples) had moved from the highest (21.9%) to almost the lowest (11.4%) poverty rates. Individual elderly (mostly widows) still had in 1984 the highest prevalence of low income of all groups, but the percentage had declined from two thirds to less than half within a five-year period while rising in all other age groups (Metropolitan Toronto District Health Council, 1988).

Social Services

One of the most prevalent issues noted by key informants (Schwenger, 1985) was the lack of harmony between so-called health and social services, which apparently occurs everywhere in the western world.

Competition between provincial departments of health and social services, or between the medical and social models (even where the departments are amalgamated) was described as destructive and a terrible waste of time. Health services were criticized by social services as being insufficiently imbued with a philosophy of community care. The social model was described by those on the health side, as having an image of poverty and a means-test mentality. Lip service was given to the various so-called home support services in this country. Meals on Wheels, friendly visiting, and even homemakers (home helps) were considered to be almost frills by respondents in departments of health. They were referred to as soft services in many places, not in any way as important as the so-called harder and more important medical, nursing, and other health care therapies.

Studies of the effectiveness and efficiency of home care in both its social and medical aspects were considered almost everywhere to be top priority. Such studies have been carried out in the United States and the United Kingdom. There are some very skeptical people in Canada who still assume that home care, and particularly home support, are not cost-effective.

Official health departments throughout Canada are seen to have an institutional bias by almost everyone else, whereas departments of social services appear to have much more of a community orientation (e.g., the Ontario Ministry of Community & Social Services or COMSOC). Also, more left wing governments appear to favor a philosophy of community care and the social model, compared with the more institutional and medical model orientation of more right wing regimes. This has certainly been the case in Ontario where the Liberals, supported by the New Democratic Party, took power in 1985 after some 40 years of Conservative control. The change has been dramatic and has continued since the Liberal landslide in 1987. COMSOC has a new lease on life, invigorated by exciting new leadership both politically and in the civil service. Considerably more money has been allocated, with the likelihood of future control and even more resources transferred from the Ontario Ministry of Health. The fact that social services funding for the elderly has tripled over the last three years is, however, less impressive in the context of the initial measly allotment. Nor does it necessarily signify a reallocation to social services.

Housing

There was an increasing recognition in the study I did for Health & Welfare (Schwenger, 1985) of the significance of suitable housing as an alternative to premature institutional care throughout the country. This was a higher priority on the part of social services than health.

A growing variety, but a pathetically inadequate quantity, of new types of development existed in all provinces and territories. The bricks-and-mortar mentality of a good many housing authorities at provincial and local levels, and the difficulty of getting coordinated efforts between health, housing, and social service authorities, were major barriers to change.

Insufficient recognition has been paid by health and social services personnel to the crucial relationship of housing, health, and social services. Elderly accommodation is often more important than health services in keeping people out of institutions. We need a much greater variety and, particularly, quantity of sheltered (or congregate) housing, shared (or communal) housing, foster home care, granny flats, retirement communities, and geriatric campuses (or multilevel care facilities) throughout the country.

Although most people live in the community, their ability to do so can depend as much on the kind of accommodation they occupy as the support they receive—what does emerge from a number of British studies is that, given adequate support and appropriate housing, a number of elderly people currently in institutional accommodation could live independently (Butler, 1986).

Health organizations generally, and at all levels in Canada, are beginning to recognize the importance of housing, but are as yet insufficiently aware of what is going on in the housing field, and the influence that this has had on (especially old) people's health. Examples of this include at the federal level, the lack of emphasis on housing until recently by Health and Welfare; at the provincial level, the lower priority given to housing compared with health and social services within the Ontario government (e.g., Ontario Office for Senior Citizens' Affairs, A New Agenda, 1986); and in the Metro Toronto District Health Council and its Long Term Care Committee, a lack of representation from the housing field and no work to date on this topic (Metropolitan Toronto District Health Council, 1988).

Living Arrangements of the Elderly

There has been a greater tendency in this country for older Canadians to live alone or in "collectives" according to Gordon Priest (1984). Between 1971 and 1981, living alone and in collectives went up (from one fourth to one third). Living with relatives has, however, gone down over the same period (from 11% to 8%). Older people want their privacy and will live alone if economic circumstances permit.

One of the leading risk factors of the elderly is living alone, which puts them at risk of loneliness with its potentially damaging effects, e.g., inability to handle an emergency on their own; not having a caregiver available to help them; and risk of premature institutionalization.

A much larger proportion of elderly (65 and older) in Metro Toronto live alone (38%) than for Canada as a whole (24%). This group poses an enormous challenge to future social services, health, and housing agencies. Another trend is the very large number and proportion living in apartments (43.1%). It is estimated that, for Ontario as a whole, 67% are living in their own homes (mostly owned) and 33% are renting (virtually all apartments). This trend to apartment living and living alone will continue, leading to ever-greater anonymity and lack of community support unless special efforts are made to prevent this from happening (Metropolitan Toronto District Health Council, 1988).

The Task Force considered a greater range of housing alternatives to be desirable. Traditionally, the elderly have been viewed either as completely independent or completely dependent, with relatively little in between; a continuum from one to the other is obviously a more desirable goal. The status of the elderly is dynamic, and they should be able to move up and down a continuum of services depending on their needs, as shown in Figure 1.

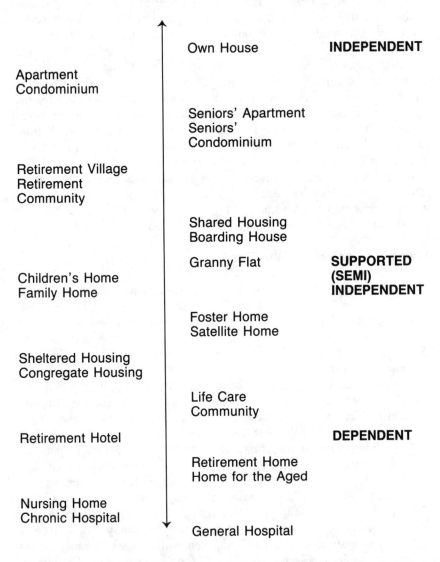

Figure 1. Shelter and care continuum. (From Metropolitan Toronto District Health Council, 1988.)

Although there is an increase in variety of supported semiindependent living in Ontario, there is still relatively little quantity. Very few provincial resources have been allocated to this sector. In Ontario in 1982/83, $80 million (2.4%) out of a total budget of $3.3 billion spent on the elderly was allocated to housing. Corke and Rusiecki (1985), in a paper presented to the Canadian Association on Gerontology, estimated that in 1983/84 less than $2 million of the Ontario elderly housing budget was allocated to innovative semiindependent housing (Metropolitan Toronto District Health Council, 1988).

Institutionalization of Elderly Ontarians

The home is, for many older people, their sole arena, in which eating, sleeping, socializing with friends and relatives and entertainment must be conducted. People in later life tend, as a group, to spend more of their time at home—the move to an institution involves giving up not only a degree of independence but also the relinquishing of many of one's personal possessions, accepting a reduction in life space and loss of privacy. (Butler, 1986).

In 1984 (the most recent year data were available) there were 76,628 chronic, extended, and residential care beds in hospitals, nursing homes, homes for the aged, and retirement/rest homes in Ontario, of which 72,242 were estimated to be utilized by those 65 and older. This translates to an institutionalization rate of 7.9% (estimated 65-and-older population was 915,000).

Had the Ontario rate of institutionalization in 1981 matched that of the United Kingdom in 1982—5.0%—the province would have "saved" 25,177 beds (based on a 65-and-older population of 868,185). In 1986, 28,788 elderly Ontarians would have been at home instead of in long term institutional care (Metropolitan Toronto District Health Council, 1988).

Sheltered Housing

Sheltered housing was of particular interest and concern to the Task Force and is presented in detail. It is recognized that this is not the best solution to all housing problems; however, it does represent a viable alternative for semiindependent seniors for whom the fewest alternatives exist.

Sheltered housing in the United Kingdom is described basically as grouped dwellings, the sharing of certain facilities (dining, recreation), the 24-hour presence of a "warden" or housekeeper, and an intercommunication system. The warden is primarily available for emergency calls, serves as the residents' counselor and advocate, acts as a liaison to community support services, and encourages appropriate contact with physicians, nurses, etc.

Sheltered housing strives to achieve a balance between care and independence activities within the continuum of increasingly protected shelter options. The original sheltered housing scheme consisted simply of a group of purpose-built bungalows. This has been extended to include bungalows, flats, or terraced housing with a common room. All of these are referred to as *Category 1*.

Category 2 includes flats and common rooms linked by a heated interior corridor. *Category 2 1/2* includes individual units (bachelor or one bedroom), and all other rooms including dining are communally shared. Category 2 or 2 1/2 may be linked to an old people's home (Part III Accommodation).

Very sheltered (extra care) housing is for more dependent elderly with an extra element of care, e.g., additional wardens, provision of meals, care assistants, and extra communal facilities. Around 1 in 5 local authorities in England provide very sheltered housing and 1 in 10 has a housing association which specializes in housing for older people (Department of Environment, 1987). Sheltered housing does not include any health professionals on the staff. These are used, as necessary, from the regular ranks of the National Health Service.

The original objective of seeking a balance of active and frail residents has been extended to each category of sheltered housing. In this way the residents help each other, thus retaining maximum independence and mutual support within the group and reduced labor for the service providers.

A key program element in Britain appears to be the resident housekeeper—typically a young to middle-aged housewife who lives with her family in a private apartment or house, attached or adjacent to the sheltered housing scheme. Usually no special skills or training are required to be eligible beyond a loving and caring nature, self-confidence, and common sense.

Visits to sheltered housing schemes over the years have left impressions of the comfort, coziness, and "homeyness" of the arrangements. They are in no way institutional, even in the very sheltered or extra care sections. Another impression is the sense of autonomy of each project—no evidence of stultifying and centralized, or even local, bureaucratic rigidities. Also important is the emphasis on local autonomy of the residents with as much independence as possible maintained at all levels. Lastly, one cannot help but be impressed with how the housing is imbedded into the local community, which provides the residents, the staff, and the seeming multitude of volunteers.

The United Kingdom has provided an extraordinary amount of sheltered housing over the years. Recent figures from the Department of Environment (1987) show that by 1986 in England alone 392,000 sheltered dwellings had been provided for the elderly in addition to 326,000 other specially designed or adapted dwellings. Anthea Tinker (1984) has estimated that around 5%

of the elderly population in the United Kingdom is living in sheltered housing.

The great majority of people in the United Kingdom remain in their own homes for as long as possible, rather than move to specialized housing. Often all that is needed is some home improvement and perhaps some help from health and social services. For those who need to move, the next option is often an ordinary small, easy-to-run house, flat, or bungalow, or for some older people perhaps a "granny annex" with relatives. However for those needing more support, sheltered and eventually very sheltered housing can help them keep their privacy and independence rather than become dependent on institutional care. Residents of sheltered housing do not have the same inducement to enter Part III Accommodation (residential care), nursing homes, or hospitals. The vast majority of residents die in sheltered housing perhaps with the residents' warden holding their hand at the end.

There seems no doubt that the very large quantity of sheltered housing in the United Kingdom is in part responsible for the relatively low rate of institutional care and institutionalization in the United Kingdom. Although we have a variety in Canada, we still have a pathetically small quantity of such assisted accommodation.

REFERENCES

Barer, M. L., Evans, R. G., Hertzman, C., & Lomas, J. (1987). Aging and health care utilization: New evidence on old fallacies. *Social Science and Medicine, 24*(10).

Butler, A. (1986, summer). Housing and health in Europe. *Social Policy and Administration, 20*(2).

Callahan, D. (1987). *Setting limits: Medical goals in an aging society.* Toronto: Simon & Schuster.

Canadian Medical Association. (1984). *Health: A need for redirection.* A Task Force on the Allocation of Health Care Resources. (Chairman: Joan Watson).

Chappell, N. L., Strain, L.A., & Blandford, A. A. (1986). *Aging and health care: A social perspective.* Holt, Rinehart & Winston (Canada).

Corke, S., & Rusiecki, B. (1985, October). *Provincial housing and shelter support programs for the elderly.* Paper presented at the annual meeting of the Canadian Association on Gerontology, Hamilton.

Department of Environment. (1987, April). Correspondence with Adam Scott, Housing Division H3, London.

Epp, J. (1986). *Achieving health for all: A framework for health promotion.* Health and Welfare Canada.

Evans, J. R. (Chair). (1987, June). *Toward a shared direction for health in Ontario.* Report of the Ontario Health Resources panel. Ontario Ministry of Health.

Evans, R.G. (1984). *Strained mercy.* Toronto: Butterworths.

Gross, M. J., & Schwenger, C. W. (1981). *Health care costs for the elderly in Ontario 1976–2026*. Ontario Economic Council.

Metropolitan Toronto District Health Council. (1988, April). *Report of the Task Force on Housing and the Health of the Elderly*.

Neugarten, B. L. (1982). *Age or need? Public policies for older people*. Beverly Hills: Gage Publications.

Ontario Office for Senior Citizens' Affairs. (1986, June). *A new agenda: Health and social service strategies for Ontario seniors*. Toronto: Queen's Printer.

Podgorski, S. (Chair). (1987). *Health promotion matters in Ontario: A report of the Minister's Advisory Group on Health Promotion*. Ontario Ministry of Health.

Priest, G. (1984, November). *Living arrangements of Canada's elderly. Changing demographic and economic factors*. Simon Fraser University.

Roos, N. P., Shapiro, E., & Havens, H. (1987). Aging with limited resources: What should we really be worried about? In In *Aging with limited health resources, proceedings of a colloquium on health care, May 1986* (pp. 50–56). Ottawa: Canadian Government Publishing Centre, Supply and Services Canada.

Schwenger, C. W. (1985, January). *Health care for elderly Canadians: A new role for Health and Welfare Canada?* a) Complete report, 206 pages (mimeographed); b) Summary of conclusions and recommendations, 24 pages (mimeographed). Ottawa: Health and Welfare Canada.

Spasoff, R. A. (Chair). (1987, August). *Health for all Ontario: Report of the Panel on Health Goals for Ontario*. Toronto: Ontario Ministry of Health.

Tinker, A. (1984). *The elderly in modern society* (2nd ed.). London: Longman.

Walker, A. (1987). Meeting the needs of Canada's elderly with limited health resources: Some observations based on British experience. In *Aging with limited health resources, proceedings of a colloquium on health care, May 1986* (pp. 27–39). Ottawa: Canadian Government Publishing Centre, Supply and Services Canada.

World Health Organization. (1984). *Health promotion: A discussion document on the concept and principles*. Copenhagen.

22. Demography, Economy, and the Future of the Health System for the Elderly: A European Perspective

ANTON AMANN

INTRODUCTION

In this chapter I will examine a number of factors that influence both the aging process of society and prospects for the aged themselves. By 2025, developing nations will account for 83% of the world population (of a projected 8.2 billion), but only 29% of those 60 and over. Conversely, industrialized countries will comprise only 17% of the population, but 71% of those 60 and over (Schade & Kühne, 1986, p. 80). To provide at least a general overview of the complexity of the aging process, I will address structural and individual issues and incorporate demographic and economic information as well as some considerations about the role of the labor market.

Beginning in the 1970s, there was a general European policy of extending early retirement measures to treat labor market problems, which now influences the cost load of the social security system. Besides, the ever-rising pressure on welfare budgets has resulted in another phenomenon already observable in welfare states: "The prime objective is to cut back statutory social services and to encourage whenever possible the hand over of welfare support to the private and voluntary sectors: this means a yet greater social division of welfare ... and an even heavier burden placed on an already overburdened informal caring sector" (Taylor, 1984, pp. 40–41). These strategies could lead to a reduction of the level of public expenditure by

Aging and Health: Linking Research and Public Policy, © 1989 Lewis Publishers, Inc., Chelsea, Michigan 48118. Printed in U.S.A.

cutting benefits, limiting entitlements, and reducing health and social services funding below the levels of actual demand.

The labor market, social security system, retirement process, and social and health care system are therefore highly interdependent. The "culture of aging" and demographic factors will also influence the future health system for the elderly.

THE AGING OF THE POPULATION AND RETIREMENT POLICIES

The labor force will undergo marked changes in the future. Almost no one will be able to remain in the same occupation or carry it out in the same way until retirement. Technology will create four main effects: loss of jobs, creation of jobs, professional devaluation, and improvement of skills. All of these changes will create uncertainty for older workers and their prospects. Many governments have implemented early retirement policies and incentives, resulting in a general lowering of retirement age. The very generous systems of old age pensions and other entitlements (early eligibility, relaxed sickness and disability definitions, etc.) implemented in a number of European countries were based on (1) the assumption of unlimited or at least uninterrupted economic growth, and (2) ignorance of demographic trends. Countries such as Austria have in recent years experienced higher demands on pension insurance. Since 1975 economic growth has slowed down, but so has the long term rise in labor force participation rates. These experiences have led to policy discussions oscillating between two alternatives: a gradual scaling-down of benefits in order not to provoke potential criticism on the one hand and complete restructuring of the systems on the other. Yet by and large, most Western countries continue to provide incentives for early retirement, but in some of them the discussion about raising the retirement age has already started.

One result of these developments has been that a diminishing number of younger and middle-aged persons support a growing number of aging persons who cease to be economically productive around their late 50s. The young and middle-aged may question their support of an increasing affluent older population (Morrison, 1986, p. 345); there may emerge the demand for a new contract between the generations. The perspective on retirement itself will change because the social definition of *age* is undergoing significant changes.

We cannot predict the attitudes and behavior patterns of older people 30 or 40 years from now. They will have more education and, probably, different attitudes toward the state and authority in general. While numerous studies reveal a deferential and obedient attitude among the elderly learned from world wars and economic recessions, one would hardly predict that the situation will remain the same in the coming decades (see Amann, 1984).

The aging of the population has particularly important implications for every nation's health sector. Aging increases the frequency of chronic illnesses, disabilities, and frailty, as well as the demand for health and long term care services. These escalations lead to consideration of scaling down benefits, which seems a cruel blow given the so recently achieved improvements in the welfare state system. "It is a direct thrust at a basic dream of an aging society: that old age and good health are biologically compatible and financially affordable. It may turn out to be no less unsettling morally, forcing choices that could well corrode values and principles that are centrally important and deeply cherished" (Callahan, 1986, p. 319).

The epidemiology and health status of the very old and their importance to the health care system are relatively uncharted on the map of empirical gerontology. However, we know from several studies that between one fourth and one third of those over 70 suffer from at least three chronic conditions. The average age of clients of some types of community care services, and in most types of institutional care, is around 80. If these trends continue, there will be significant economic and social implications, because the proportion of the population aged 80 and over will have risen between the years 1980 and 2000 by from 17% to over 60% in most industrialized nations (Amann, 1985; George & Perreault, 1985). That the elderly suffer from chronic and degenerative conditions has implications for the kind of health care they receive and how much it costs.

By 2020 or 2025, between 17% and 21% of the population in European countries will be 65 and over (Amann, 1985). According to one low-growth population projection, by 2020, 23.9% of the Canadian population will be 65 and over (George & Perreault, 1985, p. 48). In absolute terms, the Canadian population over 65 by 2031 (all of whom have been born) will rise to 7 million, over double the present number.

At the same time, the number of children in school will remain virtually the same, but in some countries—Austria, Belgium, Denmark, Federal Republic of Germany, Italy, Luxembourg—the numbers of children and students will decline considerably (Amann, 1985, Tables 4 and 8). More directly related to the future of the aged is a predictable change in the working population, especially the older component aged 45 to 64. From 1990 to 2010, this age group will increase in number among all member states of the Council of Europe, and by over 20% in seven of them. Hence it is appropriate to speak of an aging working population (Amann, 1985, Tables 5 and 6).

Finally, the changes in population among those 75 and over are especially significant; more important than the overall changes in the 65-and-over population will be the demographically supported notion of a *new class of the very old*. Furthermore, there will continue to be a preponderance of women in the higher age groups (Amann, 1981). In the Federal Republic of Germany in the year 2000, for every 100 women aged 70–75, 80–85, and 90 and over, there will be 69, 37, and 29 men, respectively (*Altwerden in der Bundesrepublik Deutschland,* 1987, Vol. 3, Table 8).

Older women face two difficulties as they age. First, because of their greater longevity and predilection to marrying men older than themselves, they tend to be widowed during the "high risk" years of old age—75 and over. Second, women's family and caregiving roles result in more erratic patterns of labor force participation, leading to lower social security benefits during their retirement years and, often, no entitlements to an occupational pension in their own right (Hoskins, 1987, p. 5).

THE LABOR MARKET AND THE SOCIAL SECURITY SYSTEM

One important question often ignored in social policy studies is: How in recent decades did older workers become increasingly a target group for labor market policies? According to Marx and Weber, the labor market has to fulfill a double-allocating function in modern capitalist societies: (1) the total labor force has to be allocated to specific activities and production processes, and (2) the income from labor has to be distributed among those active and those legitimately not participating in the work force. There is historical evidence that the market has been unable to fulfill this double allocating role on its own. Accordingly, the market system has been linked to the social security system to compensate for the deficiencies of allocative market structures.

The attempt to integrate people into, and retain them in, the labor market simultaneously leads to the release of certain groups from that market, for example, older persons, poorly qualified workers, foreign workers, etc. The release occurs unequally among the labor force according to the particular characteristics of the groups in question. We can therefore speak of an unequally distributed risk to be released—"labor market risk." The labor market risks associated with the elderly are impaired health; diminished achievement; lack of adaptability; poor qualifications; and even so-called age-dependent inabilities—stereotypes—which prevent employers from investments in human capital.

Labor market risk can be seen as a problem of unsuccessful allocation of work to the labor force, insofar as certain groups have less chance of being offered a job according to their age, sex, and qualification characteristics. Two distinct and theoretically important forces are at work here (Amann, 1983). First, there is an obvious and systematic accumulation of deprivations among certain groups. Second, there are numerous specific labor policy measures in European countries directed toward groups with certain characteristics. Indeed, specific, targeted labor policies have seemed to supplant more generally applicable policies. The result is an even greater distortion of the labor force among various groups and characteristics than the labor market would create.

Labor power can only present itself in constrained configurations. The members of a cohort entering the labor market are not able to reduce or increase their numbers according to the demands for labor power; otherwise it would be easy to escape youth unemployment. Also, suppliers of labor power differ in their qualifications and occupational experiences; they may not be able to wait for optimal opportunities to sell their labor power, because they would lack the means for subsistence otherwise (Offe & Hinrichs, 1984). These constraints are particularly prominent among older workers, who can vary the quality and quantity of their labor only within limits and have to rely on external (political) support in some instances to remain competitive.

COMPENSATION FOR UNFAVORABLE DEMAND CIRCUMSTANCES

Trade unions, associations for blue and white collar workers and employers, social security schemes, and so on are institutions—external to the labor market—which provide partial compensations for unfavorable demand circumstances. Pensions have come to play an increasingly prominent compensatory role in this regard. More generally, early retirement due to the fulfillment of pension requirements, unemployment, disability, and invalidity—all considerably increased recently in Europe—comprise external measures that compensate for the particular qualities of the labor market.

These measures are particularly important for older workers. Social security has expanded to guarantee the subsistence of suppliers of labor no longer able to meet actual demands. The linking of the labor market system to social security has channeled one of the most vulnerable labor market groups into the status of pensioners. Among significant measures are those that help older workers remain in the labor market until of pensionable age; the release of older workers from the labor market after interruption of gainful employment; and integration into one of the subsystems of social security. These measures have been termed integrative, reintegrative, and compensatory. These measures do not have undifferentiated effects on the labor force. White collar workers experience a loss of status and income through early retirement, resulting in dissatisfaction with the process. Blue collar workers, on the other hand, in many cases welcome early retirement as an opportunity to leave a physically exhausting job (Amann et al., 1986).

PREPARATION FOR RETIREMENT AND OLD AGE

Rosenmayr (1983, p. 244) lists three elements of a general preparation for age and retirement: (1) becoming conscious and critically self-aware; (2) establishing and developing a societally oriented consciousness about aging; and (3) developing means of access to support should it become necessary. He reports that attitudes to and preparation for retirement are inversely correlated and differ according to class. The upper class has a negative attitude toward retirement but prepares for it rather assiduously; conversely, the lower classes look forward to retirement but do little in preparation.

In order to discover attitudes toward retirement, I undertook a study involving qualitative interviews with 24 Austrian steelworkers. In 1983, the Austrian Ministry of Social Affairs implemented a regulation whereby women in the steel-making industry would retire at 52, and men at 57. This regulation is an example of a "compensatory equivalent" which created new opportunities for the steelworkers.

The study gathered biographical information, information on the work circumstances, private and family relationships, and so on. With these data as a foundation, we explored a number of key issues, including:

1. the level of consciousness of social policy problems related to the labor market, retirement policy, and compensatory mechanism, such as early retirement, reduced work week, and so on
2. an assessment of their current life situation, changes expected with retirement, plans and expectations in relation to the plant, work and occupation, family, social connections, and so on
3. the possible influence of discussions about early retirement and shortened working hours in selected media on the current perception of life and expectations for the future

The results presented here focused on the second area of examination. We studied everyday experiences and the perceptions, perspectives, and attitudes of the subjects, rather than limiting ourselves (and them) to standard "objective" data.

Three important institutions influence or even control orientations, expectations, and individual actions. First is the *occupational or work world,* involving formation through production, the organization of work, and control of performance. The second is *family and partnership.* The third is *"free" social connections,* which in contrast to the two others involves fewer institutionalized and unavoidable regulations.

People have to divide their strength and energy among these areas, considering what is demanded and what they wish. They must achieve a balance among the various elements of coercion and freedom—that is, they have to do what I conceptualize as *balance work.* In the group under study, the work world has dominated and has influenced their capacities to conform and adapt as well as oppose and resist. They have accomplished this by doing the balance work required. The work world siphons off energy from the other areas, which are considered interference with the working process and in opposition to the occupational world. Pressure for economic security assigns the occupational world primary importance. In this hierarchy, the realm of free social relations is relegated to the lowest status. However, engagement and investment in the three areas may change over time (for example, when starting a family, overcoming a crisis in partnership, caring for ill family members, becoming a volunteer in a care institution), although the work world seldom loses its hold on the individual. Retirement, then, constitutes a remarkable change in the performance of balance work in that it cancels all at once the obligations and demands of the occupational world.

At this point, there emerges a changing and complex range of opportunities, requiring planning, renunciation, choosing, deciding—in other words, balance work must be done. National legislation for early retirement, introduced at a specific time, changes the *opportunity structure* for older workers immensely. But these opportunities and options do not arrive in a vacuum; they emerge in the context of *learned patterns* of successful actions, experience, and habit. For example, people acquire the structures and habits of time, and the rhythms of getting up and going to work, having lunch, leaving work, weeks and weekends, and so on. The loss of this structure often provokes psychic difficulties among the unemployed. There are well-known distinctions among social relations in the plant, the family, and other intimate groups. The cessation of work at one stroke cancels a number of obligatory and institutionalized regulations and opportunities and highlights others by contrast. It is widely acknowledged that after six months, or a year at longest, contact with former working colleagues dies off.

The structurally created risk to be released from the labor market and to be channeled into the retirement system (the external perspective) complements the risk of having to change one's balance work and to suddenly adapt plans and actions (the internal perspective) to new, and often worse, situations. The expectations and orientations learned over a long period of time and integrated into one's personality persist after retirement. These acquired characteristics result in expectations of retirement almost identical to expectations of working life. They also lead to the persistence of certain behaviors even though they are no longer required. Leisure activities are frequently the same both pre- and postretirement. In the sample studied, we observed optimists, pessimists, and pragmatists in their anticipation of retirement.

Three of the 24 subjects were euphoric about the prospect of retirement and revealed numerous ideas about things they were going to do and how little fear they had that retirement would be boring or dull. Six respondents fit the description of expectation-pessimist, for whom retirement meant only stopping work, with no notion of exciting new activities, except that stress and burdens might diminish and one might experience some pleasure if health permits.

The majority of respondents (15 of the 24) can be termed expectation-pragmatists. They intend to do in retirement what they already do—devote themselves to children and grandchildren, improve the house and repair it, travel, and pursue hobbies—but only with more time no longer taken up by work. The question arises whether retirement is simply the extension of the life course thus far. For many, the plans for retirement are generally shaped by habits engraved by doing and learning over a long period of time. In this view, they will be able to do justice to activities constrained by the demands of work.

We explored the area of the gulf between dreams and the achievable. Travel forms an important part of the prospective retiree's plans. The goals reflect the effective marketing by modern tourism of expectations, invitations to experience exotic destinations, and so forth. But the respondents reduce the dreams to a realizable level by considering the money required, the state of health, and the balance between these and other objects of attainment. This "reality principle" is so pervasive that even in thinking about travel in the abstract, the dream is reduced step by step until the concretely achievable triumphs over the exotic. Almost everywhere, the limitations of what is possible become visible. In the context of diminished life energy, unpredictability about the future leads to cautious planning that embodies the notion retiring is desirable because of a drained life that has earned a right to peace. This perception results in a somewhat ambivalent view of pensions: on the one hand they are seen as charity, and on the other they are considered something deserved by one who has "served his time."

THE FUTURE OF OLD AGE

Are there, after all, indications that life will be entirely different in retirement, that people are prepared to lead a retirement life suitable to the promotion of health, the prevention of disease, and the maintenance of functional capacities?

Two themes run through the interviews of the steelworkers: the palette of potential future activities will derive from the repertory of current habits and limitations, and new "hopes" are simply old ones with a little more time. There are no expectations of or designs for a new world—what has been determines what will be. Although we cannot draw conclusions about the future, three fundamental and provocative questions arise:

1. Does the release of millions of people in their 50s and early 60s from the labor market lead to the fuller use of physical, mental, social, spiritual, and environmental capacities and opportunities leading to improved overall

well-being? Or does it simply fulfill the original intent of relief from the labor market, divorced from concerns about whether and how people would make use of additional time?

2. Are we misled by a health care system so heavily disease-oriented and so little engaged in health education and prevention that we spend even more money, but people do not become healthier?

3. Previously, many had to work until their 70th year to receive pensions, and many others died before retirement or reached it already in bad health. Are we now in a position to provide for retirement years with fewer handicaps, relief of pain, maintenance of lucidity, comfort, and dignity, and reacquisition of functional capacities?

THE DEMAND FOR SOCIAL AND HEALTH CARE

The developments of recent decades show an increasing interpenetration and expansion of professional institutional responsibilities in the health and social sectors. What is extremely difficult is to describe accurately the health status of and the service system for the elderly, due to a severe lack of statistical and epidemiological data. The restriction of financing of welfare benefits in many countries seems also to have led to a diminished capacity for social and gerontological research. Because of these research deficits, two very general proxies are used to provide an initial overview of the demand for care in old age.

The first is that mortality, displayed in a curve, could indeed become rectangularized (see Figure 1)—the phase of relatively good health status has lengthened, and without accidents, suicide, and self-harm we could approach an estimated ideal physiological life expectancy.

The second deals with the distribution of illness by age. Illnesses occur more frequently beginning from age 45 (see Figure 2). From existing data, we can infer some important findings: (1) the frequency of illness increases generally with age; (2) the average duration of illnesses increases with age; (3) the proportion of chronically ill increases with age; (4) the number of people with multiple disorders increases with age; and (5) frequency and duration of stay in hospitals increases with age.

It has been well documented that the elderly are very high users of acute care and long term care services both in Europe and in North America. Institutionalization rates vary from country to country and according to the service configurations in place. Several studies have pointed out that a substantial number of elderly people, in severe or moderate need of help, do not receive any form of assistance (*Altwerden in der Bundesrepublik Deutschland*, 1987, Vol. 3, p. 725). In almost all of the statistics on help for the elderly there are large proportions of "don't know" and "no answer" re-

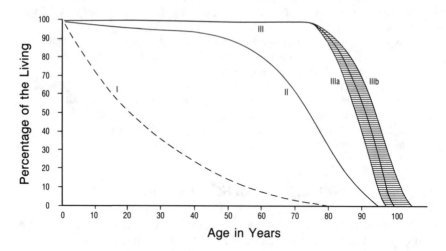

Figure 1. Mortality in the ancient world, in the present, and in an estimated ideal case. I = mortality in the ancient world; II = mortality in developed countries; III = estimated ideal physiological mortality; IIIa<en>IIIb = estimated range of genetic variance. (Adapted from *Altwerden in der Bundesrepublic Deutschland* [2nd ed., Vol. 2, p. 708], 1987, Berlin: Deutsches Zentrum für Altersfragen.)

sponses from surveys, which is reason to suspect that the numbers requiring but not receiving care are generally underestimated.

It would be risky to project future demands for old age care and financing given the incompleteness of data. However, we can propose practically relevant hypotheses. First, utilization of the full capacities of social services and their infrastructure—from kindergarten to old age homes—depends primarily on the absolute number of potential users (Amann, 1980). This is quite distinct from the question of the financing of individual and collective assistance, in which case the relative numbers of the various groups are important. For example, in the Federal Republic of Germany the numbers of people aged 75 and over will rise and fall over the next 40 years (see Table 1).

Would it be sensible to produce hospital and long term care beds on the basis of the population peaks anticipated for 1990 or 2020? Probably not, because the result might be the financing of beds which are not needed or people being influenced to use the beds despite their being the second-best solution to their needs. Furthermore, one could not create the new beds by 1990 in any case because of traditionally long planning and construction phases. I endorse the suggestion of the authors of *Altwerden in der Bundesrepublik* that to meet peak demands we must establish more outpatient and

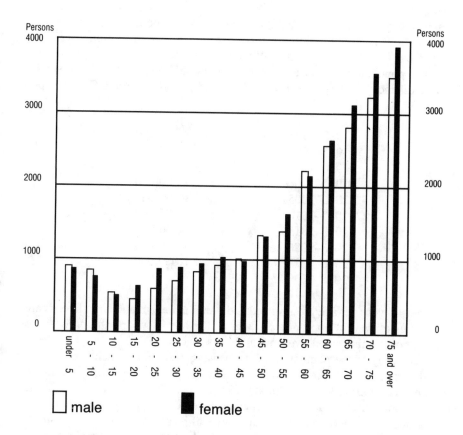

Figure 2. Sick persons according to age groups—microcensus May 1976 per 10,000 inhabitants, Federal Republic of Germany. (Adapted from *Altwerden in der Bundesrepublik Deutschland* [2nd ed., Vol. 2, p. 710], 1987, Berlin: Deutsches Zentrum für Altersfragen.)

Table 1. Changes in Population Aged 75 and Over in the Federal Republic of Germany, 1980–2030, in Thousands

1980	1990	2000	2010	2020	2030
3498.1	4082.3	3526.3	3640.2	4113.8	3734.9
	(+584.2)	(−556.0)	(−113.9)	(+473.6)	(−378.9)

Source: Own calculation from *Altwerden in der Bundesrepublik* (1987, Vol. 3, Table 8).

ambulatory facilities, such as day care centers. At present, they are insufficiently developed but are more flexible in supply than institutional services. They can be established faster and reduced easier.

The population growth among the "young old"—aged 60–75—shows its own distinct trend (*Altwerden in der Bundesrepublik,* 1987, Vol. 2, pp. 820–821):

1980–1985	−100,000
1985–1990	−100,000
1990–1995	+ 700,000
1995–2000	+ 700,000
2000–2005	+ 400,000
2005–2010	−500,000
2010–2015	−500,000
2015–2020	+ 100,000
2020–2025	+ 1,000,000
2025–2030	+ 500,000

As a rule, younger age groups need and prefer ambulant and ambulatory care facilities as well as appropriate housing. This also supports the proposal to favor community-based over institutional services.

The aging of the population leads to rising costs in the social sector, but with important variations. Social expenditures in the future will continue to concentrate on the lower and upper age groups. The younger benefit in the family and educational sectors, whereas the older get pensions and consume disproportionately high amounts and types of health care. Here the absolute numbers in each group become important: Austria, for instance, saw a decline in the school-age population by 300,000 between 1975 and 1985. However, there is a remarkable asymmetry in use between age groups: an adult over 60 on average consumes 5 times as many social sector benefits as an adult between 20 and 60.

Many questions need to be answered for effective planning to take place. We can project demographics, but do we know what type of health care needs will chiefly occur, health manpower training requirements, or the epidemiological prognosis in geriatric medicine? How can we grasp the issue of a changing family structure and division of responsibilities in relation to a state that tends to rely more and more upon the family for caregiving? Do politicians have accurate cost analyses at their disposal in order to make cost-effective allocations between institutional and community-based care? Obviously, moral, political, and administrative considerations will come into play in the resolution of these questions.

Finally, many discussions, including perhaps my own at the beginning of this chapter, sometimes leave the impression that to be very old means to be ill, and that a steep increase in the number of very old people in the near future will create an expenditure explosion in the health system. This is not the case based on available evidence.

Among the very old, many people are not severely ill. They rather suffer from sensory impairments, have difficulties with stairs, going shopping, carrying bags, and so on (Amann, 1980). Although there is a strong correlation between advanced age and multiple and chronic illnesses, a considerable number of the very old do not require continuous care. Often home care allows them to remain in their private homes. One, and not the weakest, explanation lies in the concept of "survivors"; among the very old are those who for physiological, environmental, and behavioral reasons, have outlived their contemporaries, who died "too early." We must consider that many very old people need health care less than they need social care, an insight documented already by Shanas et al. (1968).

In addition, despite general impressions, many studies show that the proportion of those who need permanent health care are still a minority—even among the very old. The age-dependent expenditure profile for health care shows an expected picture: there is a positive correlation between health expenditures per capita and age. However, the curve, which rises in a virtually linear pattern between the ages of 30 and 80, flattens out at that point. This is due to a shift from health to social care expenditures. We are dealing with a multifaceted problem: increasing numbers of very old people will require greater expenditures in the social care system, not necessarily in health care more narrowly defined.

In conclusion, let me quote from the *Vienna International Plan of Action* of the World Assembly on Aging, 1982: "The control of the lives of the aging should not be left solely to health, social service and other caring personnel [or, we might add, scientists], since aging people themselves usually know best what is needed and how it should be carried out."

REFERENCES

Altwerden in der Bundesrepublik Deutschland: Geschichte— *Situationen—Perspektiven* [Aging in the Federal Republic of Germany: History—situations—perspectives] (2nd ed., Vols. 1–3). (1987). Berlin: Deutsches Zentrum für Altersfragen.

Amann, A. (1980). *Open care for the elderly in seven European countries. A pilot study in the possibilities and limits of care.* Oxford: Pergamon Press.

Amann, A. (1981). *The status and prospects of the aging in Western Europe.* Vienna: European Center for Social Welfare Training and Research.

Amann, A. (1983). *Lebenslage und Sozialarbeit. Elemente zu einer Soziologie von Hilfe und Kontrolle* [State of living and social work. Elements for a sociology of help and control]. Berlin: Duncher & Humblot.

Amann, A. (Ed.). (1984). *Social-gerontological research in European countries. History and current trends.* Berlin (West): Deutsches Zentrum für Altersfragen; Vienna: Ludwig-Boltzmann-Institut für Sozialgerontologie.

Amann, A. (1985). *The changing age structure of the population and future policy* (Population Studies, No. 18). Strasbourg: Council of Europe.

Amann, A., Böhm, M., Kolland, F., & Penz, O. (1986). *Zum Glück Frühpension?* [Early retirement: A matter of good luck?] Unpublished manuscript, Vienna.

Callahan, D. (1986). Health care in the aging society: A moral dilemma. In A. Pifer & L. Bronte (Eds.), *Our aging society. Paradox and promise* (pp. 319–339). New York, London: W. W. Norton & Co.

George, M. V., & Perreault, J. (1985). *Population projections for Canada, provinces and territories 1984–2006.* Ottawa, Canada: Minister of Supply and Services.

Hoskins, I. (1987). Intergenerational equity: An overview of a public policy debate in the United States. *Ageing International, 14*(1), p. 5.

Morrison, M. H. (1986). Work and retirement in an older society. In A. Pifer & L. Bronte (Eds.), *Our changing society. Paradox and promise* (pp. 341–365). New York, London: W. W. Norton & Co.

Offe, C., & Hinrichs, K. (1984). Die Zukunft des Arbeitsmarktes. Zur Ergänzungsbedürftigkeit eines versagenden Allokationsprinzips [The future of the labor market. On the necessary completion of a failing allocation-principle]. In C. Offe (Ed.), *"Arbeitsgesellschaft." Strukturoprobleme und Zukunftsperspektiven* ["Labor-society." Structural problems and perspectives of the future] (pp. 87–117). Frankfurt, New York: Campus.

Rosenmayr, L. (1983). *Die späte Freiheit. Das Alter—Ein Stück bewußt gelebten Lebens* [Late freedom. Aging—a piece of consciously led life]. Berlin: Severin & Siedler.

Schade, B., und Kühne, S. (1986). Altern in Entwicklungsländern [Aging in developing countries]. *Zeitschrift für Gerontologie, 19*(2), 77–81.

Shanas, E., Townsend, P., Wedderburn, D., Friis, H., Milhoj, P., & Stehouwer, J. (1968). *Old people in three industrial societies.* London: Routledge & Kegan Paul.

Taylor, H. (1984). Welfare policy for the elderly. The politics of the periphery? In D. B. Bromley (Ed.), *Gerontology. Social and behavioural perspectives* (pp. 39–47). London, Sydney: Croom Helm.

23. Health and Aging from a Dutch Health Policy Perspective

HANNEKE M. TH. VAN MAANEN

PERSPECTIVES ON HEALTH CARE

Canada and the Netherlands appear to have many commonalities in their philosophy on health and well-being, reflected in the planning and organization of health care services. Historic ties and appreciation for each other's democracy may have strengthened the liaison between the countries and influenced certain developments, including advances in health care. In the Netherlands and in Canada there is a strong interest in the Health for All (HFA) strategy promoted by the World Health Organization. Its major components are health promotion throughout all phases of health and illness conditions, health maintenance, and consumer participation at the ground level of the health care system, that is, the community. This movement does not deny the occurrence of disease and illness, but seeks to redress the imbalance between sickness care and health care. According to van London (1987), the emphasis should shift from health care services to health policy strategies. It seems as if acute care services have become the main focus of advanced health care systems, with less emphasis on basic health care services (primary care of a general nature).

Without abandoning the gains of medical technology, the HFA strategy reemphasizes the value of community health services as the entry into the health system and as a screening mechanism for routine health issues. This ground-level health care ought to be easily accessible, of good quality, and provided at the cost a country can afford (World Health Organization/ UNICEF, 1978). In comparing reports from panels of experts in Canada such as Lalonde (1974), Epp (1986), Evans (1987), Spasoff (1987), Podborski (1987), and the *Ottawa Charter for Health Promotion* (1986) to

Aging and Health: Linking Research and Public Policy, © 1989 Lewis Publishers, Inc., Chelsea, Michigan 48118. Printed in U.S.A.

publications in the Netherlands such as the *Structuur Nota Hendriks* on the structure of the Dutch health care system (Ministry of Health and Environmental Hygiene [VOMIL], 1974); the *Nota 2000* (Ministry of Welfare, Public Health and Culture, 1986), a policy document of the Dutch Government issued in response to the Health for All (HFA) ideology of the World Health Organization; and most recently the Dekker Report, *Bereidheid tot verandering* (Commissie, 1987) with its recommendations for a radical change of the Dutch health care system, one may observe a great deal of similarity in the identification of health challenges and problems, and in the planning of health care trajectories for the future. Not all reports are clear in their definition of preventive health, health maintenance, and health promotion. There appears to be a tendency to emphasize health while focusing on the absence of disease and, by doing so, to conform to a medical model rather than a concept of health. One reason could be that for so long, medical care and health services have been used interchangeably.

NEEDS OF THE ELDERLY

This perspective has also governed the nature of care for the aging population. Under the influence of the biological and medical sciences, the process of aging has been described as the gradual deterioration of bodily function, resulting in dysfunction, disability, and disease. The potential for health, well-being, and functional ability has been undervalued and even grossly ignored. Our health care services focus primarily on the sick. The achievements of old age, such as wisdom, empathy, and the art of reflecting on life experiences, have hardly been unveiled (van Maanen, 1985). The ability to identify and to meet the health needs of the elderly, in particular the over-85 population, is still limited and primarily determined by knowledge and experience of younger adult populations, since neither the older nor the younger adults have ever been socialized with and exposed to the very old.

The Netherlands has already identified a group of over 550 centenarians (Centraal Bureau voor de Statistiek, 1986) and their number is steadily increasing. The growing number of near-centenarians challenges the health planners and policymakers to learn more about the upcoming generation of the very strong, the "SUR"vivors, and to meet the health needs of these elderly in a holistic and comprehensive manner. Acute care hospitals are not equipped to render the services the elderly need. Study findings among elderly people admitted to a large medical center in Denmark indicated— upon three measurements throughout the course of their stay—that patients' psychological health status deteriorated. The elderly expressed concerns that health professionals did not seem to listen to their health problems and that they appeared to be treated for other complaints than those indicated for admission (Lorensen, 1982). The iatrogenic effect of a "high-tech" environment ought to be modified into a therapeutic "high-touch" community that focuses on the delivery of comprehensive medical and nursing services that are safe and sound (International Council of Nurses, 1986).

Under the pressure of economic restraints, the Netherlands is facing continuing policy and planning changes. The welfare state of the '70s has gone through a systematic evaluation of its health care services. Despite the rapidly rising costs and the proliferation of health care programs, the health status of the population has not improved objectively; therefore, reallocation of scarce resources seems to be indicated (Commissie, 1987; Ministry of Welfare, Public Health and Culture [WVC], 1986).

LEVELS OF PLANNING AND ORGANIZATION OF HEALTH CARE

The Dutch nonprofit health care system is complex and unique. Although social insurance legislation is of considerable importance, the large private sector provides 25% of the resources of all health services. The majority of ambulatory (extramural) and institutional (intramural) services are rendered by independent corporate bodies, administered by independent private boards. The Sickness Funds that implement the social insurance legislation are independent juridical corporate bodies.

The extravagant cost increase, the unbalanced growth of the system, and the lack of cohesion among health services have resulted in increasing government regulation and intervention (Commissie, 1987; Rutten & van der Werff, 1982; van der Werff, 1982; WVC, 1986). The key problem at present is how to balance demand and supply. The Dutch have high expectations of a health care system that over the years has achieved a level of excellence that can no longer be maintained during a time of recession. The government is aiming at a reduction of supply; however, the Dutch people have difficulty accepting the use of regulatory mechanisms.

Changes at the governmental level have resulted in an "amalgamation" between the ministries responsible for health care and social services. Health services in the future will be organized and distributed under the legislation of the Provisions Public Health Act, the Public Health Insurance Act, and the Public Health Charges Act. Special councils will be responsible for a balanced distribution of services. More responsibility is delegated to the provinces and municipalities; the trend is to focus on deregulation and intersectoral collaboration. However, this delegation of responsibility is constrained by strict government guidelines such as volume, quality, price, cost, and financing regulations.

Traditionally, private enterprise has been very important in the Netherlands, reflecting personality characteristics of the Dutch: the urge for independence, individuality, and religious freedom (Hegyvary, 1982). Historically, the task of government was limited to the organization and financing of those factors that were beyond the control of individuals (Rutten & van der Werff, 1982). The government facilitated the conditions that enabled the private sector to plan and implement health services. Costs were established through a bargaining process between the providers and the Sickness Funds.

Quality control is one of the cornerstones of the health care system. Government inspections at the national, regional, and local levels are a guarantee to the public that quality care is delivered.

FINANCING OF HEALTH CARE SERVICES

Allocation of Resources

Public resources finance more than 75% of the total health expenditure (GNP 8.3% in 1986) (WVC, 1986). The expenditures represent direct payments from financing agencies to health care facilities, whereas private payments are covered by social insurance. Financing is regulated by legislation. Two important acts are the *Sickness Funds Insurance Act* (Ziekenfondswet [ZFW], 1964), which replaced the *Sickness Funds Decree* of 1941 and the *General Special Sickness Expenses Act* (Algemene Wet Bijzondere Ziektekosten [AWBZ], 1967).

Private insurance companies offer a broad range of insurance policies. People with incomes below Dfl. 49,650 in 1988 (approximately $33,100/ year) are insured with the Sickness Funds supervised by the Sickness Funds Council (Ziekenfondsraad). Individuals with income levels above Dfl. 49,650 must acquire private insurance against health care expenditures. The self-employed may subscribe to the public insurance on a voluntary basis. The premium is a fixed percentage of personal income—in 1988, 10.2%—to a maximum of Dfl. 3350 per year ($2233) for income levels up to Dfl. 35,000. Other rates apply for the income group of Dfl. 35,000 to Dfl. 49,650. Premiums are covered jointly by employer and the employee. All the members of a family are covered at no extra cost. Single persons pay the same contribution as a family (Groeneveld, 1988).

The *General Special Sickness Expenses Act* covers the risk of exceptional expenses such as those for long term care patients and the physically or mentally handicapped. Community nursing services since 1980 and ambulatory mental health services since 1982 have been covered by the same act. The premium is covered by the employer. Hospital, ambulatory, and professional health services are covered by either a tariff system or budget financing, or by a combination of both. Physicians' services fees are paid through a fixed amount of money per capita per year for those people who are publicly insured; private patients pay a fee for service reimbursed by the insurance. The fees are uniform throughout the entire country. Entry into the health care system is through the general practitioner, who is the only health professional who can refer a patient to a specialist or ambulatory services.

Financing of Health Care Services for the Elderly

Each Dutch citizen 65 years and over receives a basic pension upon retirement (General Old Age Pensions Act, 1957), which for most is complemented by a pension based on the previous salary (Blommenstijn, 1977). Retired elderly people enjoy the same benefits as other age groups.

In the past, if the elderly person's income fell below a minimum level, the Government would subsidize the insurance premium. However, recent changes (January 1987) in the social security system have resulted in a termination of the compulsory elderly insurance. If the recommendations of the "Dekker Report" (Commissie, 1987) are adopted, senior citizens will be entitled to basic health insurance that covers all Dutch citizens. This policy will not come into effect until 1990. This insurance, as it stands now, excludes services such as prescription drugs, medical appliances, and paramedical services in the community. Therefore, additional insurance is recommended.

It is expected that elderly people, whose disposable income decreased by almost 13% after 1981, following the recession, will not likely be able to afford additional insurance unless their income is supplemented by a regular pension. The Federation of Organizations of Senior Citizens (Centraal Orgaan Samenwerkende Bonden van Ouderen) has recommended the establishment of another compulsory health insurance scheme with premiums based on the individual's income in order to assure full coverage of health services regardless of the financial resources and objective health status of the elderly person (Centraal Orgaan, 1987; Landelijk Platform, 1987).

PERSONNEL

The care of the elderly is partially provided by health care personnel and partially by personnel employed by social services agencies. Community nursing services are staffed by qualified community health nurses (CHN) who are assisted with routine care by vocational nurses (VN) (6 CHN:1 VN). It includes the provision of hands-on care services as well as health counseling and guidance and health education.

Nursing homes are staffed by professional nurses in leadership positions and by vocational nurses trained in a two-year program in the care of the chronically ill and rehabilitation. Nursing auxiliaries are not officially employed in the Netherlands. However, under the current budget constraints, health care institutions tend to complement the limited staff with an increasing number of volunteers. Each nursing home has at least one full-time employed physician and a wide range of allied health professionals.

Hospitals are staffed by professional nurses who, in general, are trained in hospital-based nursing programs (four years). The limited number of independent nursing schools and colleges for medium level and higher education do not yet affect the size of the nursing work force.

The social service agencies are responsible for the training and employment of gerontological vocational helpers and aides. They are trained in either two- or one-year programs to provide community care to the elderly. These programs focus on the maintenance of self-care and independent living.

DELIVERY OF HEALTH SERVICES

Levels of Care

Health services are well developed at the primary, secondary, and tertiary levels of care. Cost control is not supposed to affect the accessibility or acceptability of services. Each citizen, including the elderly person, has free access to all health services. Since the country is so small, health facilities are within the reach of all citizens. Home calls are made by general practitioners, community health nurses, and those allied health professionals who practice in the community. Medical specialists consult at home only at the request of the general practitioner.

Since each health care institution has to meet minimal standards of quality care and operates within certain organizational and financial boundaries, the differences between facilities cannot be extreme. The health status indexes are high, but in the Netherlands, as in Canada, lower income groups show a higher prevalence of mortality and morbidity (WVC, 1986; Spasoff, 1987; Syme & Berkmann, 1976).

About 90% of the Dutch elderly live at home and about 10% receive institutional care under the health and social services systems. The average age of a nursing home resident has increased considerably over the last decade. Nursing homes, whether established as homes for the physically ill, for psychogeriatric patients, or for a combination of both, have three major functions: rehabilitation, care of the chronically ill, and care of the terminally ill. However, regardless of classification, all are entitled to the full range of required rehabilitation services.

A MODEL FOR THE INTEGRATION OF HEALTH SERVICES

The change in primary emphasis from sickness care to health promotion will have particular consequences for the elderly, who should be entitled to preventive health services at an earlier stage. It is an injustice to the senior citizens to ignore preliminary signs and symptoms of declining independence—frequently communicated in rather vague clues and symbols—and to postpone early intervention to the point that problems occur which require more extensive medical involvement. Building from the HFA strategy, a community-based model has been developed grounded in the integration of health and welfare services vital to maintaining the independence of senior citizens at home (see Figure 1). Emphasis is placed on preventive health services and health education for the well elderly within a 24-hour on-call availability of the support and professional services.

An example of 24-hour integrated services is the Dutch experiment in Tholen/St. Philipsland (Aertsen, 1987). Elderly persons who live independently in the community, but who could benefit from support services to maintain their self-care, should be entitled to some kind of "umbrella services" or sheltered care. The community is engaged in a more active outreach in order to facilitate people to maintain an independent household. Examples of such services are assistance with shopping, the availability of a centrally located alarm system, and friendly visiting (Valentijn, personal communication, September 1987).

If the elderly are entering an "at-risk zone," a home for the aged may be indicated, with emphasis on the maintenance of self-care rather than on the mastery of new skills. In the Netherlands, a so-called indication commission

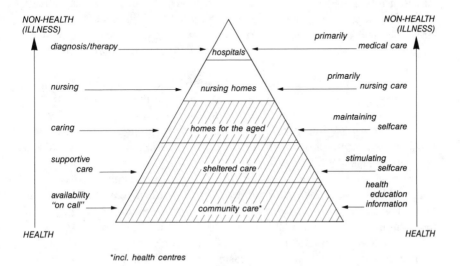

Figure 1. Structured health care services for the aged based on a health perspective.

will assess any senior citizen—upon his or her own request—who feels entitled to a caring institutional environment such as a home for the aged. The screening team, coordinated by local community authorities (town hall), includes a social worker, a general practitioner, and a community health nurse. From a health care perspective, professional help is available upon request and, in fact, strengthens the potential of health in the individual. The high-risk senior whose independence is at stake may sooner or later benefit from nursing home care with an emphasis on high-touch caring. Again, several modalities are possible, such as day- or night-care homes, outpatient rehabilitation programs, and respite care.

The frailer the elderly person, the higher the chance that a medical assessment is indicated and that the person has to be admitted to an acute care setting. In general, hospitals are not well equipped to serve the needs of the very old. The establishment of geriatric assessment units in general hospitals is a sincere effort to offer integrated, comprehensive health services from a multidisciplinary perspective. Medical diagnosis and treatment are offered with the goal that the quality of life should prevail over extending life with years. An example is the improvement in mobility after a total hip replacement (van Mansvelt, 1987). High-tech intervention could benefit many elderly if it is provided in an environment geared toward the specific needs of an aging population.

Under the current financial limitations, some hospitals have initiated plans to extend their services to the community. A similar suggestion has been presented in Canada by the Evans Committee (1987). However, in the Dutch situation this model is not congruent with modern concepts of the delivery of health instead of medical services only. If implemented, it would strengthen the medical approach to health services and suggest that the norm is hospital care rather than basic health care delivered from within the community.

To maintain health and independence (self-care, supportive care, professional care), many semi-institutional facilities have developed over the last 10 years, varying from day care centers to sheltered housing. A priority goal is to reestablish 24-hour accessible services and to strengthen the collaboration between community health and social services ("closed circuit") (Mootz & Timmermans, 1982).

However, satisfaction is not determined only by the quality of services rendered but also by the opportunities to implement change in living conditions. It may be true that elderly people in the Netherlands have been able to maintain rather comfortable lifestyles and that their desire for social change is less significant than peoples' in other countries. However, the change in social benefits, the increasing costs of living, and taxation will bring many of them close to or below the minimum income (Groeneveld, 1988). Organizations of elderly are expanding and developing more action programs. Health authorities and health professionals have to ensure that in a time of decreasing resources the elimination of health and welfare programs does not affect the well-being of the senior citizens.

Are they not the trendsetters of our own future?

REFERENCES

Aertsen, A. F. (1987, January). *De volumebeheersing in de subregio door middel van het experiment Tholen Sint/ Philipsland.* [Volume control in the sub-region by means of the experiment Tholen Sint/Philipsland.] Paper presented at the symposium "Volumebeheersing in de gezondheidszorg," Middleburg, Stichting Verpleeg—en Rusthuizen Zeeland.

Blommenstijn, P. J. (1977). *Contribution to the research project on open care for the elderly* (East-West comparison). The Hague: European Centre for Social Welfare Training and Research.

Centraal Bureau voor de Statistiek (CBS) [Central Bureau of Statistics]. (1986). The Hague: Staatsuitgeverij.

Centraal Orgaan Samenwerkende Bonden van Ouderen in Nederland (COSBO-Nederland). (1987). *Commentary to the Report Cie. Dekker presented to the members of the House of Commons of the Dutch Parliament by the Federation of Organizations of Senior Citizens* (Nr. G-87–488 B4723/PR/SR). The Hague: Tweede Kamer.

Commissie Structuur en Financiering Gezondheidszorg [Committee on Structure and Financing of Health Care]. (1987). *Bereidheid tot verandering* [Intention to change] (Report Cie. Dekker). The Hague: Staatsuitgeverij.

Epp, J. (1986). *Achieving health for all: A framework for health promotion.* Ottawa: Health and Welfare Canada.

Evans, J. (1987). *Toward a shared direction for health in Ontario.* (Report of the Ontario Health Review Panel). Toronto.

Groeneveld, F. (1988, January). Analysis of policy changes in the Dutch health care system. *NRC/Handelsblad,* Overzeese editie.

Hegyvary, S. T. (1982). *The change to primary nursing: A cross-cultural view of professional nursing practice.* St. Louis, MO: Mosby.

International Council of Nurses. (1986, June). *Mobilizing nursing leadership for primary health care.* ICN/86/157, (Workshop) Malaga, Spain. Geneva: ICN.

Lalonde, M. (1974). *A new perspective on the health of Canadians.* Ottawa: Information Canada.

Landelijk Platform van Consumenten (LPC). (1987). *Commentary to the Report Cie. Dekker presented to the members of the House of Commons of the Dutch Parliament by the National Patients/Consumers Platform* (Nr. 6–87–437, 2386/C 1003-Gn/gvm). The Hague: Tweede Kamer.

Lorensen, M. (1982, June). *Evaluation of the elderly person's need for nursing and health care in order to optimize the self-care potential and capability.* HOPE/INI. Paper presented at the First International Conference on Innovative Nursing Approaches in PHC of the Elderly, Millwood, VA.

Ministry of Health and Environmental Hygiene (VOMIL). (1974). *Structuur Nota* [Structure Document] (Report Hendriks). The Hague: Staatsuitgeverij.

Ministry of Welfare, Public Health and Culture (WVC). (1986). *Nota 2000 over de ontwikkeling van het gezondheidsbeleid: Feiten, beschouwingen en beleidsvoornemens* [Nota 2000 on the development of health policy: Facts, reflections and policy intentions]. The Hague: Staatsuitgeverij.

Mootz, M., & Timmermans, J. (1982). *Zorgen voor later, desiderata voor een toekomstig ouderenbeleid* [Caring for old age, criteria for future care of the aging] (SCP cahier nr. 26). Rijswijk: Sociaal en Cultureel Planbureau.

Ottawa Charter for Health Promotion (1986). Ottawa: Public Health Association. Ottawa: Canada.

Podborski. (1987). *Health promotion matters in Ontario* (A report of the Ministry Advisory Group on Health Promotion). Toronto: Ministry of Health.

Rutten, F., & van der Werff, A. (1982). *Health policy in the Netherlands at the crossroads* (Contribution to a comparative study of regulatory mechanisms in the health services). London: Nuffield Provincial Hospitals Trust.

Spasoff, R. A. (1987). *Health for all Ontario: Report of the Panel on Health Goals for Ontario*. Toronto: Ontario Ministry of Health.

Syme, S. L., & Berkmann, L. F. (1976). Reviews and complementary social class, susceptibility and sickness. *American Journal of Epidemiology, 104*(1), 1–7.

van London, J. (1987). Beschouwing over gezondheidsbeleid: Departmentale voordracht [Reflection on health policy: A departmental perspective]. In F. Schrameijer, J. M. Boot, E. Jurg, H. Saan, C. Tonnaer, & J. van der Velden (Eds.), *De Nota 2000 ter discussie* [The Nota 2000 discussion] (pp. 11–14). Reeks Gezondheidsbeleid, Alphen aan den Rijn: Samsom Stafleu.

van Maanen, J. M. Th. (1985). *Health as perceived by the aged.* Unpublished doctoral dissertation, University of California, San Francisco. San Francisco, CA.

van Mansvelt, J. (January, 1987). *De gevolgen van de regionale volume-ontwikkeling tegen de achtergrond van de vergrijzing* [The consequences of regional volume development with the context of graying of the population]. Paper presented at the symposium "Volumebeheersing in de gezondheidszorg," Middelburg, Stichting Verpleeg—en Rusthuizen Zeeland.

van der Werff, A. (February, 1982). *Overheidsbeleid, wetgeving en hun gevolgen voor de herstructurering van het kruiswerk* [Government policy legislation and their implications for the restructuring of the community health organization]. Paper presented at the Board conference "Restructuring of the Community Health Organization," Garderen, The Netherlands.

World Health Organization/UNICEF. (1978). *Primary Health Care.* ISBN 92 4 154350. Alma Ata, Geneva: WHO/UNICEF.

24. Private Versus Public Financing of Long Term Care in the United States

THOMAS N. TAYLOR

INTRODUCTION

Long term care encompasses a wide range of medical, social, and personal care services provided to those whose ability to care for themselves has been impaired by chronic physical or mental illness. These services include nursing home and home health care services in addition to a host of social and personal care services. Although the majority of long term care services are provided by family and friends in a residential setting, increasing numbers of elderly Americans are incurring the financial burden of home care services and extended stays in nursing homes.

Unlike short term medical care services, the majority of the expenditures on long term care are financed by the individuals (or their relatives) receiving care. Public funding for long term care for the elderly has concentrated on financing nursing home care for the elderly poor through the Medicaid program. Medicare, which covers approximately half of the elderly's total personal health care needs, provides little financial support for long term care. Moreover, private insurance for long term care services plays only a minor role, covering a scant 1% of total nursing home care expenses in 1985 (National Center for Health Statistics, 1986, Table 97).

The aging of the population has heightened interest in issues concerning the future financing of long term care in the United States. Increases, realized and expected, in life expectancy at all ages are expected to cause a dramatic increase in the demand for long term care services. This is particularly so for the oldest old, those aged 85 and over, who are the fastest growing among all age groups in the United States and who are most likely to need nursing home care. This demographic trend, combined with economic pressure to

Aging and Health: Linking Research and Public Policy, © 1989 Lewis Publishers, Inc., Chelsea, Michigan 48118. Printed in U.S.A.

shift patients from publicly financed acute care settings into residential and nursing home care settings is expected to contribute to a rapid rise in expenditures on long term care services.

Despite the general awareness of the problems concerning the financing of long term care, the United States Congress has been unwilling to support major new spending initiatives in this area. Projected deficits for Medicare's Hospitalization Insurance trust fund (HI) make further expansion of the Medicare program questionable, though not impossible in light of the expected passage of legislation providing coverage for catastrophic illness (Rovner, 1987a). Moreover, attempts to introduce any major new spending program are in direct competition with efforts to reduce the federal government's budget deficit (Rovner, 1987b). As a result, there has been increasing interest in efforts to encourage private financing for long term care services. The purpose of this chapter is to examine the implications of alternative funding mechanisms for long term care services.

FINANCING LONG TERM CARE IN THE UNITED STATES

Long term care, particularly nursing home care, is an expensive item for those who need it. Nursing home care is a catastrophic expense for most, averaging over $20,000 per year (Doty, Liu, & Weiner, 1985). Although only 5% of the elderly population in the United States currently resides in nursing homes, it has been estimated that for every nursing home resident there are two people with similar needs (Doty, Liu, & Weiner, 1985).

The present system of financing long term care in the United States relies on a combination of private and public funding sources. Over 50% of the $35.2 billion spent on nursing home care in 1985 was paid for out-of-pocket by the elderly or their relatives. Medicaid, the federal-state program designed to provide medical care for the poor, accounted for nearly 42%. Medicare, the federal program covering medical care expenses of the elderly, accounted for less than 2% of all nursing home care expenditures. Private insurance accounted for a meager 1%. These statistics exclude any measure of the value of care provided by family members, the single most important source of care provided to individuals with long term disabilities (Hughes, 1986, pp. 53–54).

Private Sources

The principal source of financing for long term care services remains individuals' out-of-pocket payments. Such payments may be financed out of current after-tax income (including pension and Social Security income) or by drawing upon wealth such as savings, housing, and other assets. Since average monthly nursing home charges exceed average monthly disposable income for the majority of elderly households, it is not uncommon for the elderly to have to use up their assets until their income and wealth has been reduced to levels qualifying for Medicaid assistance. This impoverishment of the elderly is one of the more contentious issues concerning the public financing of long term care in the United States today. One way in which the elderly in some states are able to avoid this predicament is by transferring wealth to family members in order to satisfy the spend-down requirements. This transfer, of course, merely shifts the burden of financing long term care from the family to the general population—it does not reduce it (Hughes, 1986, p. 187).

Private insurance for long term care is virtually nonexistent. Though a majority of the elderly have some form of nursing home coverage, these policies generally only extend existing Medicare coverage by paying deductibles and copayments and, in some instances, extending the coverage beyond Medicare's 100-day limit (Meiners, 1984). Since very few people qualify for Medicare's nursing home coverage, these "Medigap" plans provide little effective coverage for long term care.

Though there have been a number of new plans introduced in the last year or so, private insurance financing of long term care remains in its infancy. There are a number of reasons for this. Frequently cited is the problem of adverse selection, whereby those most in need of nursing home care are likely to purchase coverage, driving rates up and healthier enrollees away. Second, insurers claim that the presence of Medicaid prohibits the development of competing private insurance plans. In addition, insurers argue that uncertainty over future costs, difficulties in defining levels and types of care, and the impact of induced demand hinders the growth of these plans.

Public Sources

Public financing of health care took a monumental leap with the 1965 passage of the Medicare and Medicaid amendments to the Social Security Act of 1935. Since their passage, the public sector's share of personal health care expenditures has nearly doubled, rising from 22% in 1965 to 40% in 1985. More important, the federal and state governments have become full partners in the health sector. Because Medicaid and Medicare are entitlement programs—anyone qualifying for eligibility is legally entitled to the benefits—opportunities for controlling expenditures are limited. With rapidly rising expenditures absorbing more and more of the nation's resources, budget-weary legislators have renewed efforts to restrain the growth of expenditures in both programs.

Medicaid

The Medicaid program was established as a joint federal-state program to provide financing for acute and long term care for the elderly and nonelderly poor. The responsibility for administering the program rests with the individual states, with general guidelines and minimum standards set by the federal government. In 1985, the Medicaid program spent $39.8 billion in providing medical assistance to 21.1 million people, about 9% of the U.S. population (National Center for Health Statistics, 1986, Table 106).

Medicaid eligibility is means tested. Individuals are eligible for Medicaid benefits if they qualify for cash assistance such as Aid to Families with Dependent Children (AFDC). In addition, states have the option of extending Medicaid eligibility to the "medically needy," those who do not meet the strict income requirements of the cash assistance programs, but whose income after medical expenses falls within the program requirements. As of 1983 this spend-down option had been provided by 30 states (Davis & Rowland, 1986).

The program is financed out of general revenue by the states and by federal grants-in-aid (also from general revenues) determined by a formula based on state per capita income. The federal share ranged from 50% to 78% of total program expenditures in 1984 (Rabin & Stockton, 1987).

Medicaid provides financial relief for long term care expenses for those elderly meeting the eligibility guidelines. Spending on long term care services accounted for 37% of all Medicaid expenditures in 1985. Though accounting for only 14% of all Medicaid recipients, the aged accounted for nearly 38% of Medicaid expenditures in 1985.

Medicare

The Medicare program was designed to provide coverage primarily for the acute care needs of the elderly and disabled population. It provides only limited coverage of long term care expenses. Medicare is an entirely federally funded and administered program. Unlike the Medicaid program, which allows for considerable variation between states, Medicare eligibility requirements and the benefit structure are the same for all eligible Americans.

In 1985, Medicare spent $70.5 billion in providing coverage to 31.1 million enrollees (National Center for Health Statistics, 1986, Table 106). Medicare payments in 1984 covered 49% of the health care expenses of the elderly (Medicaid contributed 13% and other government programs another 6%). In 1984, out-of-pocket payments for health care averaged $1130 for the elderly versus $753 for the nonelderly population (Davis, 1987).

Medicare provides insurance coverage for acute care under two parts. Part A, or Hospital Insurance (HI), covers short term hospital care, limited skilled nursing home care, and limited home health care services. Part A coverage is available to all persons 65 and over who qualify for Social Security or Railroad Retirement benefits (about 95% of the elderly population) (Davis, 1987). It is funded by a 1.45% payroll tax levied on both the employer and the employee on earnings up to $43,800.

Although Medicare, like the Social Security system, is a pay-as-you-go transfer program, revenue from the payroll tax is accumulated in the Hospital Insurance trust fund for future disbursement. Current projections of revenue and expenses indicate that the HI trust fund will become exhausted around the turn of the century (Klees & Warfield, 1987). Although these estimates are sensitive to assumptions concerning (1) the performance of the economy, (2) labor force participation and earnings, and (3) future health expenditures, the growth of the retired population relative to the working-age population will make it increasingly difficult for the payroll tax to provide sufficient revenue to finance HI expenditures.

Part B, or Supplementary Medical Insurance (SMI), covers physician, hospital outpatient, and some additional home health and ambulatory care services. Unlike Part A, SMI is optional, though most people eligible for Part A coverage elect to receive Part B as well. Part B is financed by a combination of premiums and general revenue funding. Premiums are determined by Congress and provide approximately 25% of the revenue necessary to finance Part B expenditures. The remainder is financed by general revenues. Unlike Part A, there is no "solvency" problem with Part B financing, because any shortfall must be covered by general revenues. Given existing pressures to reduce the overall federal government budget deficit, however, increased attention is being paid to the rapid growth in the general fund contributions to Part B.

As mentioned above, Medicare provides very little coverage for long term care expenses. The nursing home and home health care coverage that does exist is for skilled care. Medicare (partially) covers 100 days of care in a Medicare-certified skilled nursing facility (SNF) for patients who had been hospitalized for at least three days for the same illness or injury. The average recipient of this benefit in 1981 was covered for only 27 days (Meiners & Gollub, 1984). This same approach of covering skilled care follow-up for acute illness and accidents applies to the home health care provisions.

Other Public Programs

There are a number of additional federal, state, and local programs supporting long term care for the elderly. The Veterans' Administration provides limited support for nursing home care for veterans. The Older Americans' Act provides support for in-home services such as home-delivered meals and personal care services. Title XX of the Social Security Act provides block grants to states to support community care services. These programs and others provide important services to the elderly and others in need of long term care, though their expenditures are small in comparison to Medicare and Medicaid.

HOW THE CURRENT SYSTEM RATES

The current system of financing long term care for the elderly relies heavily on out-of-pocket payments by those requiring nursing and home health care services. Medicaid provides a form of social safety net for the elderly poor and those impoverished by long term care expenses. As such, the burden of financing long term care services falls primarily on those unfortunate enough to need (primarily institutional) care.

From an efficiency standpoint, the current system's greatest shortcoming lies in its failure to provide effective insurance against catastrophic long term care expenses. Although the Medicaid system provides insurance against the possibility of not receiving needed care, it does not provide insurance against large financial losses. Nor does this appear to be a failure of demand. The elderly have demonstrated a willingness to purchase long term care insurance, even though these policies are of limited practical value.

The system must also be given low marks from an equity perspective. The current heavy emphasis on out-of-pocket payments for long term care, though consistent with the benefits principle, places heavy burdens on those who need care irrespective of their ability to pay. Moreover, the reliance of Medicaid on general revenue funding (though itself mildly progressive) places the burden of this financing on the current working population. Because the elderly as a whole (though certainly not the elderly qualifying for Medicaid) now have a lower poverty rate than the nonelderly population, it is no longer clear that intergenerational transfers from the nonelderly to the elderly population are consistent with the ability-to-pay principle. To be sure, the current nonelderly population will eventually become the elderly population, but demographic forces make it questionable whether future generations will be able to finance even the level of benefits currently provided. Either the current nonelderly population will face the prospect of reduced real health care benefits, or their children will be forced to assume a still greater burden of long term care financing.

HOW THE ALTERNATIVES RATE

Whereas many choose to view the debate over private versus public financing of long term care services as pitting a choice between two clear alternatives, whatever the mix of private and public sources of financing, it is individuals who must ultimately pay. Moreover, in some cases distinctions between private and public financing of health care may mean little, if anything at all. For example, it makes little difference whether workers' health insurance is financed "publicly" through payroll taxes or "privately" through mandatory coverage paid by the employer. In either case, most economists would agree that the ultimate burden of financing such activities would fall on workers in the form of reduced after-tax wages.

Private Sources of Finance

Private Insurance

Private insurance coverage for long term care services, though not currently an important source of financing, is expected to play a much more important role in the near future. Although it remains to be seen which type of long term care policies will stand the test of the marketplace, two basic types of policies are most frequently discussed. Individual coverage is generally designed for the young elderly (under age 75) and marketed to individuals. Group coverage, also often for those aged 75 and under, is now being marketed to employers to be included with postretirement health benefits (Burda, 1987).

There are a number of potential advantages to private insurance coverage. First, as insurance, these plans provide protection against the catastrophic expenses of nursing home care. Second, because employee benefits are not taxed, employer-financed long term care insurance may be viewed by both employers and employees as an attractive alternative to wage and salary increases.

There are, however, a number of potential disadvantages. First, premiums rise rapidly with age, so that those facing the greatest risk of incurring catastrophic nursing home expenses are least likely to be able to afford insurance. Second, the potential financial burden on employers is great, which in itself is likely to prevent most employers from offering such coverage. Moreover, given that such coverage would not have to be "pre-funded" as are pension funds, the burden of financing these benefits would fall on the current labor force. The growth of the retired relative to the working population will cause the same fiscal problems currently faced by Medicare. Third, even under the most optimistic assumptions, a large percentage of the elderly population will not have employer-provided insurance, and many of these will be unable to afford individual plan rates. Finally, the potential is great for "cream-skimming," wherein employer-sponsored long term care programs cover the healthy, low risk population. If these group plans were to cover those least likely to need nursing home care, the individual rates for the rest of the elderly population would become prohibitively high.

Home Equity Conversions

Home equity conversions are schemes to tap a principal source of the elderly's wealth—the equity in their homes—to provide funds for long term care services. A "reverse mortgage" is one such arrangement, whereby home equity is used to secure an agreement from a bank or savings institution, which provides monthly payments to the homeowner in exchange for a promise to repay the "loan" though proceeds from the eventual sale of the house (Jacobs & Weissert, 1986). The stream of income generated from the home equity could then be used to finance long term care insurance or to pay for home health care services.

Freeing up private wealth to finance the long term care needs of the elderly has some advantages. First, there is a large and potentially growing share of the elderly population who could use home equity conversion to finance at least part of their long term care needs (perhaps one third to one half of the elderly with high risk of home care needs) (U.S. House of Representatives, 1986). Second, home equity as a source of finance for long term care services will grow with the aging of the population. Third, home equity conversions provide an opportunity for the elderly in need of assistance to remain in their homes for a longer period of time than would otherwise be possible. Finally, as a private source of finance, home equity conversions are likely to be viewed favorably during times of fiscal austerity.

Home equity conversion has a number of shortcomings. First, the small number of home equity conversions attempted to date reflects a reluctance on the part of both homeowners and financial institutions to pursue this option. Homeowners appear to be leery of making a commitment involving the eventual liquidation of their single largest asset. Bankers appear to be reluctant to offer such arrangements because of a lack of mortgage insurance, the problem of foreclosing on elderly who have exhausted the equity in their homes, and the lack of appreciation of older homes (U.S. House of Representatives, 1986).

Life Care Communities

Life care communities are formal arrangements providing housing, meals, housekeeping, and social and personal services for the elderly for the remainder of their years. These communities, frequently nonprofit and church affiliated, agree to provide a set of services for members for a large entrance fee ($4000 to cover $100,000 in 1984) and monthly payments (averaging $562 per month in 1981) (U.S. House of Representatives, 1986). Many elderly use the equity in their homes to pay the steep entrance fees and apply pension and Social Security income to the monthly charges. Still, for many elderly, life care communities are beyond their financial means.

Life care communities offer a combination of insurance against long term care needs and an integrated approach to providing health, social, and personal care services. As such, they represent one of the few means by which the elderly can protect themselves against the catastrophic expenses of long term care. For many elderly who wish to remain in their homes, however, life care communities, with their emphasis on centralized living arrangements, are not likely to be very appealing.

Public Financing Options

The public financing options examined below include only alternative revenue sources. Public policies such as tax incentives for privately purchased insurance coverage or premium subsidies are not explicitly examined. Such policies, however, entail either direct (subsidies) or indirect (tax incentives) funding. Although the nature of these policies is not explicitly discussed here, the major revenue sources to finance them are.

Payroll Tax

Currently, the principal source of finance for the Medicare program, the payroll tax, could conceivably provide the financing for long term care. Such a measure would require overcoming substantial political opposition. Medicare's funding woes, combined with concern over the budget deficit, make it doubtful that rate increases or a broadening of the base (e.g., eliminating the earnings ceiling) would be used for anything other than restoring solvency to the HI trust fund.

Even if political opposition could be overcome, it is not clear that it would be desirable to use the payroll tax to finance long term care. First, the payroll tax is more or less regressive. Whereas it is progressive at low incomes because transfer payments are not counted as earnings, it becomes regressive for higher income earners because of the earnings ceiling ($43,800) and because unearned income (interest, dividends, capital gains, etc.) escapes taxation.

Moreover, increases in the age-dependency ratio mean that long run growth in earnings is unlikely to keep pace with the long term care needs of the elderly population over the next 50 years or so. This lag means an increasing share of the burden of financing long term care would be shifted onto the young. Although administrative costs may be relatively low, the payroll tax would appear to be a poor choice for funding long term care needs.

General Revenue Taxes

Individual and corporate income, excise, and other revenue sources constitute general revenues. These are likely to play an increasingly important role in financing long term care, if only because they are the source of the federal share of Medicaid expenses. Political pressure to reduce the federal budget deficit makes it somewhat difficult to commit additional general revenue funds to finance additional long term care expenditures. General revenue sources are probably the most progressive source of funding, however. Moreover, because the tax base for general revenues is so broad, its growth can be expected to match the pace of overall economic growth. Although overall administrative costs are not low, the additional administrative cost is likely to be trivial.

Select Excise Taxes

Long and Smeeding (1984) have proposed increasing the excise taxes on tobacco products and alcoholic beverages. They argue that in addition to raising revenue, such corrective taxes would reduce activities known to contribute to illness and injury. Though increasing taxes on tobacco and alcohol sounds like a good idea, the strength of these revenue sources over the long run is questionable. First, substantial tax increases are likely to add to the decline in cigarette and alcohol consumption. Although this is undoubtedly desirable, it reduces the revenue yield from these sources. Moreover, though it is clear that society would benefit from reduced cigarette and alcohol consumption, it is not clear that such reductions would lead to reduced health expenditures. Indeed, to the extent that reduced cigarette and alcohol consumption increases life expectancy, one would expect to see an increase in long term care expenses.

Estate and Gift Taxes

Estate taxes are levied on property holdings at the time of death. Gift taxes are levied on transfers of property from one individual to another. Since 1977, federal estate and gift taxes have been integrated under the Unified Transfer Tax. Federal estate and gift taxes accounted for less than 1% of total federal revenue collected in 1984 (Browning & Browning, 1987, Tables 1–3).

Estate and gift taxes offer some advantages as a potential source of funding for long term care services. First, as a relatively untapped revenue source, they represent a politically more appealing target than some of the more heavily used alternatives. Second, estate and gift taxes are likely to be one of the faster growing revenue sources as the population ages. Third, the rate structure for estate and gift taxes is the most progressive (at least in design) of all the taxes.

The efficiency effects of estate and gift taxes are not clear. Because estate taxes lower the net value of bequests, some argue that they would tend to discourage the accumulation of wealth. On the other hand, estate taxes may encourage the accumulation of wealth among those who are concerned with providing a given after-tax bequest. Unfortunately, little is known about the behavioral effects of estate and gift taxes.

SUMMARY AND CONCLUSIONS

This chapter has pointed out the financial burden faced by elderly Americans in need of formal long term care assistance. The current system of relying more or less equally on private out-of-pocket payments and Medicaid coverage for the poor and near-poor elderly leaves much to be desired. Reliance on out-of-pocket payments places relatively greater burdens on lower income groups. Moreover, both the public sector and the private sector have failed to provide adequate insurance against the risk of severe financial loss, although recent developments in private long term care insurance appear promising.

Among the options considered potential new private sources of financing for long term care services, private insurance coverage appears to hold the most promise. Whether in the form of (1) individual policies, (2) group policies offered through employers, or (3) insurance embodied in life care communities, private long term care insurance appears to be ready to play a larger role in long term care financing.

While private provision of long term care insurance would lessen the pressure for public financing, it will never provide coverage for all Americans. Individual policies are expensive to market and difficult to design to minimize the adverse selection problem. Group policies would be cheaper, but if provided by employers, would shift the burden of financing onto employees. With international competition putting pressure on businesses to reduce the costs of production, it seems unlikely that employers will flock to provide long term care insurance. Similarly, opportunities to insure against long term care expenses with life care communities are limited by the reliance of those communities on centralized living arrangements.

Although opportunities for expanded private initiatives clearly exist (and are being pursued), a need for substantial public financing of long term care services will continue to exist. If the public sector's role in financing long term care services is to be expanded, the revenue generated will have to be sufficient to meet the future needs of the elderly population. It would appear that existing and future funding needs will preclude the use of the payroll tax as a major source of long term care financing. Similarly, the many competing demands on general revenue sources (individual and corporate income taxes especially) may make it difficult to tap these sources as well. Although excise taxes on cigarettes and alcohol are desirable on efficiency grounds, they are unlikely to provide the kind of growing tax base necessary to support future long term care financing needs. A value-added tax could provide the necessary revenue, though it would probably be regressive. Estate and gift taxes, on the other hand, would appear to be a viable source of funding for long term care needs, though probably with substantial increases in the rates.

REFERENCES

Browning, E. K., & Browning, J. M. (1987). *Public finance and the price system.* New York: Macmillan.

Burda, D. (1987, September 20). The nation looks for new ways to finance care for the aged. *Hospitals,* 48–54.

Davis, K. (1987, Winter). Medicare financing and beneficiary income. *Inquiry, 24,* 312.

Davis, K., & Rowland, D. (1986). *Medicare policy: New directions for health and long term care* (pp. 51–55). Baltimore: Johns Hopkins University Press.

Doty, P., Liu, K., & Weiner, J. (1985, Spring). An overview of long term care. *Health Care Financing Review, 6,* 74.

Hughes, S. (1986). *Long term care: Options in an expanding market.* Homewood, IL: Dow Jones-Irwin.

Jacobs, B. & Weissert, W. G., (1986, Winter). Helping protect the elderly and the public against the catastrophic cost of long term care. *Journal of Policy Analysis and Management, 5,* 378–83.

Klees, B., & Warfield, C. (1987, June). Actuarial status of the HI and SMI Trust Funds. *Social Security Bulletin, 50,* 11–20.

Long, S. H., & Smeeding, T. (1984, spring). Alternative Medicare financing sources. *Milbank Memorial Fund Quarterly/Health and Society, 62,* 325–348.

Meiners, M. R. (1984, January). The state of the art in long term care insurance. In U.S. Department of Health and Human Services, Health Care Financing Administration, *Long Term Care Financing and Delivery Systems: Exploring Some Alternatives, Conference Proceedings.* Washington, DC.

Meiners, M. R., & Gollub, J. O. (1984, March). Long term care insurance: The edge of an emerging market. *Healthcare Financing Management,* 58–62.

National Center for Health Statistics. (1986, December). *Health, United States, 1986* (DHHS Publication No. PHS 87–1232).

Rabin, D. L., & Stockton, P. (1987). *Long term care for the elderly: A factbook.* New York: Oxford University Press.

Rovner, J. (1987, October 31). Catastrophic-costs measure back on track despite delays. *Congressional Quarterly,* 2677–2682.

Rovner, J. (1987, November 21). Pepper wins a round on long term care bill. *Congressional Quarterly,* 2874–2875.

U.S. House of Representatives. (1986, July). *Long term care services for the elderly: Background materials on financing and delivery of long term care services for the elderly* (pp. 40–44). Washington, DC: U.S. Government Printing Office.

PART III

Performing Effective Gerontological Research

25. Research, Policy, and the Delivery of Care to the Elderly

MALCOLM L. JOHNSON

INTRODUCTION

The challenges which arise from the demographic revolution are undeniable. In Canada, as in Britain, the expectation of life at birth has grown by half since the turn of the century. Twenty-five years has been added to the average life span. It is a spectacular achievement, not least because it is—plagues and nuclear war apart—a permanent gain for human kind. The number of people over 85 in both our societies will double by the year 2005. More than a million British will be octogenarians, and older as we enter the third millennium. In Britain, the number of people living beyond 100 years has increased 10-fold in the last decade, from 300 to 3000.

In our right minds, we would be hanging out the bunting and celebrating this magnificent shift from a population that throughout history has been stunted and curtailed by sickness, disability, and premature death. Our demographic profile moves from a pyramid to a rather shapely barrel—from an artificially young population to one that is for the first time in recorded history properly mature. Having one fifth to one fourth of our number beyond the age of 60 is a *normality* we have failed to achieve before.

How do we respond to such news? In most of the developed Western societies, the predominant cry has been a wail about the burden of an aging population. Governments and their apologists see only the costs and none of the benefits. Their pained pronouncements are replete with projections of dependency ratios, increases in health, social care, and social security budgets. Britain and the United States have been in the forefront of the approach I will call a historical economic barbarism. By that, I mean an approach to the needs of older people which is ignorant of or misinformed about history,

Aging and Health: Linking Research and Public Policy, © 1989 Lewis Publishers, Inc., Chelsea, Michigan 48118. Printed in U.S.A.

which assumes that the current distribution of resources across the generations is the limit of what can be afforded.

As Peter Laslett (1987) has pointed out in his article "The Emergence of the Third Age," Britain is in the second division in the international league of life expectancy—Canada is in the first (75 years and over)—with expectancies at birth of 70–74 years, sharing its position with countries as diverse as Italy, Israel, and Puerto Rico, only 1 point ahead of Costa Rica, Jamaica, and Taiwan. It is interesting and instructive that countries like these which observe a new dimension of longevity, but are not yet overwhelmed with an aged population (a situation that pertains in Canada, with less than 10% over 65) are making more intelligent, less hysterical plans for lifelong caring services.

It is encouraging to know that China, which imminently faces an elderly population of staggering size, has opened itself to learning from and adapting the experience of other societies. Here in Canada, which has its share of prophets of the elderly-induced apocalypse, there is a calmer and more mature approach. Robert and Rosalie Kane (1985), in their detailed comparative study of long term care in Ontario, British Columbia, and Manitoba, drawing out lessons for the United States, wrote:

> The aging of the United States population has been looked upon as a fiscal crisis. The effectiveness of programs is measured by their ability to control costs. . . . Public and scientific statements in Canada are calmer than the crisis-oriented pronouncements in the United States. . . . Canadian analysts make frequent references to offsetting reductions in the number of other dependent groups, especially children.

Perhaps the virtual absence of Canadian analyses of aging by political scientists and by economists, rightly lamented by Victor Marshall in his Introduction to *Aging in Canada* (1987), has benefits after all!

RESEARCH AND POLICY

The problems that undoubtedly accompany longer life—both for individuals and for societies—will find no solution in contemporary policies strapped by financial controls. Research has a profoundly important role in helping societies and their policymakers to properly understand the social, psychological, and medical correlates of aging. At the same time, we need to provide a clearer picture of old age in earlier times, the nature of intergenerational relationships, and the distribution of wealth and income among the old. Being old is not a pathology; it is normal. Like earlier life stages, it contains patterns of health and welfare, poverty and wealth that are also normal. Until we have a confident sense of what normal aging is *throughout the life span,* there will be no intelligent use of caring and support services.

Regarding policy and service delivery, two distinct but interrelated modes of research are essential. First and foremost is the body of knowledge (1) about the processes of aging and old age, and (2) about the social and organizational settings in which they take place and in which care and support are provided. Well-grounded decisions about services cannot be made unless we have reliable theory and data about such matters as population change, the epidemiology of late-life illnesses, family and friendship patterns, the history of multigenerational family units as opposed to other living arrangements, the extent and nature of religious observance, or the way memory functioning changes throughout the life span.

Those things we choose to call *services* only become so when some needed and wanted assistance is rendered in an acceptable form. Not infrequently, what is intended to be a service fails to meet these criteria. A study I conducted on Meals on Wheels and luncheon clubs some years ago (Johnson, di Gregorio, & Harrison, 1981) revealed how comprehensively this provision failed to meet its objectives. Yet they continued to operate on a vast scale because older people did not complain and professionals continued to assume they knew what was good for them. It represented a lack of research-based knowledge about the eating patterns of elderly people at the outset and a failure to evaluate on the other.

Thus, it is important in the framing of new services to draw upon what the general corpus of research tells us about the subject area. In retrospect, it seems ludicrous that professional people should send no-choice meals around the countryside, keep them warm in a tin box by heat of a candle for an average of one and one half hours, and expect they were providing a valued nutritional service.

By the same token, many vaunted beliefs about the all-embracing three-generational cohabiting family of the 19th century and its care for its older members are myths. Despite this, family care represents 80% of all personal care, and as Neena Chappell (1983) has shown, many older people prefer help from their nonrelated age peers rather than from their children. Also, the Swedish researcher Alvar Svanborg (1987) has shown that 60% of people over 80 have no evidence of coronary heart disease and that joint and back complaints do not increase after age 70.

Both policy and service innovation can spring from well-meaning but untutored personal prejudice. As yet, too few policymakers or practitioners are in command of the body of knowledge, with the consequence that commonsense innovations can become established practices. Straightforward research of a kind that may have no policy objectives remains vitally important. The current emphasis on policy relevance represents an overcorrection of previously anarchic patterns of inquiry.

Once new policies and services are put into practice, the common experience is for them to be reproduced and disseminated on the basis of enthusiastic advocacy of their effectiveness. Meals on Wheels is a good example. Until recent times, homemaker services excluded dusting the tops of cupboards, cleaning windows, and shopping—all tasks much required by the disabled elderly person. Evaluation and reformulation in a portable form are increasingly recognized as indispensable ingredients in service development. Such testing will teach us as much about what *not* to do as what is truly effective in recreating health and independence. Both are important.

THE GLOUCESTER PROJECT

To narrow down the discussion further, let us consider the problems facing a typical Health Authority in the United Kingdom. It is likely to serve a population of 350,000 people and contain one large district general hospital and a number of smaller hospitals, some of which provide for elderly long-stay patients. In addition, it is linked with primary health care teams in each locality. A common size for these teams would be four primary care physicians with associated home nurses, health visitors, a social worker, and practice manager. Together they will serve about 9000 people of all ages, 1 in 5 of whom will be over retirement age.

Health Authority managers will be concerned about provision for older people and will observe within their district the following:

- expensive and not very well used geriatric services
- "bed blockage" by elderly patients whose delayed recovery or multiple illnesses prevent discharge
- appalling discharge arrangements with very little community follow-through
- too many hospital admissions, because both health and social care in the community is poorly organized
- primary health care teams good at routine medicine, but with no links to social services departments, voluntary bodies, or informal caregivers

This not uncommon depiction was present in the city and district of Gloucester in 1984, when the District General Manager approached me to help construct a more appropriate strategy and to evaluate it. The opportunity was an uncommon one because it is rare for such service organizations in Britain to set aside large sums of money for research or to engage with a university academic department. To ensure that a wider range of knowledge and skills was available, I drew in two colleagues to form a research team—one a gerontologist and social worker by background, the other a policy analyst with experience in consulting. Later a postdoctoral Research Fellow joined the team, physically based in Gloucester.

I intend to provide a description of this project—now halfway through its three-year life—not because it is a model of research and policy in practice, but because it is a suitable case study, where we have tried to implement certain self-imposed rules and procedures.

Before any staff were employed on the project, the core research team spent a year gathering local information and discussing ideas and problems with the District Management Group. They fed in the problems, and we contributed our knowledge of the literature. What resulted was a joint product, containing highly specific practical problems and knotty academic issues. From the outset, the objective was to find ways of improving the health of older people at home—especially those at risk of hospitalization or transfer to a residential home. Five elements became central:

1. that primary health care teams should be the focal area of service delivery;
2. that special attention should be given to devising more sensitive and effective ways of understanding (diagnosing) the treatable needs and requirements of older people;
3. that for purposes of the project, specialist care workers (later called care coordinators) would be located in primary health care teams;
4. that there should be innovation in the creation and monitoring of individualized packages of care which transcend traditional boundaries;
5. that the resulting changes in practice should be systematically monitored and, as far as possible, evaluated and costed.

These elements include the adaptation of several already evaluated innovations (e.g., use of *keyworkers* and creation of *packages of care*) as well as entirely new approaches (e.g., *biographically based assessment interviews*). Our concern was to integrate knowledge as well as to extend innovation.

THE SCHEME

The scheme centers around three care coordinators. They were appointed for the life of the project to work as members of three primary health care teams (PHCTs) in the Gloucester area which volunteered to help with the project. They come from different backgrounds: one is a district nurse on secondment, another is a graduate teacher and social work assistant, and the third has a degree and experience as a cardiographer and nursing auxiliary. Personal abilities rather than a particular background were sought, and all three have integrated well into their PHCT without being assumed to be part of any particular professional group.

The care coordinators were given a dual role. They were asked to be researchers, finding out about the needs of elderly people in the practice areas, about what services were available, and how those services were being used and might be used. They were also asked to take on a caseload and work with individual elderly people to assess their needs and then put together a package of care to assist them.

The PHCTs were asked to refer elderly people whom they felt were at risk of no longer being able to cope in their own homes. The research team provided a list of at-risk indicators that had been derived from the literature. It was important to identify elderly people who were at risk before a major crisis challenged their independence. The list of indicators was revised in the light of the first few months' experience as follows:

- elderly people living alone, with a caregiver or family, any of whom are showing signs of stress
- elderly people suffering from senile dementia or whose confusion may indicate senile dementia
- elderly people under pressure to move from their own home or who are thinking of giving up their home for any other reason
- elderly people who are experiencing social isolation, resulting in distress or depression
- elderly people with significant health or social needs who are refusing offers of service or support
- elderly people who have recently had a fall

ASSESSMENT

An important feature of the project is an attempt to devise new approaches to the assessment of need. Much work has gone into constructing and refining a biographically based assessment tool. Early work began with guided reading and a series of training workshops conducted by myself and Brian Gearing. Our purpose was to explain the rationale behind life history interviews and to develop skills required in a listening and noninterrogative approach.

At first the care coordinators conducted full-length biographical interviews, which were tape recorded and transcribed for group analysis. To help them, I devised the Lifetime Chart as a short-form guide to the interview. This has proved a durable part of the exercise nearly 200 cases later. To accompany it, we produced a Biographical Record, which summarizes the essential detail for other care workers to see in the file.

The biographical approach involves an assessment that begins with the person. A rapport is established in which the care coordinator knows something about the client and can relate the past life with current needs. Current needs can then be discussed with the elderly person and any caregivers involved on the basis of a sympathetic relationship. The individual's needs are considered before selection of services.

As the process of using life histories for assessment became more refined and therefore less lengthy, a companion Assessment Checklist was devised to incorporate the best features of existing functional assessment schemes.

PACKAGE OF CARE

The elderly person agrees to a plan proposed by the care coordinator. The aim is to establish a package of care in which support and assistance from different sources are fitted together to help maintain the elderly person in the home and maximize independence. This may include, for example, district nursing, home care (perhaps from a private agency), a volunteer visitor, or regular visits to day centers. It may also include things like renewing old friendships, visits to a family center, or joining a craft center. The care coordinator will also be able to coordinate the use of these services with the support caregivers or relatives give.

The principal role of the care coordinator is to coordinate existing services, but they do provide two important direct services: counseling elderly people about their situation and providing information, advice, and help in claiming benefits. By establishing their interest in the person early on, care coordinators often become particularly trusted. The role of counselor also extends to caregivers—care coordinators are often sought out by caregivers looking for someone who can understand their problems and who knows what practical solutions are available. All three care coordinators have become involved in local caregivers' support groups. The rules and procedures surrounding the various benefits are complex, and advice centers do not provide a domiciliary service. Besides advising people about their entitlements, the care coordinators also assist in filling out forms and writing letters.

The care coordinators have very small budgets to provide instant cash to assist people, though the budgets are not to be used to make up shortfalls in social security. An important use has been to unlock other sources of funding, e.g., to finance laundry payments while the claim for laundry costs is established. The payments can then be reclaimed and returned to the budget.

RESEARCH

Because the service being developed was exploratory rather than a model service, it was decided early on that a systematic experimental evaluation with a control group would be inappropriate. Instead, the research component of the project has been developed as "action research," making it a virtue that the exact nature of the care coordinator role was not settled when the project started. The role has developed with the project. For example, whereas care coordinators put effort into working with groups in the early months of the project, they now concentrate more on individuals referred by the PHCT.

The care coordinators keep diaries of their activities so that their developing role can be studied in retrospect. We also require them to keep far more detailed notes on their work with individual elderly people than would be practical for a normal service. Checklists designed so that information can be coded and transferred to computer for quantitative analysis are completed for each individual. The checklists include basic factual information about the individuals' present situations and their apparent needs. Besides being used for research purposes, these forms are also the basis for a case review held at six-month intervals on the work done with and for that person. The aim is to have a systematic component in the case recording process that will complement the fuller, person-centered biographical notes.

In addition to gathering data on the work of the care coordinators, the research team is also gathering data on the work of PHCTs in the area and the relative costs of different community services for elderly people at home. Before the project is complete, consumers and professionals who have been in contact with it will be interviewed to find out how useful they feel the approach being developed is.

IMPLEMENTATION

The Health Authority included development funds for community services for elderly people in its strategic plan at the same time that the research project was set up. While the research project has been developing, the Health Authority has been reviewing its services for elderly people in consultation with the Social Services Department, Housing Department, Family Practitioner Committee, Community Health Council, and voluntary organizations. This review has resulted in a report by the District General Manager proposing a strategy with specific recommendations. The Care for Elderly People at Home project was able to feed into the review both by publishing working papers and by having a member of the research team on the review group.

What are we able to say to policymakers at this stage? There are four main messages that we have fed from the field research back to the managers and policymakers:

1. There seems to be a role for a keyworker to work with elderly people in the community at risk of no longer being able to stay in their homes. There seems no compelling reason why the key role should be played by any particular professional or, indeed, by a professional worker at all. (It might be an appropriate role for a relative or a home care assistant without formal training or qualifications.)

2. If the idea of having keyworkers with elderly people is to work, keyworkers must be part of a wide team of professionals in the community and be accepted by them as the key point of communication about the person they are all working with. This means the development of teamwork, both within the PHCT and in a broader context across the boundary between health and social services workers.

3. Developing the notion of *keyworker* with elderly people and the conditions for multidisciplinary work requires an improvement in the flow of information between workers in the community. New approaches have to be developed, such as transferring information common to different assessments at the time a person is referred, and joint training that fosters a reciprocal understanding of professional roles and skills and encourages respect and understanding of the rights and wishes of elderly people.

4. Although there are resource problems in specific areas (e.g., insufficient day centers, transport, district nurses, or home care assistants), these are well recognized by managers and are being tackled as well as they can be in a climate of chronic underfunding. The problems much more difficult to identify, and sometimes even more difficult to tackle, have to do with communication between (1) hospital and community staff, (2) health and social services staff, (3) the voluntary sector and the public services sector, and (4) the professional caregivers and the informal, unpaid, and often unrecognized caregivers. In all these relationships, there are effects on both the long term planning and development of services and the everyday care of particular elderly people.

All four of these messages have been recognized in the review of services for elderly people, and the research team will be represented on the group implementing recommendations arising from the review.

CONCLUSION

These descriptions of a project in process are, I hope, of interest in themselves. But they serve principally to illustrate earlier themes about the desirable links between research, policy, and practice. In such a formulation, we have found a wide range of research problems—ethical concerns about life history data and others about the meaning, interpretation, and veracity of these personal accounts. These are intimately linked with the problems of everyday practice and professional credibility faced by our coworkers, the care coordinators.

Our action research orientation requires the research team to constantly feed back its findings to senior management and to other professionals, who are both curious and threatened. This very involvement is what guarantees access to and involvement in the policy process. Our work has already helped to shape priorities and patterns of work for the next decade.

Despite this influence we refuse to recommend the role of care coordinators to others who would admire and initiate. It is an important principle that we should not promote our ideas until they have been fully evaluated. Indeed, it already looks likely that the care coordinators will prove too costly an option, so we are working on a distillation of the role in order to provide a training manual for existing staff to take on the keyworker tasks.

It is by adopting more self-critical approaches and more consumer-centered modes of caring support, that professional caregivers can become more cost-effective in enhancing the health of older people. In this process, both fundamental and evaluative research is an indispensable component. But equally important is its transmission into usable policy and workable practice. We as researchers need increasingly to be interpreters, policy analysts, and teachers if good and tested ideas are to change the way we support our elders.

REFERENCES

Chappell, N. (1983). Informal support networks among the elderly. *Research on Aging, 5*(1).

Johnson, M. L., di Gregorio, S., & Harrison, B. (1981). *Ageing, needs and nutrition.* London: Policy Studies Institute.

Kane, R., & Kane, R. (1985). *A will and a way: What the United States can learn from Canada about caring for the elderly.* New York: Columbia University Press.

Laslett, P. (1987, June). The emergence of the third age. *Aging and Society, 7*(2).

Marshall, V. (1987). *Aging in Canada: Social perspectives.* Markham, ON: Fitzhenry & Whiteside.

Svanborg, A. (1987, September). Sandoz prizewinner's address given at the Conference of the European region of the International Association of Gerontology, Brighton, England.

26. Linking Theory, Research, Practice, and Policy

BETTY HAVENS

While many of us have participated in either research or policy-oriented conferences, CONNECTIONS '88 is designed to bring together communities and perspectives that are all too often fragmented. Our symposium seeks to promote discussion and debate among program managers, researchers, public policymakers, health practitioners, and consumers. The crucial question is: How can far-reaching decisions best incorporate the insights of sound research?

The health system for the elderly is expensive, complex, and increasingly subject to economic constraints, changing expectations, and the pressures and possibilities of new technologies. Never has it been so crucial to ensure that the research and policy-making processes are properly linked. Yet policies frequently lack a solid research foundation, while researchers are not always sensitive to the needs of and dilemmas confronting policymakers. It is the research/policy chasm that CONNECTIONS '88 seeks to overcome.

From the CONNECTIONS '88 brochure

Some people claim that no chasm between research and policy exists; however, our language belies such a claim. That is, we refer to academic and nonacademic gerontologists and health professionals. In fact, health professionals are often subdivided into health scientists and health practitioners. Presumably, researchers in the area of health and aging are academic scientists, and policymakers are nonacademic practitioners. Nonacademic research and, by inference, nonacademic researchers, being primarily concerned with applied research, are assumed to be somehow less than scientific, or atheoretical. Similarly, academic research and, by inference, aca-

Aging and Health: Linking Research and Public Policy, © 1989 Lewis Publishers, Inc., Chelsea, Michigan 48118. Printed in U.S.A.

demic researchers, being primarily concerned with theory testing (or basic research), are assumed to be somehow less than practice- and policy-oriented, or irrelevant.

Both of these assumptions are potentially damaging—in fact, damning—and less than accurate. However, they stem from long histories of fragmentation in all of our disciplines, fields of practice, and policy arenas. The multidisciplinarity of aging and health intensifies that history of fragmentation and the resultant problems, but it also provides an even greater challenge. If and when researchers, practitioners, and policymakers become truly collaborative and cooperative, the benefits to aging Canadians and to our collective enterprises will be great.

RELEVANCE ISSUES

To begin to deal with the issues surrounding relevance, three potential stumbling blocks must be addressed: (1) the perceived gap between academic research and the broader community; (2) determining what is relevant to whom; and (3) listening to those with whom our research is concerned—that is, listening to senior citizens.

The Gap Between Research and Practice

A major problem for researchers is the lack of feedback from service providers, from program administrators and evaluators, and from policy- and decisionmakers. Without this feedback, how will we ever bridge the moat between academic and community service? We are quick to jump all over the ivory-towered academic who doesn't tell us what we need to know, but we are sadly negligent at the other end in not using standardized measures and in not reporting back to the field. We rationalize these omissions by being too busy "doing" to report findings.

The academician must be made aware of the real constraints under which our delivery systems function. The first call on money must be the provision of services and, in fact, research is likely to be given the lowest priority. Nevertheless, policymakers require options or alternative strategies; administrators require program evaluations; both require information on which to base allocation of resources; service providers require needs assessments—and all of these were essential yesterday. We cannot wait for six months for a study design to be completed and another year or three for the information to be collated and analyzed and even more time before the results can be disseminated or used—if they are not completely stale.

Unless we are willing on both sides of the moat to build the bridges between academia and practice, we will not progress. We will perpetuate the same problems. Both our older population and our students will suffer. If we can be alerted to this problem of potentially differing though not conflicting aims, gerontology and health research in Canada should be able to develop many bridges and, in the process, to eliminate or reduce the gap.

There are few social and health researchers in Canada concerned primarily with the process of aging. Although we bewail this paucity of researchers as a problem, we must recognize and herald the benefits. That is, few Canadian health scientists or gerontologists exclusively do research; most are also teaching a broad range of courses to a wider range of students. Many of these same researchers are also either directly or indirectly involved with programs and policymakers whose primary foci are senior citizens. How better to bridge a gap than to realize that you are talking to yourself across a meaningless abyss?

Determining What Research Is Relevant to Whom

Certain research must be relevant to policymakers, to program administrators, to practitioners, and to senior citizens, but must *also* be relevant to evolving knowledge and theories in our various disciplines, to those who teach, and to our students. It is possible, on rare occasions, for a single research endeavor to be relevant to all these sectors, but even in this unusual circumstance, a single finding of such a project cannot be equally relevant to all sectors.

Researchers must stipulate clearly to whom their research will be relevant, then deliver to the designated consumers. Similarly, consumers must communicate their interests and priorities to researchers. For example, many policymakers today are concerned with the economic implications to the labor force—and hence to tax revenues and social benefits—of the changing age structure in our society. How many policymakers have asked researchers to undertake studies to answer these questions, and of those few who have asked, how many have designated research funds for this purpose? How many gerontologists have developed research plans to answer these questions and have made it their business to communicate the relevance of such findings to policymakers?

The special research program on population aging of the Social Sciences and Humanities Research Council of Canada (SSHRC) was one attempt by some policymakers both to communicate relevance and to fund the gerontological research community. In the course of that program, fewer than one fifth of the funded proposals and an even smaller portion of all proposals submitted had any potential relevance to the macro-level concerns of these policymakers. Most addressed micro-level (individual) aging issues, which, although included in the terms of reference of the program, were not expected to predominate. Similarly, the proposals generated by the National Health Research and Development Program (NHRDP) of Health and Welfare Canada's one-time special competition on aging concentrated at the micro level and fell short of the more macro health policy concerns, which the policymakers had hoped to stimulate.

All too frequently, inappropriate and even harmful decisions result from an insufficient factual or research base. The research community challenges such decisions; senior citizens either join the challenge or give up in despair. In the long run no one, including the decisionmaker, is satisfied with the results. However, given a lack of attention to relevance and timeliness, we leave decisions to that old, if inaccurate, premise that we know best—especially for someone else.

The 1950s and 1960s

The ad hoc, intuitive, fragmented, single-problem and single-discipline oriented research and planning of the '50s and '60s was productive at a time when very few resources existed. Some excellent facilities and services resulted, but the basic issues remained.

The 1970s

The scene in 1970 was one of questioning. Where do we go from here? What opportunities are now needed to assure older persons their rightful place in society?

For planners, there was the problem of determining which facilities, programs, and services should be developed. Questions were raised about the adequate range of resources, about the need for employment and social outlets, about the proper balance between institutional and noninstitutional care, and about the levels of care and services necessary to assure continuity in service delivery to older persons.

The desirability of making facilities and services both available and accessible raised issues about the location of and the appropriate combinations of resources. The need to assure reasonable alternatives to the older person while making the most appropriate use of resources raised the problem of assessment for utilization of facilities and services. The setting of standards, generally, and the supervision of standards, specifically, became a matter for public concern. And there was the problem of costs—costs to the older persons and costs to the public, which was implicit within, and resulted from the questions and answers to, all other problems.

The 1980s

The concern with costs of services and cost containment has become the major theme in health and aging during the '80s. One jurisdiction after another virtually worldwide and certainly across Canada has frozen one program or benefit after another in efforts to balance budgets. In some instances, seniors have rallied to the challenge and precluded enforcing such freezes, as in the recent proposed deindexing of pensions in Canada. In other cases, health professionals and older Canadians have formed coalitions that have effectively delayed and perhaps precluded a rollback in services, such as the recent maintenance of the urban foot care service in Manitoba. But, essentially the message has been to do more for more people (and to do so in the community, not in institutions) with fewer resources at lower cost.

These problems, both of aging Canadians and of planners and policymakers, cover a broad spectrum of needs and resources. Any planning approach to such problems requires (1) knowledge of the needs and priorities of the elderly population; (2) concern for a total range of facilities and services; (3) examination of the social and resource structures of the community; (4) a multidisciplinary planning capability; and (5) a deliberate capacity for continuous review and evaluation to accommodate these plans to the ever-changing needs and requirements of our aging society.

As a corollary, an elderly population generally reports a better health status than most people assume. Many of those making this assumption are the service providers, who are steeped in a system trying to stretch insufficient resources to a seemingly limitless number of consumers. It is easy to understand the origins of such a misconception. If there are 100,000 noninstitutionalized people over age 64 and 5% of these people could be helped by some particular service, then those dealing with the problems of the 5000 are likely to conclude that those 5000 people are representative of the whole 100,000. Unmistakably, 5000 people in need of services is a lot of people and represents much individual suffering and hardship: there are still 95,000 other older people who do not require anything from this service sector. In a period of scant fiscal resources, it is especially critical to gauge accurately the need for service expenditures.

At a time total expenditures for services are insufficient, the advocate or provider who overestimates the constituents' needs and secures a disproportionately large share of the expenditures does so at the expense of other constituents with as much or more need, but less skilled advocates. Just how deplorable that type of situation would be serves to reinforce the fundamental need for a reliable and valid quantitative information base from which comprehensive, rational, and systematic planning can be accomplished.

Our Failure to Listen to Senior Citizens

In a field that claims to study a population that is articulate and thoughtful both about itself and society, it is a particular tragedy that researchers and practitioners have spent so little time listening to the concerns of the subjects of their study and practice.

BUILDING BRIDGES

Given that we can agree that the schisms identified earlier do exist, and given that these schisms have both historical disciplinary and professional roots as well as contemporary discrepancies in relevance, we are left with the necessity of spanning these chasms. In other words, we must build the bridges between theory and practice, between research and policymaking.

Four mechanisms from within the fields of health and aging to reduce these gaps by building bridges are (1) the evaluation of health programs and policies by academic researchers; (2) the development of an iterative process between researchers and consumers (whether policymakers, practitioners, other academics, students, or seniors); (3) the active provision of data and subjects for theory-testing research by programs and practitioners; and (4) the exchange of personnel, including students, across these gaps (i.e., applied fellowships for academics, teaching assignments for practitioners, and student internships in health and aging services).

Health Program and Policy Evaluations by Academics

Professor Malcolm Johnson's evaluation of the Gloucester Home Services programs (Chapter 25) provides an excellent example. He and his team of evaluators are academics working in the applied field of health service evaluation and making policy recommendations to the local Health Authority. He also noted the work in Kent of Bleddyn Davies and his Canterbury University colleagues.

Professor Johnson's Open University research team has been involved in various iterations with the local Health Authority (i.e., the policymakers and program managers) and with the professional staff (i.e., the practitioners) who work for the Health Authority. The evaluation instruments were modified to capture the same content as the practitioners did, and to foster comparability and ease of instrument use, even though the changes rendered some small research goals more difficult. The success of the project was certainly enhanced by these iterations.

Wim Van den Heuvel and his colleagues at Groningen, Utrecht, and Nijmegen universities in the Netherlands (Ministry of Welfare, Health and Cultural Affairs, 1987) have developed the health and aging scenarios for the Dutch government policymakers. These scenarios are based on needs assessments, program evaluations, and policy analyses and have been developed to assist the policymakers in establishing policies that will meet the WHO goal of Health for All (including the elderly population) in the Netherlands by the year 2000. A governmental committee of policymakers was involved in vetting each step in producing the scenarios. The most policy-relevant and politically viable were eventually published.

Neena Chappell and her colleagues at the Centre on Aging at the University of Manitoba have produced evaluations of, among others, the Adult Day Care Program; the Day Hospitals; a sample of those receiving Home Care as compared to a matched sample of Manitobans not receiving these services; and, more recently, a specific Support Services project.

In all of these cases, the government has initiated the requests for the evaluations and, with the exception of the comparison of Home Care users and nonusers, all were government funded. (The Home Care project was publicly funded by another level of government.) In addition, all of these evaluations have provided learning opportunities for students and have been theory-productive.

Iteration Between Researchers and Consumers

In the Centre on Aging evaluations, two and often three iterative processes take place. Neena and the project teams always sit down with the consumers (often a government committee) prior to submitting the research proposal and after funding is received, but prior to the actual project start-up, to ensure that the aims of the project are mutually understood and that the desired results are addressed. This same consultative process occurs at several stages during the evaluation process, but most notably when the draft report has been prepared. The final report therefore includes the analyses and interpretations of data as produced by the researchers and as vetted by the practitioners and administrators. This process ensures that the policy implications become a collaborative product.

The second iterative process involves a panel of consumers (i.e., seniors) to determine exactly how the study subjects will understand the content of any interviews or questionnaires. This iteration has the further goal of determining the relevance of the research to the consumers of services. The process, applied in a recent study to assess the needs of urban elderly Native Canadians in Manitoba, revealed cultural differences, resulting in some extremely interesting changes in the project instrumentation.

In some cases, the third iterative process is the consulting with colleagues and graduate students about a project. Sometimes this simply takes the form of the usual university collegial consultations; however, in some cases the proposal or the instrument, or the preliminary results (or some combination of these) are shared in an informal seminar of colleagues—from the university and the community, i.e., practitioners—and of students.

The building of bridges as highlighted by these examples crosses a wide range of chasms. Disciplinary boundaries, practice or policy and academic boundaries, researcher and consumer and subject boundaries, and theory and practice boundaries are all crossed and recrossed many times in the process of these research projects.

Provision of Data or Subjects for Theory Testing by Community Agencies and Practitioners

All of the examples referred to earlier have produced data for the researchers to use in two ways: (1) as the basis for the evaluation report and (2) in generating knowledge and testing theory. Professor Johnson will be able to pursue his theory testing relative to biography as a mechanism for understanding the aging process. Dr. Chappell has continued to test theories relative to support networks and care giving as they relate to well-aging versus ill-aging processes.

One of the most poignant comments in the Dutch scenarios report was a plea for appropriate and adequate access to health service data by the researchers. The Dutch data are renowned worldwide for their excellence, reliability, and comprehensiveness, but they are virtually inaccessible to the research community, which is a tragic loss—loss of a main span to the bridge between policy and research in the Netherlands.

The access to data in Manitoba has been a boon to researchers in health and aging. This access, of course, protects the confidentiality of the service consumer and provider, but is actively provided to researchers for legitimate research endeavors. We consider ourselves very fortunate to have such a structurally sound bridge across this potential gap. On both sides of the gap, we would actively encourage other jurisdictions to be as enabling and productive.

The Exchange of Personnel

The applied fellowships as established by the Gerontological Society of America provide one model for this bridge. Academics are eligible for fellowships to work in an applied setting evaluating programs or analyzing policy, with fiscal support from the host agency and the Society. The opposite direction on this bridge is for universities to encourage part-time (or intermittent) teaching and research by practitioners. Some schools and some disciplines do a better job of this than others.

Student internships provide another similar and often successful model, if carefully undertaken. In a 1974 article (pp. 528–529), Hickey and Spinetta describe what can occur:

It is our intention that we initiate our professional careers with this dichotomy present within ourselves; but as we progress in our professions, one side or other of the dichotomy seems to take precedence. As we begin to devote our time to, and professionally emphasize either the digital (basic researchers) or the analog (practitioner), we become similarly committed in attitude, value judgment, and personal and professional preference. In the static model, we become polarized at either end of the dichotomy. As a result, when communication does take place between the poles of research and practice, it is often accomplished through a student with a half-load of classwork at the university under the direction of a researcher, and the other half of his semester hours in field work at a local facility under the tutelage of a practitioner; the student himself often becomes the bridge and finds himself stretched across a chasm so wide that he has to struggle to keep from falling in.

POTENTIAL OUTCOMES

In many instances, the academic goal of theory testing may only be possible when practice data or subjects are available from the community outside the academy. The policy and practice goals of answering practical and relevant questions can often best be undertaken with the expertise of the academic who moves into—or, at least, studies—the applied setting.

Therefore, there should be ample stimulus to establish a viable functional reciprocity (across these bridges in the aging and health fields) that should serve to strengthen the structure of not only those specific bridges, but all similar bridges over time. This functional reciprocity would seem to be especially necessary in these multidisciplinary fields. That is, if the most appropriate data and subjects come from multiple relevant practices and if the most appropriate research and evaluation skills come from multiple academic disciplines, how can we possibly ignore the other sides of the many chasms? Collaboration is essentially the only way to build theory, provide adequate program evaluations, enhance effective practice, respond to seniors' needs, and to train students in these multidisciplinary fields.

Functional reciprocity may be essential but, given the present situation, establishing effective symbiosis within the fields of health and aging may become critical. In fact, symbiotic bridges may be the only ones to survive. Symbiosis may become the sole mechanism, in an era of severe fiscal constraints, to accomplish the goals stated above from the perspective of establishing functional reciprocity. In times of constraint, competitiveness among the components will shortchange all components willy-nilly.

RESULTS OF LACK OF COLLABORATION

The ultimate policy and fiscal response to a lack of collaboration across the various chasms identified earlier is the potential elimination of all health and aging related research and theory building and, hence, ineffective practice and uninformed policymaking. That is, competition is just too costly to all aspects of the field. In the long term, these costs will jeopardize present and future consumers of health and aging services, i.e., older Canadians. As a spin-off, these costs will jeopardize our students in the health and aging fields, which could ultimately affect each one of us quite personally, when *we* are the consumers of those services. The health and aging field will be jeopardized if our students are ill-prepared or employed in health and aging programs that are (1) based on ineffective practice (i.e., neither theoretically grounded nor adequately evaluated), (2) produced from inadequate research (i.e., neither theoretically nor practice-relevant), and (3) derived from insufficient theoretical knowledge (i.e., neither adequately tested nor practice-relevant).

One of the concrete steps we can take to protect our collaborative efforts and preclude such a dreary future is to make sure that we build and maintain the ordinary little bridges across the relatively small gaps within our own disciplines and professions. We should not assume that every bridge has to be as dramatic as a "fixed link" between Prince Edward Island and the Mainland. We need not be faced with chasms (or schisms) that could only be spanned by the likes of a fixed link.

CONCLUSION

Given that the health and aging research community is faced with limited funds and often meets resistance from funders—based on general societal negativism relative to aging and to sickness and a consequent lower funding priority—it is essential for this community to cooperate in pursuing research goals both within and across disciplines locally and nationally. This position invites certain difficulties: it is more difficult to cooperate across disciplines and across our broad geographic expanses. However, if we cannot develop such cooperative strategies, funding competitions rather than research will consume our time, leaving relevant questions unanswered—few rest within a single discipline or a limited geographic or social context. We must encourage practitioners to be fully recognized participants in the health and aging research community. We must encourage academics to be fully recognized participants in our practices and policymaking. We must learn to speak in a timely fashion to each other and to policymakers, and we must learn to listen to senior citizens.

If we are willing to operate within a cooperative and collaborative framework, we will address each issue from three major perspectives: (1) Which discipline(s) are the most appropriate to deal with the issue, and where do we find that expertise? (2) To whom and to what extent is the issue relevant and under what time constraints? and (3) What is the best approach to, or methodology for (identifying alternatives where appropriate), addressing the issue to service the greatest number of sectors—the aging population, policymakers, program administrators, practitioners, academics, students, and our varied disciplines?

Given that we can agree on the foregoing guidelines, we are left with two major tasks, which I hope will become personal and collective commitments on an ongoing basis. Each must ask, (1) How can I help to make each research project not just better, but the best by building the appropriate little bridges, and how completely can I commit myself to each issue? and (2) What are the major priorities for health and aging research for the next year, 3 years, 5 years, and 10 years?

It is up to each one of us as we return to our usual settings and familiar "ruts" to make sure that we carry out our commitments to cooperation, collaboration, and collegial assistance and that we create an expanding network or cadre of professionals in our local areas which can span these same issues. If there is a challenge to us for the late '80s and early '90s, it is to accomplish the rational solutions to the issues identified here before we run out of time to be rational and have to give serious consideration to numerous ventures of the scope of a fixed link.

REFERENCES

Hickey, T., & Spinetta, J. J. (1974). Bridging research and application. *Gerontologist, 14*(6).

Ministry of Welfare, Health and Cultural Affairs. (1987). *Health as a focal point: An abridged version of the memorandum Health 2000, The Netherlands.* The Hague: Government Printing.

SUGGESTED READING

Blandford, A. A., & Chappell, N. L. (1986). Elderly native Indian women—An at risk group. *Canadian Association on Gerontology,* Quebec City, Quebec.

Carley, M., Dant, T., Gearing, B., & Johnson, M. (1987). *Care for elderly people in the community: A review of the issues and the research* (Project Paper No. 1). Milton Keynes, UK: Policy Studies Institute, The Open University.

Chappell, N. L. (1981, June). *Value of research to practitioners in work with the elderly.* Keynote address, conference of the Alberta Association on Gerontology, Calgary, Alberta.

Chappell, N. L. (1982a). *An evaluation of adult day care in Manitoba—Phase I* (Final Report). Winnipeg: Manitoba Health Services Commission.

Chappell, N. L. (1982b). The value of research to practitioners in work with the elderly. *Canadian Journal on Aging, 1*(1&2), 62–65.

Chappell, N. L. (1983a). Who benefits from adult day care: Changes in functional ability and mental functioning during attendance. *Canadian Journal on Aging, 2*(1), 9–26.

Chappell, N. L. (1983b). *Adult day care and change in the utilization of medical and inpatient hospital services* (Final Report). Winnipeg: Manitoba Health Services Commission.

Chappell, N. L. (1985). Social support and the receipt of home care services. *Gerontologist, 25*(1), 47–54.

Chappell, N. L. (1988). Long-term care in Canada. In E. Rathbone-McCuan & B. Havens (Eds.), *North American elders: United States and Canadian comparisons* (pp. 73–88). Westport, CT: Greenwood Press.

Chappell, N. L., & Blandford, A. A. (1983). *Adult day care: Its impact on the utilization of other health services and on quality of life* (Final Report). Ottawa: NHRDP, Health and Welfare Canada.

Chappell, N. L., & Blandford, A. A. (1987a). Adult day care and medical and hospital claims. *Gerontologist, 27*(6), 773–779.

Chappell, N. L., & Blandford, A. A. (1987b). Health service utilization by elderly persons. *Canadian Journal of Sociology, 12*(3), 195–215.

Chappell, N. L., & Horne, J. (1987). *Housing and supportive services for elderly persons in Manitoba* (Final Report). Ottawa: Canada Mortgage and Housing; Winnipeg: The Winnipeg Foundation.

Chappell, N. L., Segall, A., & Lewis, D. (1987, October). *Helping networks among day hospital and senior centre participants.* Paper presented at the conference of the Canadian Association on Gerontology, Calgary, Alberta.

Dant, T., Carley, M., Gearing, B., & Johnson, M. (1987). *Identifying, assessing, and monitoring the needs of elderly people at home* (Project Paper No. 2). Milton Keynes, U.K.: Policy Studies Institute, The Open University.

Grant, K. R., & Chappell, N. L. (1983). What is reasonable is true. . . . Life satisfaction and functional disability among day hospital participants. *Social Science and Medicine, 17*(2), 71–78.

Greene, J. C. (1987). Stakeholder participation in evaluation design: Is it worth the effort? *Evaluation and Program Planning, 10,* 379–94.

Havens, B. (1980). The relevance of social science research in aging. In *Towards a Maturing Society Proceedings* (pp. 121ff.). Winnipeg: University of Manitoba.

Havens, B. (1981). *Sociologists in government: At the boundaries building bridges.* Paper presented at Midwest Sociological Society Meetings, Minneapolis, MN.

Health and Social Development. (1973–77). *Aging in Manitoba: Needs and resources for the elderly.* Winnipeg: Government of Manitoba.

Penning, M. J., & Chappell, N. L. (1987). Ethnicity and informal supports among older adults. *Journal of Aging Studies, 1*(2), 145–160.

Strain, L. A., & Chappell, N. L. (1982). Problems and strategies: Ethical concerns in survey research with the elderly. *Gerontologist, 11*(6), 526–531.

Strain, L. A., & Chappell, N. L. (1983). Rural-urban differences among participants of adult day care in Manitoba. *Canadian Journal on Aging, 2*(4), 197–209.

Strain, L. A., & Chappell, N. L. (1984, November). *Social support among elderly Canadian natives: A comparison with elderly non-natives.* Paper presented at the conference of the Canadian Association on Gerontology, Vancouver, British Columbia.

Strain, L. A., Chappell, N. L., & Blandford, A. A. (1987). Changes in life satisfaction among participants of adult day care and their informal caregivers. *Journal of Gerontological Social Work, 11*(3/4), 115–129.

Commentary

SHEILA M. NEYSMITH

I want to take up Betty Havens' metaphor of chasms—she argued for building bridges between academic researchers, consumers, and policymakers/planners/service providers—but explore them from a different angle. Johnson's and Davies' work in England, Chappell's in Manitoba, and the Dutch scenarios are good examples of where this model is being effected. However, those examples are outstanding *because* they are succeeding. Put differently, they are the exception, rather than the rule. My immediate conclusion after reading Havens' paper was that someone should be studying the dynamics of bridge building. I would like to make a start in that direction by examining why it doesn't happen.

I am assuming we all agree that not only should these bridges be built, but also it is imperative to do so in order to improve the quality of our knowledge and resource usage, i.e., in the interest of effectiveness and efficiency. However, my second premise is that good will and/or exhortation will not build them. Like most cooperative efforts in life, there has to be an incentive to join or cooperate. This may be in the form of a stick, a carrot, or a little bit of both, but it must be there. Certainly the social service field is riddled with aborted efforts to coordinate services to reduce overlap, ensure coverage, and do effective planning. Unfortunately this rational planning model approach only works if resources are tied to cooperation, that is, if an important part of an institution's funding, access to clients, or some other important resource is dependent upon cooperation. The explanation is quite simple. Organizations, be they university departments, social service agencies, or seniors' groups, have differing purposes. They are engaged in pursuing different institutional goals. Therefore, simple prioritizing means that efforts that do not impinge directly on an organization's primary goals get a secondary place on the agenda.

My third assumption is that universities, government planning departments, service agencies, and consumer groups are going to continue to march to different drummers in the future. I have no difficulty with that. The thought of service providers shaping the agenda of citizen advocacy groups, senior citizens designing university research projects, or researchers delivering social services boggles the mind! (Although I would be willing to back a six-month experiment for pure consciousness-raising purposes.)

The most compelling reason for the continued separation of the spheres, however, is that each sees the world differently; consequently, each raises different questions and pushes competing priorities. The service system is concerned with delivery—ensuring at a minimum that entitlements are honored and, one hopes, that need is being met. Incidentally, the rewards and sanctions in that system correspond to this mandate. The academic researcher's goal is to build knowledge—she, or he, is rewarded for this. Research grants are assessed for originality, methodological rigor, and so on. Peer-reviewed journals use these same criteria for deciding what gets published. Not surprisingly, promotion within the university is based on success in this area, i.e., publish or perish. The mission of consumer groups is to advocate for the needs of their members—not to evaluate the relative merits of their claims against those of competing groups. That is the task of policy developers.

Given these dynamics, if I were trying to assess why Havens' examples work when so many do not, I would probably start from a perspective very familiar to gerontologists—exchange theory. Who gets what in these situations? What is the value of the resource(s) to the respective parties? What is the balance in the exchange relationship?

Havens has hinted at where some of the balances and imbalances occur. In all her model cases, interested parties were engaged in applied research. The local authority or provincial government not only made money available, but also helped negotiate the goal of the studies and the process of carrying out the research. Now the question is, Why would both parties agree? From the academic or research center's point of view, funds are made available—a large data base or a whole program becomes accessible for studying. The questions may take a different form or the program may not be the model that I, the researcher, would ideally like to test, but it surely is better than the alternative of few funds or no program.

Similarly, from the policymaker's point of view, programs do get put into place—with or without the benefit of reliable data. Necessarily, their primary focus is on running the program. At best, any routine data collected is shaped by information needs of program managers concerned with program delivery, not impact. Managers are rewarded for delivering the program. Therefore, impact assessment will be a secondary consideration. The pitfalls of going outside the service delivery institutions for research purposes have been well documented. However, it does increase the probability that different questions will be addressed, because of diminished vested interest in current practice. The difference in the questions asked is probably the gain to be realized when academic researchers and policymakers join forces. Setting up a data base capable of delivering information to both parties may be less of a challenge than ensuring relevant questions get asked.

This joint enterprise is difficult to carry out under suspicion from purists on both sides. What I am arguing is that if we want to promote these interchanges, we have to go far beyond using moral suasion. Such research undertakings must become at least as attractive and respectable as basic research.

The Social Sciences and Humanities Research Council of Canada (SSHRC) grants that Havens referred to did not do this. They provided the funds and defined the substantive areas but individual researchers chose the topics. There was no stipulation, for example, that the research was to be done in collaboration with a policy planner, or service institution, with seniors' groups, or whatever. Therefore, the research question was totally defined by the disciplines applying for funds. It seems that most academics were interested in micro questions. (As a social policy practitioner I will refrain from commenting on the ideological origins of this outcome.)

I can hear the rebuttal that what I am suggesting will give policymakers more control over the research agenda of the academic community. Yes, it will. But the other side also has an argument. These are public monies. *Who* has the right to decide where our limited research funds are spent?

Frankly, none of the players has an exclusive claim on truth and justice— for all the reasons outlined above. Unfortunately, nor do they all have equal power to enforce their relative claims. However, they do have different resources that are valuable to each other: funds, methodological expertise, data sources, community sanction, and so on. A strategy that consciously builds on exchange empowers the respective players without pretending that we are all in perfect agreement—a menu for guaranteed disaster in my opinion.

To return to Havens' metaphor: I am suggesting that the separate land masses of researchers, policymakers, and consumers will continue to exist and there are good arguments for why they should. But I prefer to see them as peninsulas with the connections big enough for some folk to live right on the pathways.

This imagery comes to mind because I am a social worker with an academic appointment. On the one hand, I find myself (as happened a few years ago) on a committee trying to convince SSHRC that research on program implementation *is* research; more recently, I have been sitting on a university committee examining the research and publication track record of our faculty. Here I have found myself arguing that dissemination of knowledge comes in many forms—refereed publications, yes, but training manuals for agencies will probably have a more substantiated impact on practice. Both SSHRC and the university have severe reservations about such arguments. On the other hand, I am confronted with students who are seeking a professional degree to qualify them to practice. The relevance of skills, techniques, and supervised practice experience is obvious to them. Acknowledged are my arguments that the foregoing may make them excellent technicians but that as professionals they must develop a critical perspective on their knowledge, but my arguments are seen as secondary to getting the job done.

These experiences have convinced me that gaps are spanned when it is clear that I need you as much as you need me. So let us start the negotiations. Compromises there will be, but funding bodies, taxpayers, and senior advocates have made it clear that isolated knowledge building and services without knowledge will no longer be tolerated.

Commentary

LINDA BAKKEN

Before I react to the presentations made by Malcolm Johnson and Betty Havens, I want to tell you a little of my role in aging, because it is from that perspective that my reactions and remarks are bred. On behalf of the provincial government, I work with community groups, health facility boards, municipal corporations, the boards of voluntary service agencies, and the providers of care. This work has been directed at solving service problems, interpreting and shaping government health policy, and developing provincial program initiatives to respond at the community level. In 1980, this program development and policy influence became focused on aging.

Action research is Malcolm Johnson's term for university-based researchers working in a collegial and collaborative manner with program staff. The values, principles, and philosophies guiding action research struck a responsive chord in my heart. He describes an evaluation design that changes as the program matures, the development of data-gathering tools that are responsible and meaningful to care providers, and a value base that states the program is the thing.

Community and government-based program and policy staff and service providers need access to the resources and dedication of researchers with Malcolm's style.

Aging is a new frontier: the program, service, and system challenges are new, ever-emerging, and immediate. We, the program/policy/problem solvers need help in designing and evaluating the new approaches that are being implemented at the field level, and we need that help on the basis of an equal, collegial, and collaborative relationship.

Although I *see* a commitment to this collegial and collaborative approach, there are some barriers that we must overcome. The first and most frustrating to me is the use of language. The academic and program worlds use different language.

Academics are neutral, program staff are passionate; academics are statistically correct, program staff are desperate for definitive answers. The statistical significance of a finding or a change is difficult to comprehend when we are asking the question, Did it work?—Did the intervention increase or decrease functional ability? Was the program more or less expensive? Does the program matter in terms of quality of life? Does quality of life matter if our objective is cost-effectiveness? We ask different questions, and therefore we are rarely satisfied with the answers.

A second barrier is the structure of research funding. Almost all research funds in the area of aging come from tax dollars. Yet the government departments that fund service delivery and program development have little to say about the relevance or timeliness of the research questions that are asked, and rarely provide funding for program evaluation as part of the program budget. Funding is not provided to hire evaluation staff, increase staff-years to dedicate collective time to program evaluation or even provide large delivery units (such as hospitals, personal care homes, regional community service structures, etc.) with program evaluation expertise.

The structure of the financing of research is keeping us apart. The values of university-based researchers control the financing of research on aging and pay insufficient attention to the issues and questions at the program and service level. Senior government officials deny program staff the funds to hire or contract for program evaluation skills, yet continue to expect new program initiatives to justify their existence.

My third concern continues the theme that we live in different worlds, with different agendas and different roles and values. My experience in "bridging the gap" between researchers and program people has been frustrated by the sense of ownership I feel for "my" programs and the data they produce. Similarly, researchers have a sense of ownership of the data produced by their evaluation design and collection efforts.

Where we have overcome the hurdles and barriers to researchers and program staff coming together around a program evaluation question, the initial project comes to an end, the formal and contracted relationship is over, yet the data and the numerous unanswered questions continue to exist. The researcher continues to massage the data, publish the findings in a variety of forums with no regard for the questions and issues of the programmers and with little reference to the skills and dedication of the program design and implementation unit. Publication of the findings from the continued mining of the data 5, 10, and 15 years after it is collected is the final insult. For as the researcher continues with new forms of analysis, combining studies and trying to answer questions raised by the original analyses, the program continues. The program has been shaped by the results of the original study, by ongoing program monitoring, by the changing needs of the target population, and by the changing nature of the delivery unit or the fiscal situation. Programs are not static, programs change, programs ask new questions; yet researchers, just by their continued involvement with old and outdated data, provide credibility to old data and the old results, making statements about "the program" that in effect no longer exists.

Havens raised the questions of timeliness and relevance. In my view, program evaluation data gathered to make a statement about a particular program or a program design constitute a snapshot in time, and the longer it takes to analyze and publish, the less applicable are conclusions to the program as it evolves. Human service programs are not static; they change in response to the multiple variables of the political, economic, and human issues of the time. Therefore "old" or dated data reworked to provide new insight, more controls, larger samples, or to test a research tool are a tragic waste of limited research and evaluation resources. The timeliness of the data, and the timeliness and relevance of the question, should be items of discussion between researchers and program staff.

However, I see evidence and am therefore convinced that there is commitment to support each other because we are united in our commitment to the senior citizens of today and tomorrow.

Strategies that may contribute to enhancing and enabling the cooperative and collegial relationship referred to by Havens and Johnson are as follows:

1. Program and policy personnel must be represented on all committees with authority to grant tax-supported research funds. The relevance and timeliness of the question must be a key factor in the approval mechanisms of governing federal and provincial research dollars. Program and policy staff are most closely in touch with the relevance of the research question.

2. Research funding authorities must encourage or mandate that the policy and practice implications of research be addressed and reported in publication. This strategy will encourage dialogue between university-based researchers and program and policy staff at the research design, analysis, and conclusion phases.

3. We must encourage research applications from practitioners. Program administrators, directors of nursing, field-level social workers, occupational therapists, and so on, should be encouraged to do their own research. Because they form the questions, the commitment to data gathering and to program change based on the outcome will increase. As field-level practitioners and program managers increase their academic training, this possibility increases.

4. Program and policy staff at all levels must collectively insist on the allocation of funds dedicated to research and evaluation within all new and existing program budgets. Program and policy staff must have the power to purchase the evaluations essential to good program monitoring and decisionmaking. This strategy will provide funds to contract with university-based expertise in the design of management information systems for programs, and over time increase the knowledge and skill in format evaluation at the program and policy level.

Program evaluation research questions provide challenges to research design and technique, as well as setting the general direction of studies. At the Long Term Care Programs Division at the Manitoba Health Services Commission (MHSC), the questions we ask fall into three categories: (1) Does it matter? (2) Is it cheaper? and (3) How will we do it?

Does It Matter? Does it matter that activity department staff have degrees in recreation? That is, is quality of life improved and does improved quality of life affect the functional level of the resident?

Is It Cheaper? Is it cheaper, more cost-effective, least intrusive, or interventionist? That is, when we introduce higher standards for pharmacy services in personal care homes, does this intervention do more than increase the quality of pharmacist services? Does it also meet our overriding objectives of cost-effectiveness?

How Will We Do It? What is the most appropriate system or model for achieving our objectives? That is, how do we increase the skills of nursing home personnel as we are faced with increasing behavior-management problems due to degenerative brain disorders? Do we provide each home with a link to an extended treatment hospital? Provide each home with a psychologist? An occupational therapist? Or do we increase staff-to-resident ratios?

The delivery system chosen is an intervention. We look to the journals for guidance in our decision, then we look for an evaluation strategy to monitor the effectiveness of our decision.

System and process questions are numerous at the program/policy level in long term care. What are the effects of a community liaison between an extended treatment unit and a community-based mental health program?

How does the organizational intervention affect the use of insured health services or the use of community programs? We have health care system objectives: cost-effective, equitable, universal, least interventionist, et cetera, et cetera—but we are challenged by the administrative and organizational models that will best meet our objectives.

Every jurisdiction in Canada is purporting to develop low cost community-based programs aimed at supporting, maintaining, and maximizing independence for seniors. The approaches, the organization models, legislative frameworks, and health system infrastructures are different. Is there commitment to evaluate the model as an intervention? To my mind, this is fruitful territory to link theory, research, and public policy.

If these questions interest the research community, what barriers will you experience if you approach us? There are research headaches in working with program and service providers which act as barriers. Service providers can be "prima donnas"—their commitment (bias) to service provision leaves little room for compromise. Turf protecting is legion; in health care, hard-won resources and mandates are difficult to compromise for research and evaluation purposes. In addition, some service providers have a high level of discomfort with research-oriented professionals and lack the confidence to form the required linkage with university expertise in evaluation design.

In conclusion, I will discuss how we at the MHSC have initiated research to answer questions, shape policy, make resource decisions, or choose an organizational model, and also some of the personal, organizational, and system problems that show the imperfections in our attempts at bridging the gap.

Planning generally begins with the question, What is happening now? In November 1985, the MHSC wanted to know who was occupying the beds in our urban acute care facilities. That is, how many geriatric patients were in medical beds (e.g., of the designated ophthalmology beds, how many were used as such and where were they located)?

The Health Department's Research and Planning Directorate, the Commission, and the urban hospitals launched a cooperative effort. Research and planning provided the design, and the nursing consultants at the Commission and nurses from hospitals did the data gathering. The results were useful at the provincial and facility level for planning and monitoring of resources. The study was repeated by one community hospital and formed the basis for significant organizational changes to ensure greater resource efficiency and appropriate care for patients. However, neither the study design nor the findings have been reported in the professional literature.

On another occasion, we were not as successful in producing a useful product, because the barriers to bridging the gap became insurmountable.

In Manitoba, we use a very simple but effective tool for assessing the level of dependency on nursing time for our personal care homes. The tool is used in the community at the time of assessment for personal care home placement, is applied annually by the MHSC to determine funding levels, and in many personal care homes is applied on a regular basis to assign internal resources. However, the tool is criticized as inadequate to measure dependency on nursing time in the psychosocial area. A "behavior assessment supplement" was required.

A research-oriented psychologist from one of our facilities, and two nurses—one from the Commission and one from a personal care home—became the project team. The initial project was unfortunately a frustrating failure. The team (1) asked the wrong questions; (2) developed a tool that was too complicated, the results of which raised more questions than provided answers; and (3) provided information that was not useful.

The failure here does not mean that the task was impossible and should not have been attempted, or that the scientific method failed or the resources were inadequate. The failure here was human: failure in leadership, vision, communication, and confidence; failure to listen and to hear; failure to be realistic in expectation; failure to feel confident about concerns; and failure to have at least one project member who could bridge the gap between the research process and the development of simple and useful information. The challenge in these circumstances is to develop research methodologies and to present findings that are practical and applicable in the field.

In aging, the management and care of incontinence is an area where published research has failed to be practical. Have any of you found any practical information regarding incontinence in the practice journals? In long term care, assuming that all medically treatable approaches have been tried, incontinence means the resident is wet and possibly smelly. The questions are very practical. How do we manage this problem? How do we keep the resident dry, smelling appropriately, and at what cost, in terms of personal dignity, staff, and supplies? Practical, basic issues deserve research energy and should be published in the most popular and prestigious journals. We must not forget the practical, day-to-day concerns in the care for the elderly.

The next example is one of our more successful, practical, low cost projects that shaped program, helped to articulate standards, and developed policy.

In 1985, our pharmacy consultant hired two students to carry out a study on the administration of medications in personal care homes. Their hypotheses or concerns were observed and shared by nursing, pharmacy, and dietary consultants at the MHSC. A simple observation study was designed; the student temporary employment program provided the salary dollars; and data were collected on medication crushing, medication administration, frequency and amount of liquid administered with the medication, documentation, and compliance with written procedures and protocol.

The study verified the hunches or hypotheses of Commission staff, and the documented results are now used regularly in standards visits. It helped articulate pharmacy and nursing standards, and the results were incorporated into our prescribing guide.

Although this project has never been published in the professional journals, the results or the impact on the articulation of standards and a specific section in the prescribing guide have fulfilled a number of research objectives. The findings have changed practice standards and procedures and have therefore contributed to the provision of higher quality care for elderly residents of personal care homes.

In closing, I would like to continue with Havens' analogy of the fixed link. My sense is that the participants at CONNECTIONS '88 are committed to a fixed link among research, theory, and practice. However, may I suggest that the fixed link be *aboveground* so that all can see it and that aging can be the prototype or model for other issues and program areas? Our link must be visible to all. Though the journey must continue, we can be proud of the existing links among research, theory, policy, and practice in aging.

27. Demystifying the Research Process

NEENA L. CHAPPELL

> *The whole of science is nothing more than a refinement of everyday thinking.*
>
> Albert Einstein

> *Science is nothing but trained and organized common sense.*
>
> T. H. Huxley

Research is nothing more than a method for the pursuit of knowledge. There are, however, specialized skills involved in science and research. Jules Henry Poincaré expressed it well when he said, "Science is built up with facts as a house is with stones. But a collection of facts is no more a science than a heap of stones is a house." Forming that heap of stones into a house requires a certain type of skill.

It is the research process, particularly applied research, that I will address. I, like Malcolm Johnson, will draw on applied research in the area of health care and the elderly. There are a couple of assumptions with which I start. These are important assumptions because they flavor one's participation within the applied research process.

1. Applied research requires a partnership between researchers and others, who include policymakers, practitioners, administrators, and the elderly themselves. A partnership requires a recognition by all of its participants of the importance and indispensability of the contribution of each. All have a particular role to play, and all bring vital information to the research process (Chappell, 1982a). The researcher brings to this partnership a particular set of specialized research skills that

Aging and Health: Linking Research and Public Policy, © 1989 Lewis Publishers, Inc., Chelsea, Michigan 48118. Printed in U.S.A.

take years of education and application to acquire and refine. Further-more, and importantly, the researcher brings a more distant (impartial) view to the question at hand. The other partners bring vital knowledge about the question at hand, and also a sense of which questions are important to ask and which ones are less important.

2. Each of the participants accepts the importance of the research process. Each, furthermore, should understand that research is not a panacea. It is important to view research as an ongoing process of knowledge accumulation. That is, a well-designed, well-executed study can pro-vide important information, but it requires several studies in several jurisdictions over time to provide conclusions in which we can have confidence. The definitive study, I believe, is a myth. Nevertheless, research can provide more reliable information than individuals' hunches and guesses about what is going on.

STAGES OF THE RESEARCH PROCESS

Stage 1: Defining the Question

The research process begins with the initial ideas and discussions that define the problem. It is not unusual for a project to begin with a general question that later becomes refined. The original question that started the process is not always recognizable.

Some Native Indian groups in Winnipeg wanted to obtain money to build a Native nursing home, or personal care home as we refer to them in Mani-toba. However, the funding agency required evidence that there was a need for such a specialized long term care institution. Not knowing how to obtain the necessary data for a needs assessment, the Natives approached the Centre on Aging, University of Manitoba. The researchers and representatives of the Native groups agreed after several discussions that a broader assessment examining a spectrum of health care needs would serve the purpose more adequately. The needs assessment would include data on whether a Native nursing home was required, but would identify other needs. It was important for the Native groups to recognize that their particular desire for a Native nursing home may not be supported by this undertaking. When the question was sufficiently defined, the Native groups asked if they could turn the money over for the Centre to conduct the research. The researchers agreed to participate only if the Native groups were full partners, because it was their understanding of their culture and their access to this group that would be vital for the conduct of the research.

Adult day care (ADC) programs were being established as part of the province-wide home care program in Manitoba. Those involved believed it important to evaluate this program when it was being established so it could be monitored appropriately. The government agreed to fund the program but not its evaluation. The researcher was approached, in this instance, by individuals with a fairly well-defined notion of what they wanted to evaluate; the problem was one of obtaining funds. They wanted a longitudinal design with baseline data prior to entering the program and follow-ups at several points thereafter to assess the individuals' mental health, social integration, and physical functioning and to relate this to utilization of various aspects of the health care system. The researcher had the skills to design the study so it could help to answer these questions.

The idea for a third study, of supportive housing, was initiated by a governmental and nongovernmental committee asked to inform provincial ministers of policy on multilevel care (MLC) facilities. They approached the Centre about the possibility of conducting such a study. After lengthy conversations, several questions arose: (1) whether individuals living in different types of accommodation differ in their health characteristics, their social integration, their mental health, and so on; (2) whether individuals enter the housing level of MLC facilities prematurely in order to ensure a place in the long term institutional component later on; (3) whether nursing homes that are part of MLC facilities accept those in their own lower levels of care over and above persons from other sources; and (4) whether there are cost differences for delivering various services in different settings.

Stage 2: Obtaining the Resources

Research is expensive if it is to be done properly, and research is time consuming. Though much can be accomplished through individual efforts to standardize, collect, codify, and analyze information, a commitment to the research process is not a spare-time hobby. Research money—particularly applied research money—is not easy to come by. Canadian researchers tend to be university based and, particularly for those of us with a social perspective, such as sociologists, the Social Sciences and Humanities Research Council of Canada in Ottawa is a major source of funds. As long as we have to apply to these types of sources, research questions frequently become phrased somewhat differently than the community interest would like. Until community groups and governments provide the money to have the questions answered that they are interested in, this is inevitable.

There are, of course, other sources of funds as well. Increasingly, there are what are known as contract research opportunities. These are calls—frequently from government—for someone to undertake research, calls which go primarily to private research firms. These contracts build in a large margin for overhead costs because private firms cannot compete without taking such financial considerations into account. The contractor also specifies the time period (usually very short) as well as the specific questions to be investigated, and the contractor owns these data. There are differing views on the appropriateness or benefits of this type of research.

At the Centre on Aging at the University of Manitoba, the major criterion for deciding whether to undertake a research project, irrespective of how it is funded, is that it meet rigorous scientific standards. The test of scientific rigor is that it is publishable in a peer-reviewed scientific journal. If it does not meet this criterion, then we are not interested in it. The difficulty involved with contract research is that frequently the percentage of the budget absorbed by overhead costs leaves an insufficient amount to conduct the research with a rigorous scientific design able to meet scholarly standards. If the research does not meet these standards, it probably is not adequate to answer the questions. In this case, it could be bad research, and bad research can be harmful, leading to changes in programs and policy which are incorrect.

There are, in addition, other sources. Several provincial granting councils exist and, not unexpectedly, the richer provinces provide more money. Private foundations or other agencies sometimes provide research funds. By and large, however, research funds tend to be scarce.

This scarcity is evident, for example, in the evaluation of the ADC program mentioned earlier, when the government funded the program but refused to allocate any money to evaluate it. The researcher wrote a proposal and submitted it to a local agency for funding. That local agency responded positively to the need for the research and to the evaluation design. However, it refused to fund it on the grounds that the government should evaluate its own programs; it even offered to make a presentation to government on the researcher's behalf. Ultimately, the evaluation of ADC turned into a series of three studies over five years. The first was funded through the Manitoba Health Services Commission (not a research funding agency), the second by Health and Welfare Canada in Ottawa in a regular research grant competition, and the third, once again, by the Manitoba Health Services Commission. In all instances, the researcher wrote the research proposal.

The needs assessment for the Natives was funded by the original group from whom they requested the money for building a Native nursing home. This group provided funds for them to conduct a needs assessment. The study of supportive housing was funded from several sources. Two local sources, the Manitoba Health Services Commission and Manitoba Housing and Renewal, each funded one third of the total after being requested by the Committee that approached the researcher. They could raise no further funds and asked the researcher to write proposals to submit to other agencies. The researcher submitted a proposal to Canada Mortgage and Housing Corporation (CMHC), which eventually funded it after the initial fiscal commitment from the two local agencies had run out. That commitment had to be reinstated. CMHC gave the maximum amount allowed by its guidelines, which proved insufficient to meet the other third required. The researcher made an appeal to a local foundation, which provided the remainder.

In other words, to fund a research project frequently requires creativity, and it always requires time, particularly on the researcher's part, to put together a research proposal. The form that proposal takes varies tremendously depending on the funding source. Assuming the necessary funds have been obtained, the research proper can start.

Stage 3: The Research Proper

By the time funds have been obtained, the research question has been defined, and the methodology has been specified. In other words, the timetable for the different phases of the study has been worked out. The researchers usually assume primary responsibility for the methodology, given the resources and questions to be answered. They have the responsibility for communicating these decisions to the nonresearchers in terms of what can meaningfully be expected from the results, the timeline, and other factors. In applied research, one is not always able to implement the design one would like. Given resource constraints, many compromises are made.

In the Native needs assessment, approximately $34,000 was provided. This allowed a one-shot, cross-sectional design in which data were collected at one point in time. Given the subcultural group we were dealing with, it was particularly important that we gain their cooperation. We therefore involved the Native groups to a great extent. People involved in the Native groups themselves searched out Native listings from which a representative sample could be drawn. The researchers trained Natives as interviewers so that Natives interviewed other Natives. One hundred and ninety-three Natives were included in the study. This study never would have been conducted were it not for the many extra hours that the Natives put in cost free. Similarly, the researchers' contributions were never reimbursed monetarily.

The Three Phases

The ADC studies were a series of three because of the difficulty in obtaining funding. The initial ADC evaluation received $16,000 to interview respondents (1) at the beginning of entering ADC, (2) four months later, and (3) one year later, retrieving their use of home care services from the noncomputerized file system for home care, and linking these data to computerized records of their utilization of physician services, inpatient hospital stays, and assessment for long term institutional care. The study included approximately 134 respondents province-wide and was conducted through heroic efforts by researchers and nonresearchers in a major cooperative effort to collect the data. The money was far too little.

The second phase was funded by the National Health Research and Development Program of Health and Welfare Canada for just under $63,000. This phase included approximately 70 respondents in Winnipeg only—those participating in ADC as well as two control groups matched on age, sex, functional disability, and illness. Earlier data from ADC plus other studies were merged, and a follow-up interview conducted. The funding was appropriate for the study.

The final phase was conducted for just under $17,000 and, because of the limited budget, was restricted to one time only, that is, a cross-sectional study. It included all users of ADC in the province after the program had been going for a number of years and incorporated computerized records only, with neither longitudinal nor interview data. The study was done adequately for that amount of money.

Evolution of the Study

Collecting the data and merging the data are primarily the researcher's responsibility. The type of study governs amount of interaction with nonresearchers during these aspects of the research. For example, in a process evaluation, frequent meetings will be held with nonresearchers both for feeding back information to them and for obtaining their reactions to what is going on with the project. During data analysis, there should be much dialogue, with researchers writing drafts of data analysis and interpretation, meeting with nonresearchers for their reactions to both the consideration of questions to be addressed and the interpretation of findings. This requires additional analyses. The ADC studies provide an example of how some of the information collected feeds back into the program during the process of the project.

Phase One. In the first phase of data analysis, it emerged that those attending ADC tended to be needy, at risk (i.e., with greater functional disability), and nonethnic. This finding led to questions, because the program had been envisioned for those prior to deterioration of functioning. The nonresearchers discovered that those who had better functioning did not want to attend because all of the programs were physically housed within long term institutions. Eventually, some programs were established in other locations. That mainly nonethnic elderly attended the ADC program related to the areas or districts in which the ADC programs were located. The nonresearchers then canvassed various ethnic communities to see whether they would utilize a program in their areas. Such findings relate to program development and provide examples of how research information can be used to help programs evolve.

Phase Two. Phase Two incorporated different control groups and matched samples. A major finding was that the greater tendency of ADC participants to be assessed and admitted to personal care homes cannot be attributed to worse functioning or greater illness. Nor do they tend to be assessed as requiring greater care. These findings resulted in a closer look at this phenomenon by those involved with the program.

However, there is a more optimistic finding. According to subjective measures, ADC participants increased their life satisfaction compared with both control groups. Objective measures of quality of life revealed ADC participants showed (1) increased social integration and (2) increases in indoor activities, outdoor activities, and church-related activities compared with both users and nonusers of other home care program services. Manitoba Home Care through the ADC program appears to be successful in meeting the objective of addressing socialization needs.

Phase Three. Phase Three, conducted after the program had been established for some time and cross-sectional in nature, showed dramatic decreases in hospital utilization by participants of ADC. Because control groups were not included in this aspect of the study, it is impossible to say whether this decrease is due to participation in ADC and whether there is a concomitant increase in home care utilization. Nevertheless, the finding is striking and warrants further study (Chappell, 1982b, 1983; Chappell & Blandford, 1983).

Analysis

In terms of policy development (as opposed to program development), this series of studies suggests ADC is meeting its goal of socialization. It is enhancing the quality of life of its participants. The methodological design of Phase Two (longitudinal and with control groups) permits the drawing of conclusions with relative certainty. However, an argument to establish such programs as a means of reducing the utilization of other services, such as hospital or physician services, has not been established in this or in other studies of ADC.

The Natives' study did not suggest overwhelming demand for a Native nursing home. It pointed to a demand for culturally congruent services, irrespective of what those services may be. It also pointed to the need for a few long term care beds, but mainly information and outreach services to Natives by Natives. As a result, a center offering information and outreach services to and by Natives with a limited number of residential suites is being built (Strain & Chappell, 1984; Driedger & Chappell, 1987).

Research is useful but not the answer to all questions. Furthermore, research inevitably leads to more questions. In ADC, another longitudinal study with appropriate control groups is necessary to establish whether the program, after operating for some time and known by others in the system, can lead to drastic reductions in hospital utilization and whether such reductions are associated with increased use of home care services. Also, although research can easily take two or three years to complete, programs are continuously changing—the initial questions may have evolved. The continuous exchange between the researchers and nonresearchers in the analysis of data results in the utilization of the information. This exchange clearly increases the researchers' time required for analyzing and reanalyzing data.

Stage 4: Conclusions and Policy Implications

The final stage after findings have been analyzed, reanalyzed, reinterpreted, and finalized, is to draw the conclusions and policy implications from applied research. The latter is primarily the responsibility of the nonresearchers. The researchers do have the role of ensuring that interpretations flow from the data and are otherwise valid as well. Examples of policy implications following from the supportive housing study include (Chappell & Horne, 1987):

1. The study found no strong support for one housing type over another; rather, each housing type has its different strengths. The ability to choose the type of housing to suit individual preferences and perceptions is important. Communities considering housing development should be made aware of the need for a variety of housing models.

2. To the extent that elderly person's housing (EPH) residents indicate economic security as the major reason for choosing that housing type, the study indicates that the Department of Housing is fulfilling its mandate to provide safe and affordable housing through its EPH units.

3. The study found no indication that multilevel care (MLC) facilities tend to "funnel" their residents from lower to higher levels of care to the exclusion of applicants from other locations. Nor was there any evidence of "premature entry," where individuals enter the lowest level of care in an MLC facility in order to ensure subsequent placement in that facility's personal care home. Such negative consequences of MLC facilities were not demonstrated. Rather, there is evidence that seniors residing in the lower level of care units within MLC facilities experience greater social integration than those living elsewhere.

   However, sponsors of MLC facilities should be aware that there is an expectation of service and support that is not currently available through their own resources. Although in many instances residents chose to reside in a MLC facility because of the perceived availability of health care, that health care is actually provided externally.

Some attention should be directed to the higher use and cost of Continuing Care nursing care by residents of MLC compared with residents of other housing models. It is to be noted, however, that these higher costs for MLC residents are concentrated in rural facilities and are based on a relatively small number of respondents. Nevertheless, these facilities might be encouraged to monitor this situation more closely.

4. Managers and sponsors of EPH(NS) must be made aware that residents of EPH(NS) have a perception of support availability that is untrue. Either that there is no service provision beyond the provincial home care program could be more publicized, or minimal supports could be developed to meet the perception of residents choosing this type of housing.

Continuous dialogue between the relevant parties also ensures continuous education of both the researcher and the nonresearcher—for the researcher, the subtleties of the world he or she is studying; for the nonresearcher, the research process. This continuous eduction, in turn, results in friends of research, that is, those who appreciate the importance and the usefulness of research in various places outside the university community.

SUMMARY

From over a decade of involvement in applied research, we have learned that:

1. It takes time.

2. It takes a nonarrogant attitude on the part of all the participants, that is, a genuine desire on everyone's part.

3. Everyone must perceive a benefit to the research, that is, contributions to knowledge (to researchers, publications; to nonresearchers, a better program).

4. Bad research can actually be harmful. Research, because of the mystique that has evolved around it, frequently carries an added weight. The added weight means added responsibility. Bad research is not neutral. Bad research can result in wrong changes to programs, the wrong implementations. It is of the utmost importance that research be conducted with care and rigor.

5. The process involves continuous education for everyone.

6. It is helpful if individuals learn to talk without jargon and, if this is

not possible, to learn one another's jargon. To learn their own applied areas, researchers will find this necessary anyway. To assist them in the most beneficial use of research findings, it is also necessary for nonresearchers. Nonresearchers have jargon just as do researchers.

In sum, this type of research, collaborative applied research, ensures that research findings do become used. The process I have discussed, I hope, shows the realistic use of research findings. They help programs evolve but are not the end-all and be-all. And despite its attendant difficulties and problems, research has its own rewards. As Lawrence Sterne said, "The desire of knowledge, like the thirst of riches, increases ever with the acquisition of it."

REFERENCES

Chappell, N. L. (1982a). The value of research to practitioners in work with the elderly. *Canadian Journal on Aging, 1*(1&2), 62-65.

Chappell, N. L. (1982b). *An evaluation of adult day care in Manitoba—Phase I* (Final Report). Winnipeg: Manitoba Health Services Commission.

Chappell, N. L. (1983). *Adult day care and change in the utilization of medical and inpatient hospital services* (Final Report). Winnipeg: Manitoba Health Services Commission.

Chappell, N. L., & Blandford, A. A. (1983). *Adult day care: Its impact on the utilization of other health care services and on quality of life* (Final Report). Ottawa: NHRDP, Health and Welfare Canada.

Chappell, N. L., & Horne, J. (1987). *Housing and supportive services for elderly persons in Manitoba* (Final Report). Ottawa: Canada Mortgage and Housing; Winnipeg: The Winnipeg Foundation.

Driedger, L., & Chappell, N. L. (1987). *Aging and ethnicity: Toward an interface.* Toronto: Butterworths.

Strain, L. A., & Chappell, N. L. (1984, November). *Social support among elderly Canadian natives: A comparison with elderly non-natives.* Paper presented at the annual meeting of the Canadian Association on Gerontology, Vancouver, British Columbia.

Commentary

GLORIA M. GUTMAN

In responding to Dr. Chappell's excellent presentation, I should like to begin by picking up and elaborating on one of her themes: specifically, the need to ensure that all participants in the research enterprise understand the importance of and need for the research. I shall use this as a vehicle to introduce *my* main theme, which is that applied research in gerontology is no mystery if one has the necessary research skills and is knowledgeable about adult development and aging.

THE IMPORTANCE OF EVERYONE'S ACCEPTING THE NEED FOR RESEARCH

In recent years, many agencies have been faced with having to include an evaluation component in their application for funding for a service and demonstration project. Many view this request with suspicion ("they" don't trust that *we* know what we are doing) and/or as a waste of time, effort and, if they have to hire an outside evaluator, precious research dollars. Frequently, one of the first tasks facing the applied researcher is to explain to the agency that has hired him/her *why* the evaluation is important. This includes explaining that *process evaluation* can enable the project to be easily replicated in another jurisdiction—thus considerably expanding its impact. A good process evaluation will describe both the successful implementation strategies and those that were not so successful. By describing the latter, it can save another agency from repeating what sometimes have been some very painful and costly mistakes.

Outcome evaluation, on the other hand, more directly benefits the agency conducting the project. An evaluation which reveals a project's tangible positive effects can provide the agency with "hard" data to use as a springboard for additional funds—funds that can allow the project to continue beyond its original time frame and perhaps become a permanent part of the spectrum of services available to the target group. Where the outcome evaluation shows the project to have had no significant effect or a negative effect, the agency (and indirectly, the taxpayer) benefits—in terms of knowing not to waste further time and money on something that "doesn't work."

The applied researcher's life would be easier if funding agencies would take it upon themselves to explicitly state the rationale when they require that an evaluation component be part of the research proposal. It would also considerably help service agencies if funders would provide some guidelines for what they should look for when advertising for and hiring a program evaluator.

SELECTING THE RIGHT RESEARCHER

These days, many people are jumping on the aging bandwagon. Service agencies need to be alerted to the fact that not everyone with a PhD can do applied research and, furthermore, that not every applied researcher, even an experienced one, has the necessary knowledge and skills to work with older people.

In the Gerontology Diploma Program which I direct at Simon Fraser University, among the first things we teach students is that in working with older people, whether in a research or practice setting, one must bear in mind that aging very often entails changes in vision, in hearing, and in information-processing abilities. When using visual materials, one has to ensure that the print is sufficiently large and distinct and the lighting in the room sufficiently intense for the material to be clearly seen by the aged eye. In the case of verbal information, one not only needs to speak more slowly and distinctly than is necessary with younger people, but also to take into consideration the high incidence of presbycusis, (i.e., high-tone loss) and the resultant need to lower the pitch of one's voice. One also needs to minimize distractions in the environment, because older persons find it more difficult than the young to ignore irrelevant aspects of the situation.

In cross-sectional studies, one also has to be very careful to minimize cohort effects: not to stack the cards against the elderly by, for example, using language that is beyond their level of comprehension (most of today's senior citizens have only, on average, a ninth-grade education). One also has to be careful not to use vocabulary unfamiliar to older people or which has different meaning than to the young. (For example, if one said someone was a "cool" person—the older person might (1) think he/she was aloof and standoffish or (2) wonder why he/she didn't just put on a sweater!)

SELECTING THE RIGHT RESEARCH INSTRUMENTS

Selection of research instruments also requires care and attention. Many people assume that because a particular instrument is well known, it may be used with any population. The fact is that many of the tests in common use in gerontological research were developed for younger people and are *not* appropriate for use with the elderly or, at least, must be interpreted differently. One such instrument is Zung's (1965) Self-Rating Depression Scale.

Blumenthal (1975) and others have suggested that certain items on this scale may have different meaning for the young than for the old. In particular, items referring to somatic symptoms are suspect. For example, while tachycardia and fatigue may indicate depression in the young, they may be symptomatic of physical disease in the old (Steuer et al., 1980). This is but one example of the problem inherent in using scales developed for other age groups in gerontological research.

ASKING THE RIGHT QUESTIONS AND SETTING THE RIGHT GOALS

Individuals inexperienced in gerontological research commonly err by setting unrealistic goals and/or asking questions that do not lend themselves to empirical test. The knowledgeable gerontological researcher, as Dr. Chappell has pointed out, can help these individuals and their sponsoring community groups or agencies to ask the "right" research questions. He/she can also help them select appropriate goals for determining the success of the proposed intervention.

The importance of doing so was brought home to me several years ago, when I was involved in a project (Gutman, Herbert, & Brown, 1977) comparing Feldenkrais with the American Red-White-and-Blue exercise program for seniors. In this study, in addition to including measures of height, weight, blood pressure, heart rate, balance, and flexibility, we included a number of questions about level of performance of activities of daily living (ADL) (e.g., bathing, dressing, grooming, mobility) and concerning level of psychosocial functioning. Much to our surprise, although the *subjective* reports of the participants identified a number of benefits from participating in the exercise programs, there was little *objective* evidence of improvements on the physiological, the ADL, or the psychosocial measures. Only after considerable soul-searching did we realize that perhaps our measures were not sufficiently sensitive to detect the very small physical changes that would likely be produced after only a six-week program of regular exercise and/or that some of the measures may have been inappropriate for the type of intervention employed in the study. (As I think back on it, it seems silly, for example, that we expected six weeks of gentle exercise to have had a major impact on participants' long-standing patterns of interaction with their children or other relatives.)

At least some of you will be in the position of contracting out research or reviewing research proposals. As I have argued elsewhere (Gutman, 1986b), it is critical that you carefully examine the proposed measures and projections (e.g., that there will be a 30% improvement in this or a 20% reduction in that) and be sure that the measures are appropriate to the intervention and the projections realistic. The latter is particularly important where the intervention is proposed as an "alternative to institutionalization." Evidence is beginning to accumulate that alternatives thought to keep seniors out of care facilities or out of subsidized housing may serve, at least in part, a population different from those who subsequently go into such settings (Borup, Lintz, & Van Orman, 1986; Varady, 1984; Zamprelli, 1985).

GUIDING DISCUSSION AND INTERPRETING FINDINGS

Knowledge of the target group, of their modal characteristics and typical patterns of behavior, is also critical in studies involving group discussion. One such methodology is the *focus group technique,* currently very much in vogue, where the group or agency is doing a needs assessment or attempting to determine the market for a particular idea or product. The focus group technique brings together a small group (8–10 individuals) with a group leader. As usually practiced, after telling the participants that there are no right and wrong answers, the group leader takes the group through a list of often vaguely defined topics or questions, stopping to pursue this or that response which *the leader* thinks is interesting or important. Following the discussion, which usually lasts an hour or two, the leader makes notes of what he/she recalls was said in the group. These notes, plus a transcript of the audiotapes of the session are the data from which a final report is subsequently written for the sponsoring agency.

In our view, based on first-hand experience with several focus group projects (Gutman, 1986a; Gutman, Milstein, & Doyle, 1987; Gutman & Milstein, 1988; Gutman, 1988), modification of the technique produces more accurate and reliable data. The modifications we have made deal with the problem of the leader's failing to cover all relevant issues and concerns; injecting his/her biases into the wording of the questions; or the possibility that he/she might forget or misinterpret what was said by the group or infer consensus when, in fact, there was none. We accomplished this in the following way:

1. We developed for the group leader a list of specific questions rather than just general topics. The leader, though not restricted to this list and encouraged to probe responses and ask additional questions, had to ask the mandatory questions. This ensured that all questions of critical interest were asked of all groups in a consistent manner, using wording that had been pretested to ensure clarity and comprehension. It also ensured that key areas were covered, which might not be the case where the leader lacks extensive knowledge of the area being explored.

2. We had two observer-coders attend each session and record, on a partially precoded form, all comments made by focus group participants as they occurred. As well, the observer-coders were instructed to record nonverbal responses such as nodding agreement with a point of view expressed by another participant. Nonverbal responses were lost in the conventional focus group methodology, because the leader was not able to keep note of such occurrences, which of course could not be reconstructed from the audiotapes.

3. We recorded responses separately for each individual in the group. This enabled us to identify, with considerably more precision than was usually the case with the focus group methodology, the extent to which there was consensus within any one group and across the various groups in the study. This key innovation guarded against the possibility of the leader highlighting, in his/her report, essentially idiosyncratic viewpoints (which we have observed to happen where the traditional focus group procedure was used).

Additionally, we gathered more personal data from focus group participants than is usually the case. These data included sociodemographic characteristics (age, sex, marital status, employment status, occupation, highest level of education completed, self-perceived health status) as well as possessions or habits of particular relevance to the topic being explored (e.g., in the case of housing studies, the size and type of dwelling they currently occupied; how long they have lived there; whether, if owners, they carried a mortgage and what they estimated their home would sell for if placed on the market that day). This enabled us to produce frequency and contingency tables in which responses to any particular focus group question were cross-tabulated by sociodemographic or other personal characteristics. Such tables were a distinct aid in interpreting findings.

FACILITATING RESEARCH

Returning once more to Dr. Chappell's paper, I should like to point out that the SFU Gerontology Research Centre, like the Centre on Aging at the University of Manitoba, has a mandate both to conduct and to foster and facilitate research on aging. In working with community groups and agencies, we provide a variety of services. These range from providing consultation on how the group or agency should go about defining the research question, identifying and recruiting subjects and selecting data collection instruments, to participating in projects as an active partner, to taking on the project on a contract or grant basis.

We use two main criteria to determine how to proceed. First, we attempt to ascertain whether the group or agency has the ability to carry out the project on its own. We recognize that although health care providers may have a keen interest in a particular topic (e.g., Alzheimer's disease) and can identify problems of importance (e.g., protecting wanderers from venturing out into traffic; reducing caregiver burden), they may lack the research skills and the *time* to carry out the needed research. Our second criterion is whether the results of the project will advance knowledge concerning aging or the aged. A *no* answer to the second criterion has led us to reject some very lucrative grants and contracts (usually for what we term "local area needs studies") and to take on several projects where there has been very limited or no financial return to the Centre.

To be sure, as Dr. Chappell has pointed out, it is important that research meets rigorous scientific standards and that research centers produce publications that will stand the scrutiny of peer review. Production of articles for peer-reviewed journals is, however, less of a priority for our Centre than generating and rapidly disseminating information that will be useful to practitioners, administrators, policymakers, and the elderly themselves. For that reason, our Centre has embarked on a vigorous in-house publication program. Additionally, a considerable number of journal articles have been produced by various of our researchers.

CONCLUSION

I should like to underscore the point made at the outset of this presentation, i.e., that gerontological research need not be mystifying if one has the requisite research skills and knows the target population. If one does not have the necessary background knowledge nor the time to acquire it, the appropriate strategy is to call in the professional gerontological researcher. There is now a network of gerontology research centers across Canada. These are resources which should be brought to the attention and utilized more fully by the health care community and others concerned with the older segment of Canada's population.

REFERENCES

Blumenthal, M. D. (1975). Measuring depressive symptomatology in a general population. *Archives of General Psychiatry, 32,* 971–978.

Borup, J. H., Lintz, L., & Van Orman, W. R. (1986, November 23). *The effects of a long-term care community based program as an alternative to nursing home care.* Paper presented at the 39th Annual Meeting of the Gerontological Society of America, Chicago, IL.

Gutman, G. M. (1986a, March). *Focus group findings and their implications for health promotion for seniors.* Report submitted to the Health Promotions Directorate, Health and Welfare Canada, Ottawa.

Gutman, G. M. (1986b, June 23). *Focus group study of the elderly—Implications for the Health Promotions Directorate*. Paper presented at a meeting of Health Promotion Directorate staff, Ottawa.

Gutman, G. M. (1988). *Focus group study of seniors reactions to the New Vista Society's community concept*. Report to the New Vista Society.

Gutman, G. M., Herbert, C. P., & Brown, S. R. (1977). Feldenkrais versus conventional exercises for the elderly. *Journal of Gerontology, 32*(5), 562–572.

Gutman, G. M., & Milstein, S. L. (1988). *Focus group study of older drivers*. Report to the Insurance Corporation of British Columbia.

Gutman, G. M., Milstein, S. L., & Doyle, V. (1987, November 30). *Attitudes of seniors to special retirement housing, life tenancy arrangements and other housing options*. Report submitted to the Canada Mortgage and Housing Corporation, Ottawa.

Steuer, J., Bank, L., Olsen, E. J., & Jarvik, L. F. (1980). Depression, physical health and somatic complaints in the elderly: A study of the Zung Self-Rating Depression Scale. *Journal of Gerontology, 35*(5), 683–688.

Varady, D. P. (1984). Determinants of interest in senior citizen housing among the community resident elderly. *Gerontologist, 24*, 392–395.

Zamprelli, J. (1985). Shelter allowances for older adults: Programs in search of a policy. In G. Gutman & N. Blackie (Eds.), *Innovations in Housing and Living Arrangements for Seniors*. Burnaby, BC: Simon Fraser University, The Gerontology Research Centre.

Zung, W. W. K. (1965). A self-rating depression scale. *Archives of General Psychiatry, 12*, 63–70.

Commentary

BRUCE A. MCFARLANE

Dr. Chappell has helped to make the research process less bewildering to all of us as well as pointing out how useful research may be as a mechanism for dispelling myths. By selecting the area of applied research and examples from her own extensive research experience, she has illustrated to us how, among other things, the interaction between those who seek the fruits of research and those who do research can be beneficial to both. Underlying this whole process, as she points out, are two basic assumptions, namely, (1) that "applied research requires a partnership between researchers and others, who include policymakers, practitioners, administrators, and the elderly themselves"; and (2) that all involved accept "the importance of the research process." To a great extent, the case studies she has cited as examples clearly illustrate that indeed these two assumptions seem to be the foundation blocks upon which the interaction of the researchers and others were built, and which lead to the success of the joint ventures.

Each instance of these case studies seems to reflect Jacques Barzun's dictum that "in a scientific culture, research is the universal solvent of problems." That is, "the hegemony of science is an accepted part of Western culture" (Barzun, 1964, p. 133). Proof by assertion is rejected by all who will be guided by science and scientific methods: "Everything must be subject to scrutiny, (and) guesswork must be replaced by exact count" and so on.

In large measure in our culture given this orientation, the findings of research are deemed to be able to eliminate "fears and spells and old wives' tales." That is, it is deemed to be a kind of "purification process of the common mind" (Barzun, 1964, p. 119).

To this end, research centers, where researchers are trained and where research is done, have grown up in universities, in institutes, and elsewhere (industry, business, associations, government). Research departments exist in any self-respecting organization or firm today. Needless to say, respect for research on this grand scale has not always existed. Between the early Hellenic times in Alexandria and modern times the only center of any note was that set up by Prince Henry the Navigator at Sagres, Portugal to study navigation, create maps, and so forth in the late 15th century. His research goal was not commercial but rather to forward the gospel to remote lands. To a great extent, of course, this lack of research enterprise in antiquity through the 15th to 18th centuries arose because of lack of sponsorship. As recently as 1870, when a research group of an island nation asked its government for £120 to keep up its research on the tides, the government of Britain turned down the British Association's application. This denial happened at a time when the Gladstone Government was spending thousands of pounds sterling per annum for paintings for the National Gallery (Barzun, 1964).

This search for money—or *funding* as we researchers prefer to call it because *money* (or *filthy lucre*) has a rather common or degrading ring to it—is not without its problems (Zakuta, 1970). Professor Horace Miner, the anthropologist, in an ironic article entitled "Researchmanship: The Feedback of Expertise" (1960) has noted: "Researching involves a well-ordered series of operations, the initial step of which is to secure the necessary funds to cover operating, living, and traveling expenses. The placing of priority on financing does not deny that in back of every research project there must be an idea but ideas should not be allowed to retard researching." He also notes that we as researchers are lucky today in this respect, because "the development of research ideas formerly consumed a great deal of research time."

As any good researcher knows, today about one fourth of the way through research on a particular project or, at least, after about one fourth of the grant funds have been spent, considerable time must be spent developing a rationale for the *next* phase of the research for the research grant applications, which must be submitted well in advance of when the funds will be required! The situation is even worse, of course, if it is contract research, because new contracts have to be secured in order to keep the research staff employed. This time spent securing funds suggests that research, as separate from science and scholarship, has taken on a life of its own.

For many years, the type of applied research as outlined by Dr. Chappell was anathema to many researchers. To them, research meant "pure" research, that is, research unsullied by any foreseen practical application (or relevance, to its detractors) but carried out for the pure joy of pushing back the frontiers of knowledge—the goal was knowledge for knowledge's sake. The struggle between the protagonists came to a head in Canada during the hearings of the Canada Senate Special Committee on Science Policy, the Lamontagne Committee. (I recommend to all of those interested in research, pure and applied, and policy to read the three-volume *Report* [1972] as well as the Hansard-type hearings reports.) I suspect that the major contribution of these hearings (in addition to making public the stands of the various vested interest groups in science and science policy) was the introduction into everyday discourse of a third type of science research, mission-directed research. (So now we have three types of research: pure, mission-directed, and applied.) This new category, it seems to me, is simply a mechanism for getting pure researchers to do applied research, with the promise of more autonomy. This attempt by government to control and organize research and use it as a tool is not new, of course. As long ago as 1969, the Secretary of the Treasury Board, Simon Reisman, giving evidence before the Lamontagne Committee (Doern, 1972, p. 74) stated:

> . . . in the eyes of the Board, science is not regarded as a thing in itself but rather as a means to an end. In general, particular scientific projects are not examined on their own merits, but rather as components of programs which have defined objectives.

This is not without interest in any study of the impact of research on public policy.

One would have thought that after the Lamontagne Committee *Report* much of this controversy would have been laid to rest, but because we are in Saskatchewan and at a meeting called "The First," I will quote from some comments made by a distinguished Canadian and Saskatchewan scientist at a meeting in 1979. Professor J. W. T. Spinks, in a talk to The *First* Conference on the History of Canadian Science and Technology (Spinks, 1980, p. 106), when discussing the organization and infrastructure of science and research said:

> The actual infrastructure which evolves around the research will depend on the goal to be achieved but whatever the goal, assuming that there is a goal, reaching the goal will certainly be helped if one knows something of the matter in hand. This begins to sound suspiciously like a systems approach and of course, that is exactly what it is. But don't worry, my name is not Glassco or Lamontagne and I am at heart a pure research scientist and have always spent a good deal of time sniffing out the most academic approach possible to whatever I happened to be doing.

But what, one may well ask, is all of this ongoing research in aid of? Who are the beneficiaries beyond the researchers who are able to spend their time doing what they have been trained to do and what they want to do and publishing their results? (Jacques Barzun [1964, p. 126] notes the following about publishing: "The Rev. Dr. Chausable was admired by Oscar Wilde's young heroine because, as she explained, ' . . . he has never written a book, so you can imagine how much he knows.' Both defects are cured by our system, which infallibly turns every researcher into an author.")

If one examines Dr. Chappell's examples carefully, it appears that the additional beneficiaries are (1) those for whom the immediate research is being carried out in order to enable them to exert some influence on public policy; and (2) those whom the foregoing groups would serve—in our case, the elderly and the aging.

Given what was said earlier about our living in a scientific and research-oriented culture, it is at this point that the role of research in the public policymaking progress becomes evident. But even here we have to be cautious, because public policymaking is part of the political process and, as most social scientists are aware, policies of this type, although claimed to be made on economic grounds, are in fact made on political grounds. That is, to support the findings and recommendations of research in public policy terms, political decisions are required, because every interest group attempts "to get its fingers into the till." A public policy decision has to be made about who should get the assistance. It is not unusual that when those who should be making the policy decision find it difficult to do so on political grounds, they ask for *more* research and may even make some money available to do so. These new research funds, of course, are perhaps less than 0.1% of what the program to be covered by the "avoided" policy would have cost.

Dr. Chappell's recognition that "bad research can actually be harmful" is particularly true when related to public policy. As Dr. Myint, the economist, has pointed out, a bad decision made in the siting of, say, a railway station or a factory, may cost a little money but it can still be closed or used as something else (a conference center?). But a bad decision in public policy, based on poor research in, say, education or health care, can have deleterious effects for a long time, even after the policy has been changed (Myint, 1964).

Dr. Chappell's comments on the controversy surrounding contract research also require a brief comment. The pressure exerted by the Mulroney Government to link research directly with industrial and business needs raises the question of who will determine the problem to be researched. Researchers will have to be very vigilant under these conditions. In addition, as Dr. Chappell notes, because the contractor "owns" the findings, their dissemination may be limited if, for example, the contractor does not like the findings. Examples should not be too difficult to imagine in the health care field.

A similar situation has arisen in the increase of government departmental task forces at the expense of royal commissions. The studies and findings of *royal commissions* become public property when they are tabled with the Commissioners' Reports in the House of Commons (the only exception that comes readily to mind was the case of the Royal Commission on Security, when it was deemed that certain evidence presented to the Commissioners would not be made public for reasons of national security). The findings of *task forces* remain under ministerial or departmental control, and hence may never be made available to other researchers, or the general public. In the first case, the bases for the Commissioners' recommendations and the public policy that follows can be examined and become part of the public discourse; in the latter case, they may only become public via a "leaked" document in a plain brown envelope slipped under the office door of an Opposition Member of Parliament or mailed anonymously to a member of the press.

Of vital interest are the varied perceptions that each of the major partici-

pants in the collaborative research has of the research process and the research area—in the case of research on aging, the elderly, and health, the
participants' perceptions not only of research but also of the elderly and their
health. If I were to take a group of professionals and/or experts to a down-
town residential street in the inner city and then ask each of them to write a
one-page description of what they saw, the impact of occupational values,
ideologies, and experiences would soon be evident. It is not too hard to
imagine that the descriptions by the architect, the social worker, the physician, the developer, the real estate agent, the public health nurse, the police-
man, and the fireman would make it appear that each was discussing a
different street; when these descriptions are compared with those of one or
more of the local residents' descriptions, the variance might become even
wider. The consequences for collaborative research are evident. Given this,
it is obvious from the success of the collaborative research at the Centre for
Aging that to Dr. Chappell's established reputation as a researcher should
also be added her success as an educator of those who want and do research
and with whom she has been associated. We are now among that fortunate
group.

REFERENCES

Barzun, J. (1964). *Science: The glorious entertainment* (esp. Chapter 6, "The cult
of research and creativity," pp. 119–142). Toronto: The University of Toronto
Press.

Canada Senate Special Committee on Science Policy, Honourable Maurice Lamontagne (Chair). (1972–73). *Report* (Three Volumes). Ottawa: Information Canada.

Doern, B. (1972). *Science and politics in Canada.* Montreal and London: McGill-
Queen's University Press.

Miner, H. (1960). Researchmanship: The feedback of expertise. *Human Organization, 19*(1): 1–3.

Myint, H. (1964). Social flexibility, social discipline and economic growth. *International Social Science Journal, 16*(2), 256.

Spinks, J. W. T. (1980). Afterscience. In R. A. Jarrell & N. R. Ball (Eds.), *Science,
technology and Canadian history/les sciences, la technologie et l'histoire
Canadienne* (pp. 106–114). Waterloo: Wilfred Laurier University Press.

Zakuta, L. (1970). On filthy lucre. In Tamotsu Shibutani (Ed.), *Human nature and
collective behaviour* (pp. 260–270). Englewood Cliffs, NJ: Prentice-Hall Inc.

28. Lessons for Gerontology from Healthy Public Policy Initiatives

VICTOR W. MARSHALL

INTRODUCTION

This chapter outlines the basic tenets of *healthy public policy* (HPP) and explores the implications of this new formulation of public policy for the field of aging and health. These implications have been almost completely unexplored in a growing literature. Three sets of implications are explored. The first concerns the use of age categorization in healthy public policy. The second deals with the implications of the emphasis on equity in health (which characterizes the healthy public policy field) for the aged as a "target group." The third examines the possibility that the emphases on multisectoral initiatives and on fostering broadly based participation which characterizes the healthy public policy field can lessen incipient medicalization of age-related concerns.

WHAT IS HEALTHY PUBLIC POLICY?

Milio (1986) refers to HPP as a "new public health . . . a new approach to promoting people's health." Hancock (1982) was among the first to use the term in the published literature. The term is frequently used interchangeably with *health promotion policy, health promoting policy,* and *public policy for health.* HPP has been variously defined as "policy of the people and their elected representatives characterized by an explicit concern for health" (in Announcing the Adelaide Conference on Healthy Public Policy); as "multisectoral policies to achieve equity in health" (*Health Promotion*, 1986,

Aging and Health: Linking Research and Public Policy, © 1989 Lewis Publishers, Inc., Chelsea, Michigan 48118. Printed in U.S.A.

p. 19); and as "public policy supportive of health" (*Health for All Ontario*, 1987, p. 92).

Most documents in the HPP field argue that, ideally, healthy public policy should be predicated on widespread public participation. The Canadian document, *Achieving Health for All* (Epp, 1986), which outlines a framework for health promotion, argues that "enhancing public participation" as well as "coordinating healthy public policy" is an implementation strategy directed toward health promotion.

In addition to its multisectoral nature, HPP is concerned largely with the determinants of health instead of the consequences of ill health.

Another important feature of the HPP literature is a concern with "equity." This was a major theme of the important WHO document, *Targets for Health for All by the Year 2000* (1985). In Ontario, a panel appointed by the Ministry of Health to formulate health goals listed as its first goal, Achieve equity in health opportunities (*Health for All Ontario*, 1987, p. 45). The panel uses the term *equity* to refer to justice or fairness, implying equal opportunities for all individuals and population groups to achieve and maintain health.

In summary, HPP is not health care policy or health care systems policy. It is consonant with health promotion policy to the extent that the latter takes a broad, multisectoral approach. For example, a good way to promote health might be to improve economic well-being, because it is known that unemployment and poverty adversely affect health. HPP is, in addition to these things, something of a social movement: it has actors, networks, a key journal (*Health Promotion*), a growing set of conferences with the development of a HPP jet set and, it appears, a growing "orthodoxy" of belief (Pederson et al., 1988).

This orthodoxy embodies the following principles:

- HPP should be multisectoral—the health of a people will be enhanced through developments in all sectors, such as the economy, nutrition, education;
- a guiding principle of HPP is equity—principles of fairness should guide efforts to promote health;
- HPP initiatives should, ideally, be participatory in scope; and
- HPP takes an ecological perspective which places humans in a broad context of the physical and social world.

HPP in many ways returns us to historically important concerns of public health, which were deeply concerned with reforms in education, housing, and sanitation (*Healthy Toronto 2000*, 1987). Its contemporary form may, however, be said to be inspired by the seminal "Lalonde Report," *A New Perspective on the Health of Canadians* (1974). Influenced by this report, the World Health Organization in 1977 endorsed a resolution that health was to be the main social goal of government—an idea put forth in the 1985 document, *Targets for Health for All.*

The European strategy for Health for All by the Year 2000 emphasized an environmental approach reminiscent of the Lalonde Report. Health promotion was one of four strategies to be used, the others being enhanced primary health care, intersectoral action, and the use of appropriate technology (*Targets for Health for All,* 1985). WHO thinking forms the major basis of the conceptualization of health promotion found in the Canadian document, *Achieving Health for All* (Epp, 1986), which serves as the current "charter document" governing HPP at the national level in Canada.

Following release of this Canadian document, Health and Welfare Canada cosponsored (with WHO and The Canadian Public Health Association) an international conference on health promotion. At the conference, the *Ottawa Charter on Health Promotion* (1986) was released, legitimating the HPP approach to health promotion. In Ontario, the government report, *Health for All Ontario* (1987), is centrally within the tradition of HPP, and currently guides strategic health planning in that province. It outlines 7 goals and 31 subgoals. Strategies to achieve these goals include economic and community development, resource allocation, legislation, management, coordination and collaboration, advocacy, appropriate use of technology, and research and information.

AGE CATEGORIZATIONS USED IN HEALTHY PUBLIC POLICY DOCUMENTS

Some of the major documents in the HPP field employ age categories as a major analytical framework, breaking the life course into qualitative life stages.

The *Healthy People* document in the United States (U.S. Department of Health, Education and Welfare, 1979) uses five age categories. These are: infants (<1); children (1–14); adolescents and young adults (15–24); adults (25–64); and older adults (65+). The report lists one major public health goal and two specific subgoals for each age group.

The document *Objective: A Health Concept in Quebec* (Task Force on Health Promotion, 1986) lists four categories: children (0–5); young people (6–24); adults (25–64); and adults aged 65 or more. However, in discussing diseases by age groups, the report (1986, pp. 23–39) uses five, not four groups. Childhood now lasts to age 14 and is followed by adolescence and the passage into adulthood (15–24); the prime of life (25–44); middle age (45 and upward); and old age (65 and upward). The distinction between middle and old age is admittedly vague: "Biologically, old age appears gradually. It is manifested by a slowdown in the individual's physical and mental functions. The decline curve varies greatly from one individual to another" (p. 29).

The Ontario Ministry of Health's working document, *Healthy Directions: A Framework for Action* (1986) employs six life stages, which were "selected on the basis of the unique developmental tasks and health status associated with each life stage. Additional considerations were compatibility with data sources and aggregations used in other studies" (1986, p. 6). The oldest stage, senior adulthood, begins at age 65. The putative unique developmental tasks are asserted to exist but are not described or explained.

The WHO and Canadian (federal) efforts, and the *Health for All Ontario* report (1987) do not employ age categorization. However, some of the WHO health targets are specific to age groups. For example, Target 10 aims for reductions in cancer mortality "in people under age 65"; Target 9 is similar, but for mortality resulting from diseases of the circulatory system; and Target 7 aims to reduce infant mortality.

In summary, some but not all health promotion documents use age categorization; however, the cutting points are dissimilar, although those that do employ age categorization group together persons aged 65 and over.

Age 65 as a Cutting Point

It is interesting that the Quebec effort, which distinguishes adults aged 25–64 from those aged 65 and older, also emphasizes the usefulness of the "years of healthy life" construct. Although men and women in Quebec can expect widely different years of life expectancy, they are essentially similar in expected years of healthy life—an average of 60 years for women and 59 for men (Task Force on Health Promotion, 1986, p. 20). Activity limitation, then, can be expected to occur at age 60 on average, which is an age not defined by the life stages employed in the Quebec exercise. This leads to the question, What is the basis for the selection of specific ages as cutting points to distinguish age groups? A related question is, How useful are the age categories selected?

None of the major reports in this area explicitly addresses the rationale for selecting specific age boundaries, nor can rationales be found in the wider corpus of HPP literature. Gerontological literature suggests that a grouping together of persons aged 65 and older into one category is not efficacious. Moreover, serious concerns have been raised about the usefulness of alternative, more fine-grained distinctions.

Age 65 has come to be the commonly used marker for discussions of the aged. This use is reasonable precisely because of the pervasiveness of retirement and its associated financial arrangements as a complex social institution. For example, financial status is greatly altered for the majority of Canadians when they turn 65; leisure pursuits can also be expected to be greatly different when comparing a 64-year-old with a 66-year-old.

However, gerontologists increasingly express dissatisfaction with the failure to recognize the diversity of persons in the age-65-and-older category. As one response to this, Bernice Neugarten introduced a distinction between the "young-old" and the "old-old." The distinction rests largely on the basis of health status, but Neugarten added income security and active pursuit of leisure interests as characteristics of the young-old. Neugarten claimed that age 75 roughly distinguished the two groups (see Neugarten, 1974; for a general discussion see Binstock, 1985).

Unfortunately, contrary to Neugarten's intentions, many journalists, professionals, and scholars in the aging field uncritically adopted age 75 as a concrete cutting point, and the two categories became reified. The distinction between the young-old and the old-old is now routinely made on the basis not of health status but of age.

In 1984, the U.S. National Institute on Aging announced that it would fund a major research initiative focused on "the oldest old," that is, on persons aged 85 and older. A set of papers presenting preliminary data from this research program has appeared in *Milbank Memorial Fund Quarterly/ Health and Society.* As Robert Binstock (1985) cautions, in an article in that issue, it is possible that this "oldest old" distinction will be reified in the same way as the young-old/old-old distinction had been, with potentially adverse policy consequences.

The dilemma of using any age categories is captured by Suzman and Riley in their introduction to the *Milbank* special issue (1985, p. 180). They first point to the dissimilarity of the oldest old from younger old people:

> . . . as every paper in this issue demonstrates, the oldest old are very dissimilar to those who have recently entered old age—say, those aged 65 to 69. Those aged 85 and over have . . . a much greater excess of females over males than any other age category. They are currently more likely to be living in institutions, less likely to be married, and more likely to have low educational attainment. Their needs, capacities, and resources are different. They consume an amount of services, benefits, and transfers far out of proportion to their numbers. . . . [B]ecause of their needs they receive a significant fraction of all the federal benefits, services, and transfers received by all those over age 65. The differentiation of the elderly population has become so marked that it is no longer useful to treat all elderly—those aged 65 and over—as a single category. . . .

On the other hand, Suzman and Riley go on to say:

> Also widely unrecognized is the pronounced diversity of the population aged 85 and over. At this age many people still function effectively, while others have outlived their social and financial supports and have become dependent upon society for their daily living.

In the Canadian context, a number of studies have shown the older population to be highly differentiated, both within and between age groups, in health status (see, e.g., Connidis, 1987; D'Arcy, 1987; Marshall, 1987; Roos, Shapiro, & Roos, 1984; Simmons-Tropea & Osborn, 1987). These reports provide data suggesting that the age 65 group needs to be crosscut both by age and by other differentiators (especially gender and social class).

It is appropriate to speak of age-related *variability* in health status, health service utilization and, no doubt, health promotion and prevention goals. Phrasing health goals in terms of age *categories* is quite another thing, carrying the dangers of stereotyping and the creation of inaccurate emphases on health needs of those in different age groups. There is great diversity in any age group, including the very old, in health status and health care needs. For research or program design purposes, it would be advisable to use a relatively fine breakdown, such as 5-year age categories, and to impose categorization empirically.

It should also be recognized that appropriate age breakdowns in one area (e.g., giving health or disease data) are not likely to be appropriate in other areas (e.g., economic or social support data). It should be apparent from this discussion that age categories are not likely to be the optimal classification around which to organize recommendations for health goals, or most policy initiatives in this health field. The use of age categories in the U.S. *Healthy People* document (U.S. Department of Health, Education and Welfare, 1979), although perhaps suited to its emphasis on prevention rather than health promotion, seems ill-advised and ought not to unduly influence other HPP efforts.

IMPLICATIONS OF EQUITY VALUES FOR THE AGED

Equity is a major value espoused by those in the HPP movement. The *Ottawa Charter on Health Promotion* (1986), says that "health promotion focuses on achieving equity in health. Health promotion action aims at reducing differences in current health status and ensuring equal opportunities and resources to **enable** all people to achieve their fullest health potential." *Achieving Health for All* (Epp, 1986) lists reducing inequities as one of the three principal health challenges. Achieving equity is also listed as the first priority goal by the Ontario Panel on Health Goals (*Health for All Ontario*, 1987).

By *equity* is meant "justice or fairness. Equity in health implies that members of all population groups have equal opportunities to achieve and maintain health" (*Health for All Ontario*, 1987, p. 45). Equity, as a moral value, is distinguished from *equality,* either of condition or opportunity. *Inequality* refers to "measurable differences in health amongst various population groups" (*Health for All Ontario*, 1987, p. 45).

From a concern for equity, designated groups might receive *unequal* re-source allocation because of their higher risks or vulnerability to health insults. The aged are one such group that might be selected for additional resource allocation in order to achieve greater fairness or justice. The Ontario Panel on Health Goals, for example, argues that a goal of providing equal opportunities to attain health implies "affirmative action to enable the disadvantaged to reach their potential."

In gerontology, the question of equity arises from the important policy question of whether resource allocation should be based on age or need (Neugarten, 1982). Advocacy based on need is usually based on concerns for equity (Neysmith, 1987, p. 587). Neysmith suggests that although such concerns are predominant among Canadian policymakers, they conflict with other values widely shared in Canada.

At a practical or political level, there are many potential dangers of needs-based policies. Etzioni (1977, p. 38) has argued that the elderly are more likely to benefit, in terms of self-esteem and their esteem in the eyes of others, when "universalistic" social policies rather than "old-age-oriented policies" are adopted to meet their needs. He believes policies that benefit a special age group foster age grading, with attendant negative labeling of the aged (1977, pp. 38–39). Activist Maggie Kuhn, head of the Gray Panthers, suggests that "age-segregated services have isolated the elders from the voting" (1984, p. 9). Kutza (1981, pp. 127–28) goes so far as to speculate that special treatment for the aged will engender a backlash against them, because "chronological age is not a good indicator of an individual's circumstances" (Kutza, 1981, p. 141). For example, though many of the aged are poor, the poorest of the poor are not aged, but people such as young, single parents and their children, for whom special socioeconomic provisions are not as adequate as existing provisions for the aged.

IMPLICATIONS OF MULTISECTORAL AND PARTICIPATORY EMPHASES FOR AGING

Two additional themes of the HPP movement have potential implications for aging and health. These are the emphasis on multisectoral approaches on enhancing widespread participation. The field of gerontology is in great, and probably increasing, danger of *medicalization*—a tendency to focus unduly on a narrow band of geriatric issues and on age-related diseases. By *medicalization*, I refer to the application of a medical model to an event. As Conrad and Schneider (1980, p. 28) point out, although medical practitioners and medical treatment are usually associated with healing the sick and comforting the afflicted, the domains to which medical expertise and jurisdiction are now extended have expanded. Whole aspects of life become medicalized, the physician comes to be considered the expert with primary responsibility in that area, and policy initiatives focus on medical issues.

One important potential implication of the HPP movement is that it may help to counter the threat of medicalization. For example, a recent Ontario health policy report suggests hospital-based community services be expanded. The alleged advantages of organizing home care from a hospital base are the facilitation of earlier hospital discharges because of closer liaison with and greater potential to use hospital services to support the home care services (*Toward a Shared Direction*, 1987, p. 58). This would enhance continuity of care and alleviate the current situation in which over 10% of Ontario acute hospital beds are inappropriately filled with geriatric patients better suited to a less-intense level of care (Aronson, Marshall, & Sulman, 1987). However, such an approach would also extend hospital control far into the community and encroach on the authority of other health professions.

Conversely, the Panel on Health Goals for Ontario argued that "the most promising approach is development of more community-based services," by which it means "noninstitutional services accountable to the local population, ideally through a community board elected specifically to oversee the services." By implication, such services would not be hospital-based or controlled.

Medicalization is countered by the HPP tenet emphasizing what the *Achieving Health for All* report (Epp, 1986) refers to as "fostering public participation" and the related strategy of "strengthening community health services." These approaches imply the importance of sources of authority in the health field other than the physician.

The HPP emphasis on multisectoral approaches should direct health policy and resource allocation away from disease-oriented geriatric care toward more broadly based issues affecting the aged, such as the provision of decent housing and income security and the strengthening of coping abilities and mutual aid (Epp, 1986; Labonte, 1987). As Milio (1986, p. 129) notes, health services alone cannot achieve equity in health. Collaboration among all policy sectors is required.

CONCLUSION

A distinctive approach to health policy, HPP revitalizes multisectoral concerns from the traditional field of public health, and takes inspiration from the environmental approach advocated in the Lalonde Report. Only some of the many international, national, and provincial developments in HPP have been reviewed in this chapter, but they allow the identification of a core of assumptions underlying HPP: a commitment to achieving equity in health status; an emphasis on multisectoral approaches; a commitment to enhancing public participation to achieve health; and the adoption of a broad, ecological framework.

The implications of HPP initiatives for the aged have not been closely considered. This chapter has discussed three sets of implications. The first concern is with the use, in a number of HPP documents, of age categories as an organizing framework for the statement of health goals or targets. There are good intellectual and political reasons to question the efficacy of such an approach. No existing set of age categories seems to adequately organize the differentiation complexities within age categories. The second concern—targeting services specifically at the aged in pursuit of equity— risks inefficient resource allocation, marginalizing the aged as a distinct social group and generating a backlash against them.

The third concern is with the relationship of HPP initiatives to medicalization. It has not been possible in this chapter to document medicalization of age-related issues in any detail. However, the multisectoral and public participation tenets of the ideology of HPP should act as a brake or check on strong tendencies to convert concerns for the health of the aged into medical or "geriatric" concerns, to focus narrowly on diseases and to emphasize hospital-based and physician-controlled care for the aged.

HPP thus has both positive and negative implications for aging policy. The principles of HPP are largely unsupported by data or by theory (Pederson et al., 1988). There is something of a social gospel flavor to HPP, the development of an orthodoxy and of a distinct interest group whose careers are closely tied to the growth of the HPP paradigm. Precisely because this approach promises so much and because it is so critical of alternative health policy approaches, it should be examined with great effort and great care.

ACKNOWLEDGMENT

I wish to thank Ann Pederson for helpful criticism of an earlier version of this chapter.

REFERENCES

Aronson, J., Marshall, V. W., & Sulman, J. (1987). Patients awaiting discharge from hospital. In V. W. Marshall (Ed.), *Aging in Canada: Social perspectives* (2nd ed.) (chap. 27, pp. 538–549). Toronto: Fitzhenry & Whiteside.

Binstock, R. (1985). The oldest old: A fresh perspective or compassionate ageism revisited? *Milbank Memorial Fund Quarterly/Health and Society, 63*(2), 420–451.

Connidis, I. (1987). Life in old age: The view from the top. In V. W. Marshall (Ed.), *Aging in Canada: Social perspectives,* (2nd ed.) (chap. 22, pp. 451–472). Toronto: Fitzhenry & Whiteside.

Conrad, P., & Schneider, J. W. (1980). *Deviance and medicalization: From badness to sickness.* St. Louis, Toronto & London: C. V. Mosby.

D'Arcy, C. (1987). Aging and mental health In V. W. Marshall (Ed.), *Aging in Canada: Social perspectives* (2nd ed.) (chap. 21, pp. 424–450). Toronto: Fitzhenry & Whiteside.

Epp, J. (1986). *Achieving health for all: A framework for health promotion.* Ottawa: Health and Welfare Canada.

Etzioni, A. (1977). Old people and public policy. In F. Riessmasn (Ed.), *Older persons: Unused resources for unmet needs* (pp. 38–51). Beverly Hills & London: Sage.

Hancock, T. (1982, August). Beyond health care. *Futurist,* pp. 4–13.

Health for All Ontario Report of the Panel on Health Goals. (1987). Toronto: Government of Ontario, Ministry of Health.

Health promotion: Concepts and principles in action, a policy framework (discussion document). (1986). Copenhagen: World Health Organization, Regional Office for Europe.

Healthy Toronto 2000. (1987). Toronto: City of Toronto Board of Health, Healthy Toronto 2000 Subcommittee.

Kuhn, M. (1984). Introduction: Challenge to a new age. In M. Minkler & C. L. Estes (Eds.), *Readings in the political economy of aging* (pp. 7–9). Farmingdale, NY: Baywood.

Kutza, E. A. (1981). *The benefits of old age: Social welfare policy for the elderly.* Chicago & London: The University of Chicago Press.

Labonte, R. (1987). Community health promotion strategies. *Health Promotion, 26*(1), 5–10, 32. (Available from Health and Welfare Canada)

Lalonde, M. (1974). *A new perspective on the health of Canadians.* Ottawa: Government of Canada.

Marshall, V. W. (1987). The health of very old people as a concern of their children. In V. W. Marshall (Ed.), *Aging in Canada: Social perspectives* (2nd ed.) (chap. 23, pp. 473–485). Toronto: Fitzhenry & Whiteside.

Milio, N. (1986). Multisectoral policy and health promotion: Where to begin? *Health Promotion, 1*(2), 129–132.

Neugarten, B. L. (1974). Age groups in American society and the rise of the young old. *Annals of the American Academy of Political and Social Science, 415,* 187–198.

Neugarten, B. L. (Ed.). (1982). *Age or need? Public policies for older people.* Beverly Hills, London & New Delhi: Sage.

Neysmith, S. M. (1987). Social policy implications of an aging society. In V. M. Marshall (Ed.), *Aging in Canada: Social perspectives* (2nd ed.) (chap. 30, pp. 586–597). Toronto: Fitzhenry & Whiteside.

Ontario Ministry of Health. (1986). *Healthy directions: A framework for action.* Toronto: Ministry of Health for Ontario, Office of Health Promotion.

Ottawa charter on health promotion. (1986). Ottawa: World Health Organization, Canadian Public Health Association, Health and Welfare Canada.

Pederson, A. P., Edwards, R. K., Marshall, V. W., Allison, K. R., & Kelner, M. (1988). *Coordinating healthy public policy. An analytic literature review and bibliography* (Document HSHB 88–1). Ottawa: Department of National Health and Welfare, Health Promotion Directorate.

Roos, N. P., Shapiro, E., & Roos, L. L. (1984). Aging and the demand for health services: Which aged and whose demand? *Gerontologist, 24*(1), 31–36.

Simmons-Tropea, D., & Osborn, R. (1987). Disease, survival and death: The health status of Canada's elderly. In V. W. Marshall (Ed.), *Aging in Canada: Social perspectives* (2nd ed.) (chap. 20, pp. 399–423). Toronto: Fitzhenry & Whiteside.

Suzman, R., & Riley, M. W. (1985). Introducing the "oldest old." *Milbank Memorial Fund Quarterly/Health and Society, 63*(2), 177-186.

Targets for health for all by the year 2000. (1985). Copenhagen: World Health Organization, Regional Office for Europe.

Task Force on Health Promotion. (1986). *Objective, a health concept in Quebec: A report of the Task Force on Health Promotion* (M. S. Gayk, Trans.). Ottawa: Canadian Hospital Association.

Toward a shared direction for health in Ontario. Report of the Ontario Health Review Panel. (1987, June). Toronto: Ontario Ministry of Health.

U.S. Department of Health, Education and Welfare. (1979). *Healthy people: The Surgeon General's report on health promotion and disease prevention.* Washington, DC: U.S. Government Printing Office.

Commentary

N. DUANE ADAMS

INTRODUCTION

I am very pleased to be able to respond to the remarks offered to you by Dr. Marshall and to add some additional thoughts from my own experience about the relation between research and public policy and the need to improve the relations between social researchers, and planners and policy decisionmakers.

I believe there exists some serious difficulty between these two sets of players which is inhibiting their optimal contribution toward policy. This difficulty has had the consequence of depressing the benefits of social policy research and is ultimately a contributing factor to suboptimal social policy.

Essentially, Dr. Marshall has confirmed for us the accepted meaning of the term *healthy public policy*. He then has spoken to two separate issues: (1) the principles and approaches that seem desirable for the development and creation of better social policy today; and (2) some methodological considerations when undertaking research on the elderly population.

Dr. Marshall highlights the current orthodoxy surrounding *healthy public policy,* which demands that policies will: (1) be multisectoral in nature; (2) apply the principle of equity; (3) utilize a participatory approach in the creation of the policy; and (4) take an ecological perspective, which places humans in a broad context of a physical and social world.

With respect to definitions, it has been noted that *healthy public policy* generally refers to "health promotion policy." I agree with Dr. Marshall that it is a waste of time to debate the labeling of public policy fads, whether or not the fad is currently in vogue within my own department.

But it is always timely to remind ourselves that social policy, whether it concerns health, the aged, the environment, or anything else, can be graded *good, bad,* or a multitude of things in between. Although the ultimate choice of the policy is usually made by elected officials, the policy choices put to these decisionmakers heavily condition the quality of the policy itself. This quality of policy choices is where you and I count greatly and where we also should have a common interest. We are not responsible for the judgment made about the social policy, but we are collectively responsible for the quality and wisdom of the choices offered to the social decisionmakers.

If we routinely expect to achieve reasonably good (or healthy, if you prefer) social policies, high quality research supporting the policy is the first ingredient. Obviously, the essential social policy issue must be meticulously defined so that the research question and methodology are framed to address quite squarely the correct issue—not an interesting tangent. From this starting point, the quality of the findings and insights of this research are conditioned directly by the adequacy and accuracy of the data that can be assembled, the excellence of the analyses and forecasting, and the wisdom of the researchers who apply insights to the work.

THE STATE OF SOCIAL POLICY RESEARCH

Although I am not qualified to assess clinical research, I am able to assess social policy research. It will come as little surprise to you that I have concluded there are huge deficiencies in the utility and the quality of this work. Not only is this a criticism of the research product, but it is an indictment of the quality of the social policy that follows. Dr. Marshall has concluded as well that there is a serious lack of theory and research to support the principles of healthy public policy.

There are a number of reasons to explain this dilemma. It is common that the social planners are not able to define with sufficient precision the social issue to be addressed or its characteristics. In some instances, this lack of precision is a reflection of lazy intellect, but more frequently it is a reflection of rapidly changing and evermore complex social conditions that have been forecasted imperfectly, where the variables in the solutions are highly subjective and only grossly measurable, where little useful early research has been completed, and where a political imperative has emerged for an early solution to the social issue.

With some very notable exceptions, little routine attention is given collectively by researchers, planners, and decisionmakers to the contemplation of the future and its issues, the definition of appropriate parameters, and the examination of the nature of the principal variables that will affect the future human condition. Without some theoretical picture of future social policy needs and goals, and with precious few valid instruments available to examine these matters, is it any wonder that social policy planners scramble from social crisis to social crisis trying to deliver credible options to the social decisionmakers while alleging that the social policy research community is generally not making an intrinsically important contribution to the policy process?

Indeed, an estrangement has emerged between the researchers and the policy planners which in my mind is mutually disadvantageous. For our society and its social policies, the estrangement is a clear liability.

This symposium is one important attempt to bring together the principal players in the social policy arena in an attempt to understand and take steps to repair our mutually dependent relationship. I understand that an underlying theme of this symposium is that "good policy follows almost invariably from sound research, and that a strong and more beneficial link between research and policy will come about as a result of conscious effort and planning rather than 'natural' circumstances."

No doubt we can accept the generality of this hypothesis, but it is probably more correct to suppose that there is a better chance of a good policy emerging if it is preconditioned by high-quality, relevant research. For me, there can be no doubt that a greater coordination and planning of efforts between these two important communities can only generate better chances of success for social policy.

My planner colleagues and I are generally very close to the decisionmakers, who must face on a daily basis incredible pressure from the public to correct currently perceived social ills within a very short time. For the social planner, all of the past imperfections in defining social issues, in measuring relevant variables, in dealing with the subjective, the conflicting social values, the ever-changing public opinion, the deficiencies in factual information and research—all must be balanced one way or another, imperfect as it may be, to deliver policy option products to our governors.

And who takes the heat when the policy advice does not rise to society's expectation? Of course, the elected official first, who then looks with extreme disappointment on the policy advice he has received from his planners.

HOW TO IMPROVE SOCIAL POLICY RESEARCH—A PLANNER'S POINT OF VIEW

But if a good social policy can derive only from a good research foundation, does the research community not share some of the responsibility for a social policy gone wrong? From the research user point of view, what seems to be the difficulty and what improvements can be suggested?

Assess Future Needs and Issues

Researchers have to initially spend more intellectual time in the *future* before they examine the present and past. Doing so will immeasurably contribute to the selection of the most socially relevant issues, defining them, and selecting the most relevant variables for examination. Moreover, spending time in the future will reinforce our awareness of the efforts we must make to improve our social measurement tools and our knowledge of interactive effects.

Provide Appropriate Research Findings When Needed

Timeliness is always a problem with researchers and decisionmakers. In the social policy context, the main problem is that research findings are lagging behind the requirement for a social policy.

Too frequently, of sheer necessity or desperation, a social policy is constructed and implemented without the benefit of any penetrating research of some of the most significant factors in the policy. To some extent, I expect this will always remain true, but we could do much to improve the present situation.

If an organized effort were made to develop a better forecast of social policy issues, and if this forecast led to a national social policy research strategy and work program, and if efforts were expended to coordinate the available talents and resources in the area, and, finally, if researchers and planners fully appreciated their mutual dependence, then there might be a reasonable expectation that appropriate research findings would be available approximately at a time when policy initiatives needed them.

Coordinate Research and Planning

A concerted effort by all parties must be made to coordinate the diverse efforts behind social research and planning in the interest of effectiveness and efficiency.

Effectiveness

More effective products may be produced when the key interest groups have reached an approximate consensus about emerging social issues and their relevance, and when diverse intellects and orientations have shared their perspectives on issues, critical variables, and viable methodologies. This required coordination then has two thrusts: one centering on the clients or research users, and the second centering on the research community itself with its diversity of perspectives and skills.

Social research cannot be successful in a cocoon. The effort to coordinate offers both researchers and planners the benefit not only of a more effective end product, but also a vehicle which may well assist in overcoming the communication problem and estrangement I have identified earlier.

Efficiency

Throughout the remainder of this century the economic condition of Western nations and the fiscal policy of governments will remain tight. During this period, there will be significantly increasing domestic pressure on social spending. It will be evermore difficult, especially for the social research community, to capture the new marginal dollar which will be available for investment in research. This financial dilemma emerges at a time when the research community demands and needs a much larger investment.

As I am advocating a larger social policy research initiative in a context which is broader, more penetrating, and consequently more expensive, the cost-investment dichotomy can be addressed only if:

(1) the research community tightens its belt to become as efficient as possible by clarifying its priorities and goals, eliminating redundancy, and eliminating underutilization of existing resources; and

(2) the research community identifies more clearly to its "user" audience the benefits of its work. Through the coordination process, it would be especially helpful if a conscious linkage could occur between the policy needs of decisionmakers and the products of the researchers. In this way, an implicit social contract could be formed which would also form a strong basis for the research community to claim a greater share of marginal available dollars.

I am confident that an instrument and process for this coordination and linkage can occur without invading the autonomy of the research and academic community and without offending the sensitivities of governments that frequently prefer to develop and consider their policy alternatives in a rather confidential environment.

Select a Research Integrator to Oversee a National Social Policy Work Program

My observations on the need for much greater coordination imply that many more actors would participate in the social research and planning process than at present, and that these actors would possess a multidisciplinary intelligence, which collectively would have the capacity to approach social policy holistically. This is also consistent with the current orthodoxy stated by Dr. Marshall that social policy ought to be "multisectoral in nature."

It may be axiomatic to state that the purview of social policy is holistic or ecological. It deals with whole people, whole social institutions, and whole societies. Social policies must respect this holistic purview. Nevertheless to be manageable, most individual research must be undertaken within a far more narrow frame of reference. Two important implications are evident:

(1) Who is to take the responsibility to ensure that all of the issues relevant to a coherent social policy are being addressed through individual research efforts? and
(2) Who is to take responsibility to integrate all the research findings into an intelligible picture?

In the clinical research field, these activities are addressed quite well by the research community itself. That is perhaps because in so many instances the researchers and the clinical decisionmakers are the same group of people. The situation is quite different in a social policy arena, where the researchers and the decisionmakers are different groups. Currently, much of the responsibility for integrating research findings is handled by the social policy planner. The responsibility to oversee a comprehensive social research program does not seem to be addressed by anyone. In our mutual interest, we need to reach a consensus about who will take the responsibility to develop and oversee a national social policy work program, and who will adopt the role of research integrator.

Adopt a Multidisciplinary, Multisectoral Approach to Research

The argument for the multisectoral approach to social policy is compelling. Although this orthodoxy has been stated in respect to the development of public policy, if the research supporting the public policy is to be optimal, then the same multisectoral approach needs to be taken to the research as well.

There is a very close analogy to be found in the research requirements for social policy and the clinical research requirements for dealing with health problems of elderly people. I am told that when you are dealing with younger people, the assumption can normally be made that the majority of human operating parts behave in a proven and predictable manner. Deviations from this predictable behavior are more easily discernible, allowing cause-and-effect relationships to be inferred with a high degree of confidence.

As the human being ages, our knowledge of the behavior of the human operating parts is less sure, especially of the interactive effects of the failing bodily functions. This fact leads to a far more complicated and less sure diagnosis of the elderly than of a younger person. In short, a symptom that is common to both an elderly and a young person may have entirely different causes.

Similarly, in social policy research the body politic is maturing day by day. Cause-and-effect relationships that have been established in the past for this body politic may no longer apply.

The most dramatic demonstration of this point is found in Western world economics in the 1980s. The economic theories, practices, and policies developed since the late 1930s simply did not hold up when confronting the economic conditions of the 1980s. By the 1980s, new variables had been added into the national economic picture which interacted with old variables in such a way as to produce an unpredictable result for the economists and economic policy decisionmakers.

The derivative lesson for social policy researchers is that social conditions now demand that research be multidisciplinary and multisectoral in nature. Considerable vigilance must be applied to ensure that variables do, in fact, remain constant in their effects and that we simply do not *assume* that they remain constant. Social researchers either have to broaden the scope of their individual research endeavors, or establish a collective and coordinated mechanism to provide an external macroscope to the individual research efforts.

Include Consequences of Policy Options Within the Basic Research

The orthodoxy that states we need to utilize a participatory approach in the creation of policy is not a condition that should be taken lightly. There is nothing so frustrating to the policy planner and decisionmaker as to find that variables critical to decisionmaking have been excluded from the research process and that other "soft" variables like social values and interest group opinions have been ignored as well. Social policy simply cannot be implemented disregarding the short- and medium-term consequences on the people they will affect.

Although it is not the job of the researcher to choose which consequences a society should bear, it does seem reasonable to insist that the consequences have been explored by the researcher and form a part of the research product. Moreover, these consequences need to be researched and measured with the same precision as the principal research question itself.

From my point of view, it is not rude to consider a political variable in a research question, and it is not crude to treat social values and interest group opinion. It is, conversely, unreasonable to define or assume these variables out of existence.

Take an Ecological Perspective of Human Beings

The final point in the social policy orthodoxy advocates "taking an ecological perspective which places humans in a broad context of the physical and social world." You must have concluded from my remarks thus far that I consider this principle an imperative that applies as much to the researchers as it does to the decisionmakers.

Allocate Money for Social Research Intelligently

Finally, we all probably regret that research programs have to chase dollars rather than dollars chase research programs. I suppose there would be nothing wrong with research programs chasing dollars if a high degree of wisdom had been applied to the targeting of the dollars in the first instance. But I find in Canada that there is no unusually insightful intelligence applied to the allocation or targeting of social research dollars. Perhaps more productive allocations would occur in future time if the other ideas I have explored today were adopted.

Meanwhile, what can be achieved is a heightened awareness among the researchers, planners, social decisionmakers, and financiers about the nature of the financial problem, the mutual interdependence of the players, and some of the options which are available to enhance everyone's satisfaction by the improvements in the efficiency and effectiveness of the whole social policy development process.

CONCLUSION

Free Trade [the U.S.-Canada accord] is in vogue today. The promise is that those who have the insight, knowledge, and energy to produce valued products most efficiently and effectively will reap hitherto unavailable rewards. In the same spirit, perhaps the time has arrived for our research and public policy community to get organized, develop and market its product, and, in so doing, capture the promised rewards.

29. *The Consumer Response to Research and Policy*

PATRICIA FULTON

COMMON MYTHS AND STEREOTYPES

Although I am here to represent the elderly, no one person can really speak for seniors. The elderly in Canada are such a diverse group—with a range of life experiences, educational backgrounds, interests, philosophies, and political beliefs—that it defies all efforts to find one category with which to define them. However, researchers often do just that: categorize the elderly as if they were a homogeneous group rather than the heterogeneous population they really are. Perhaps the best way of understanding this diversity is to consider Pogo's dictum—We have seen the future and they are us—and then to think about what, outside of professional interests, we share in common.

Sometimes we attempt to classify the elderly by denoting them as people who receive care. Yet if I tell you about one woman who is 85 years old and who has been caring for many years for a 50-year-old niece who is emotionally disabled—can you tell me who is young and who is old? Or if you think that you are safe in categorizing seniors as physically diminished, remember that team of elderly cyclists who biked across Canada.

Researchers who model a simplistic construction of reality in order to form a category called *seniors* may have fallen victim to some of the myths about aging that they will themselves want to scrupulously avoid when they cross the arbitrary demographic line between middle age and old age. Of course, not only researchers are susceptible to these myths. Often one finds stereotypes at the root of capricious policy or regulations.

One tireless consultant that I know was involved in the planning and design of long term care facilities. She argued vociferously that the bathrooms should be equipped with showers but met a wall of resistance. When she challenged the designers to make clear their objections (was it cost? space

Aging and Health: Linking Research and Public Policy, © 1989 Lewis Publishers, Inc., Chelsea, Michigan 48118. Printed in U.S.A.

problems? a question of plumbing?), they answered, "But these people don't take showers."

Why have we as a society fallen for gloomy, mocking stereotypes, what Simone de Beauvoir (1978) has characterized as a view of old age as life's parody? Part of the answer is that in the postindustrial age the value of the wealth of experience of the old no longer seems appreciated. Experience might be perceived as a hindrance in a society where a mastery of yesterday's technology does not guarantee even an understanding of today's or tomorrow's. Couple the loss of economic power with this depreciation of skills, and the ingredients are there to create a concept of the elderly that emphasizes a dependency position in relation to the rest of society.

COMMON CONCERNS OF THE ELDERLY

The grounds that bind the elderly together are (1) the struggle against the physical dependency—poverty, loss of security, the risk of homelessness, inadequate transportation; and (2) the struggle to go on pursuing ends that give our life meaning—devotion to individuals, to groups, or to causes; social, political, intellectual, or creative work (Beauvoir, 1978). How do these relate to health? The Hon. Jake Epp, Canada's Minister of Health and Welfare, in his document *Achieving Health for All* (1986), points clearly to poverty and loss of control as determinants of ill health. The health needs of seniors will not be met if we do not address these issues head on.

Bias in Research

What we need from researchers is some consolidation of all the data that relate to the health effects of marginal income, inadequate housing, and the isolation that lack of transportation brings into a meaningful, concise form that we can use to focus the attention of policymakers. What I am arguing for is problem-solving research firmly grounded in the reality of the elderly.

In a recent article, George Foster (Foster, 1987) distinguishes between a problem and a researchable problem. A *problem* is some threat to health; a *researchable problem* is a statement that provides the basis for deciding upon research design, data-gathering techniques, and data processing or interpretation. Good practical research must start out with a clear statement of the problem. Only then can appropriate methodology be worked out. In this process of defining the problem, or asking the right question, the elderly themselves should be consulted.

A young researcher that I know was dispatched to a number of nursing homes with a well-designed questionnaire in hand to interview the residents about the appropriateness of the location of these facilities. After a number of fruitless attempts to get residents to rank preferences, he sat down and just talked with them. In essence, they told him, "This place could be on the dark side of the moon. I was sick so I had to come here." However, they did raise with him a number of issues that concerned them—issues that revolved around the quality of their lives. When he took these concerns back to the research committee, they told him, "This is only your opinion. It has no scientific basis."

The bias here is obvious. The questions that the researchers wanted to ask were more important than the questions that the subjects wanted to address. Inherent in all of this are language questions that hinder the collaboration between the researcher and the researched. The needs, concerns, or aspirations of a group of people become translated into academic jargon rather than clear, concise descriptions or recommendations. Perhaps we should make it incumbent upon researchers to prove that they have consulted subjects and provided concise problem statements prior to receiving funding approval.

Bias in Policymaking

One senior politician was recently heard to say that she became interested in the particular problems of older women when she herself turned 50. Must we be thankful when personal revelation is the stimulus to policy, despite the fact that so many women have already turned 50?

Consultation with seniors must become an integral part of the policymaking process, and we must give seniors the tools to do the job. Seniors need assistance to participate (perhaps, in this regard, researchers could lend some of their writing skills), and their participation needs to be made effective through such small devices as large-print literature and accessible meeting halls, or small courtesies like adequate notice of meetings. One senior that I know received a telephone call about a week before a meeting organized by a federal government agency to discuss seniors' housing. He found it impossible to organize a delegation with such short notice, and when he called back to explain his predicament he was told, "Thanks for trying." The meeting went ahead anyway without any representation from seniors.

THE NEED FOR SYNTHESIZING RESEARCH

In order to direct policy, we need not only problem-solving research, but research that synthesizes what we already know. One example of consolidating research is the recent report prepared by the Women and Mental Health Committee of the Canadian Mental Health Association (1987), which looks at the mental health of women within the full context of women's social, economic, and cultural position and urges the active participation of women in helping to define their mental health needs. This kind of report helps seniors in particular (1) by considering the elderly woman not as a case apart but as a member of the larger community of women; (2) by drawing attention to the economic status of women as a determinant of depression and anxiety; and (3) by outlining some strategies for change for a problem that is of particularly urgent concern for seniors.

Almost 72% of all psychotropic medicines in Canada are prescribed for women, many to aging women. Thirty percent of admissions to long term care in British Columbia arise from mental or cognitive handicap, not physical impairment. It is estimated that this will rise to 50% within the next few years. Loneliness, anxiety, and depression have become synonyms for old age. Obviously, as seniors, our ability to sustain our mental health will be key to our ability to maintain independence and pursue meaningful work.

Another piece of research that points us in the right direction is the work by Morris Barer, Bob Evans, and others, which looks at aging and health care utilization (Barer et al., 1987). Their analysis reveals that the growth in the numbers of elderly will not by itself jeopardize the financing of the health care system, assuming normal rates of economic growth. However, they also point out that there has been a disproportionate growth in the use of health care services by the elderly and ask the question: Is this increased intensity of servicing an appropriate response to levels of morbidity among the elderly?

This research is important because it clears away some of the fallacies that distort the debate about the crisis in health care, and it helps us to more clearly define a problem. It is one that seniors have been aware of for a long time. We know that we make many visits to doctors, have lots of tests, and go frequently to hospital. However, we are not sure whether this behavior is on our own initiative or that of our physicians and whether in the end this is having any real effect on our health. If we can answer these questions, I think we will be in a better position to evaluate the degree to which we should promote personal responsibility and the extent to which we should commit ourselves to other than medical treatments for dealing with our health problems.

A few examples of other important areas for research are: (1) We need demonstration projects that will test the effectiveness of having short-stay units in long term care facilities. Would a periodic short stay improve the ability of an elder to maintain herself at home? (2) We need to know something about the cost and utility of family caregiving. Eighty percent of elders live and die in their own homes. How well is the Canadian family coping with this situation? (3) We need to know more about the needs and concerns of that cohort of women now between the ages of 45 and 60 who are single, marginally employed, and experiencing affordability problems and who have lost social support systems. (4) We need to devise community-based prevention programs to minimize the high incidence of falls in the elderly. This list could go on and on.

CONCLUSION

Research is important. The effectiveness of new policies depends not only on the quality of supportive research, but also on the ability of policymakers and consumers to understand it. Research results are often inaccessible because the history of the argument is difficult to penetrate. No doubt researchers encounter the same type of barrier when they delve into the literature of another discipline. Seniors themselves should be involved in designing and conducting some of this research. Indeed, their participation might help to lessen the constraints that the academic culture sometimes unconsciously imposes on the usefulness of research. The process of having to explain the argument to someone outside of the discipline, like a senior who is a core-searcher, would be a good trial run for the next step—explaining it to a policymaker.

How can we bring all of this sound problem-oriented research that I have advocated to the attention of the policymaker or the administrator? The necessary first step is that we all must know about it. It is a constant source of frustration, for example, that Health and Welfare Canada does not provide annotated bibliographies of all of the research that it funds in a given year. In the age of the computer, it would seem a simple enough thing to do, yet it is not done. Nor to my knowledge do universities routinely do this kind of summary and make it available to the general public.

Once we have good research and an information system that connects the researcher, the policymaker, and the citizen, then we need to create forums for mutual discussion. In a particularly heartening speech that the Minister of National Health and Welfare gave in New York in November 1987 (Epp, 1987), he underlined the importance of achieving collaboration from all members of the community in planning and implementing health services, especially because the decisions about resource allocation in health care are really statements of public value. In this speech, Mr. Epp quoted C. E. A. Winslow, a leader in the 20th century American public health movement, who said: "The program is far sounder if worked out in honest and open discussion, in which the experts and the public participate, than if it is prepared by the expert alone in his ivory tower." This collaboration is overdue, and I hope that this conference is but the first of many discussions.

REFERENCES

Barer, M., Evans, R., Hertzman, C., & Lomas, J. (1987). Aging and health care utilization: New evidence on old fallacies. *Social Science and Medicine, 24*(10), 851–862.

Beauvoir, S. de. (1978). *Old age.* New York: Penguin Books.

Epp, J. (1986). *Achieving health for all: A framework for health promotion*. Ottawa: Ministry of Supply and Services.

Epp, J. (1987, November 18–19). *Health care reform: The challenge for North America*. Address to the Americas Society/Canadian Affairs. Health and Welfare Canada.

Foster, G. (1987). World health organization behavioural science research: Problems and prospects. *Social Science and Medicine, 24*(9), 709–717.

Women and Mental Health Committee, Canadian Mental Health Association (1987, April). *Women and mental health in Canada: Strategies for change*. Toronto: CMHA.

30. The Consumer View of Research and Policy

DONNA L. ROSE

THE SENIOR CITIZENS COUNCIL OF ALBERTA

It is my pleasure to represent Alberta and to share with you, as best I can, what is happening in our province through our Senior Citizens Council. Our Council was formed by Ministerial Order in 1976 and reports directly to the Minister of Social Services by means of an annual report tabled in the legislature. There are 14 on the Council, and we are appointed for terms of three years. We are selected by geographical location so that all regions in the province are represented.

When I became a member of the Council, I was not the youngest member, but very close to it. On our latest turnover of members, there are now several of us in our 50s. More and more of us are becoming interested in making a contribution to the lives of the senior world, because all too soon we will be a part of that world. It is because of both altruism and selfishness that we serve and because it is so very interesting. (Our oldest member is in her 80s.)

Administration of the Council

The Senior Citizen Secretariat takes care of our administrative services. The Secretariat is an arm of the Department of Social Services that acts as a liaison between the government and the people. Information requests to the Secretariat average about 600 a month.

Many papers are prepared and distributed by the Secretariat on a wide variety of subjects of interest to seniors. Mary Engleman, the Executive Director of the Senior Citizens Secretariat, and her staff do an outstanding job of keeping senior concerns before the various government departments because of the hands-on work they do of listening and helping. A bimonthly Fact Sheet is distributed to 2800 people around the province, some of them

Aging and Health: Linking Research and Public Policy, © 1989 Lewis Publishers, Inc., Chelsea, Michigan 48118. Printed in U.S.A.

seniors and some of them interested professionals. The purpose of the Fact Sheet is to inform people of the latest news concerning seniors and government.

In 1987, after an evaluation, the Secretariat's importance was deemed to be so high that its responsibility was given over to a member of the Legislative Assembly, Mr. Harry Alger, who also became Chairman of the Council, which strengthened the ties between seniors and government even more. This new approach is working very well. Previously we met four times a year and prepared our annual reports, but the new chairman and a number of new members hit the table at the same time, and it has been a joy to see a great deal of action taking place. Whereas we were not encouraged to speak publicly before, now the province is being divided up, and we are expected to speak up about our Council and seniors in general, helping those in our area to be informed and listening to their concerns.

Functions of the Council

Annual Report

Our annual report is still the highest priority of the Council. At the moment we have upwards of a dozen topics of interest. Of course, we cannot deal with so many at once but discuss at length which ones to emphasize at a given time. One of the subjects I have enjoyed the most in the past has been foot care, which started as a joke but became a very serious subject for us.

Research Grants

Another important part of our yearly agenda is the giving of research grants in the field of aging. It became very clear to the Council some years ago that there was not enough research being done in Alberta on aging. A very *un*scientific questionnaire was sent across Canada to determine what kind of research was being done and who was doing it. We found that not a great deal was being done in Alberta as opposed to the rest of the country, and most of that had to be financed by the federal government. We then asked the provincial government for and have received $100,000 annually for this purpose. We are now in our fifth year of awarding grants, which is done totally in conjunction with the Secretariat.

At first our system of awarding grants seemed painstaking, but as we got into it, it has proved a very worthwhile project. My first response to being asked to be a part of the research committee was that it was probably tedious and I would not understand it, but that has turned out not to be so.

The Secretariat receives the applications and sends them out to our three-member subcommittee of the Council members, who go over them. We meet and decide as a group which ones will be sent out for review by researchers or knowledgeable people across Canada. Each application is reviewed by three different professionals, who say yea or nay as to the worthiness of the subject and evaluate it according to our guidelines. (These evaluations are truly enlightening, because two may agree while the third may take a very strong opposite view.)

With the reviews before us we sit down again, this time with another person knowledgeable about research grants from the Department of Advanced Education who assists us in the final decision.

We have encountered some problems with the grants. An interesting one is seeing the finished project. A requirement of funding is seeing the final report and some simply do not comply. As a result of this, we are now withholding a sizable portion of money until we see the report. We have found that studies from nonuniversity people seem to get better results. By that, I mean they finish what they start and they have interesting, far-reaching topics of study. The Lutheran Society of Edmonton did a study on shared housing for the elderly, and as a result, housing is now being built for this purpose. The senior citizens of the Peace River area did a study on the needs of seniors in their area which is now being implemented with success. We have found that academics focus large amounts of money on minute subjects, and one sees that the puzzles confronting us will be a long time in being solved at the rate things are going now.

CONFERENCE QUESTIONS

1. What do older people think about being used as research subjects?

We believe that older people do not mind being used for research, *but* researchers frequently:

- do not fully explain to senior participants the purpose behind their questions or what they are trying to achieve;
- in writing their report, use jargon that absolutely no one understands except professionals in their field;
- seldom, if ever, give any kind of results to the people who have been kind enough to participate. The most that people involved in research projects get is a letter expressing thanks. They never hear how the project turned out. There is no follow-through. This makes participants unwilling to ever be involved again.

Our seniors today are better educated than ever before in history. Explanations therefore are of the essence.

People also need to be treated with respect—not treated as "cases" or "guinea pigs." They deserve strict confidentiality. There should never be any possibility that material from a survey could be identified as to the source.

People also need to feel they are not wasting their time. Seniors are often regarded as having little to do and as being happy to see an interviewer to talk to because they are lonely. There is a difference between being lonely and alone. Most seniors are busy. They have an agenda. Their time should be respected, and they have a right to hear the outcome uses of a research project they were involved with.

2. What really can anyone say about a system that is planned by "significant" others in government?

Our system is generous, though cumbersome at times. Could our seniors run it better if they were in charge? In all probability they could, but I feel sure they do not want to, except perhaps to suggest that it could be simpler.

Also, government has a habit of deciding what care is to be provided for our seniors and where it is to be administered. In other words, the patient goes to the service once long term care is initiated. Yes, the patient/client is consulted and so is the family, but the result is the same. As a consumer, it seems to me that the care should come to the senior and not the senior to the care. I am a believer in multilevel care under one roof! If more seniors had a say, I am sure they would agree that this change is overdue.

It does seem clear that the actual delivery of the health care system is planned by those who do not use it and have not fully researched what will be done in advance of implementation. An example of this is our new single point of entry into the long term care system. One interview puts a senior into the system computer, eliminating the need for an interview at every level of care required. Seniors specifically were not consulted, but the idea was considered excellent and went ahead, and the program is good. Before province-wide implementation, a trial run took place in one area, where clients found themselves with a 28-page form to deal with. It was close to a nightmare. I believe it is now down to 14 pages, with more cuts being planned.

Government always says they give high priority to consumers, but it seems superficial at best. Often they do not consider that for the consumer:

- the location of services can be hard to get to for seniors with health problems;
- the number and length of questions on forms can be painstaking; and
- being treated like children when requesting information from workers can be a final straw—"What's the use?"

A simplification of systems would be most helpful. Sometimes one wonders exactly what does go on in our bureaucratic government. Is it a desire to help or busywork in order to keep a job?

3. Is anyone ever sure that researchers and policymakers are on the right track?

Are they behind the times or ahead of it? Are policymakers far reaching in their thinking or simply plugging holes? When consumers perceive needs to be important, how long before anyone high up listens and responds? Sometimes it takes years.

It is hard to judge what is appropriate for seniors, for they themselves are seldom asked. At the Canadian Association on Gerontology Annual Conference held in Calgary in October 1987, Dr. Carol Ryff, sociologist from the University of Wisconsin, spoke on the topic "The Challenge of Successful Aging." In summing up her speech, she stated that we know little of how old people feel about themselves. Our theories on aging have affected our study on aging. Researchers' expectations are frequently negative. We should pay greater attention to the unique resources and challenges of old age and to the continuing potential for growth. We rarely ask older people whether life satisfaction is of interest or importance to them. Positive aging is not only an individual initiative, but also a societal responsibility. Potential will not be realized unless opportunities for development are available.

I loved the description of seniors by Dr. John W. Rowe, Associate Professor of Medicine at Harvard Medical School, who says, "that the term 'normal aging' has not served us well and we should discard it." He says that studying aging is like "peeling an onion. We took off the outer coat, which was disease, and we said what we are left with, the onion without the skin, is normal aging." But according to Rowe, gerontologists jumped too soon to the conclusion that everything that was not disease was normal aging. Other layers of that onion exist that are neither disease nor normal aging—layers related to such external habits as exercise, diet, even economic status or personality traits. He goes on to say with R. L. Krohn that "within the category of normal aging, a distinction can be made between usual aging . . . and successful aging."

It is difficult to meet all the needs of every senior citizen who may feel maligned or overwhelmed by the system. Our Alberta system endeavors to keep as many senior citizens as possible in their homes as long as possible with home care and community services. Some seniors take everything they can get. Some seniors refuse any help at all. And we know there are some who do not even know what is available. There are a lot of gray areas.

Health professionals, policymakers and researchers need to listen to seniors and to their needs. It is time for researchers and policymakers to spend more time together instead of researchers heading off into any interesting subject that looks promising, with policymakers making decisions with little or no consultation as to what the needs really are.

4. Are the elderly adequately consulted about service and program development?

I believe that older people are consulted about health services in a limited way. They sit on councils and committees and work very hard to make things better, but this is a minority of interested seniors. It takes a great deal of time and commitment to have government act on suggestions that we as consumers make to them, because when all is said and done, government is seldom wrong in what it believes is right.

I shudder now when any organization or business says that government should or must step in and legislate something. We live in a democratic society, but we are governed beyond our wildest imagination. We have asked to be governed and we are, but it is hard now to make policymakers hear us when needed.

For me as a consumer, the biggest problem before us on every level is dissemination of information and learning to really listen to what the older people themselves are saying:

- listen carefully
- gather information openly and widely
- decide wisely
- disseminate everywhere

We require both a broad view of the perceived future and then narrower views of the broad picture so that we can focus accurately on, rather than guessing, what our health care system can and will do for us in the years to come.

31. A Consumer's View of Research and Policy in Aging and Health

JOHN OUSSOREN

I speak not only as a 47-year-old working myself through my life and faith journey, but also as a surrogate spokesperson, attempting to speak on behalf of some of the older adults I work with in the Seniors' Education Centre at the University of Regina. That target group is part of the 90% 65-and-over population which is not institutionalized and managing quite nicely on its own with lots of self-reliance and dignity.

First of all, I want to portray the Seniors' Education Centre as one small but significant attempt to integrate some older adult learning, research, policy, and practice. Second, I will respond to the five questions given to each panelist.

THE SENIORS' EDUCATION CENTRE AS PART OF THE UNIVERSITY EXTENSION AT THE UNIVERSITY OF REGINA

I view the Seniors' Education Centre as a rudimentary demonstration project or prototype of integrated research, policy, and practice in preventive health and aging. Philosophically, programmatically, and administratively, the Centre builds in maximum involvement of older adults. The Centre's stated purpose is "to provide opportunities whereby the quality of life is improved by activities which are stimulating and educational."

In its 10th year of operation, the Centre's Senior University Group Inc. Board sets overall fiscal, program, and administration policy in close liaison with the two University Extension staff members.

Annually, approximately 1500 older adult registrants are involved in 60 courses, including nutrition and lifestyle, world religions, Saskatchewan his-

Aging and Health: Linking Research and Public Policy, © 1989 Lewis Publishers, Inc., Chelsea, Michigan 48118. Printed in U.S.A.

tory, conversational French, and word processing. These noncredit programs are delivered on and off campus by a variety of traditional and innovative means.

Currently active and retired University professors, plus community instructors, offer University-level topics as identified by the course participants and the Education Committee.

The participants tend to be females aged 60–75, with a number of older persons. One third have finished elementary school or some high school; the other two thirds have completed high school, taken some university courses, or attained a diploma or degree.

The approximately $90,000 Centre budget comes equally from the government, the University, and the seniors themselves. The seniors have an active fund-raising program, whose target has been oversubscribed during the last two years.

In addition to the Board and Education, and Finance Committees, the seniors also control or administer the registration days, course orientations and evaluations, the Newsletter, and the Distinguished Canadian Award dinner which in recent years recognized four distinguished Canadians: T. C. Douglas; Judge Emmett Hall; Dr. Irene Spry; and Dr. John Archer.

A volunteer bank listing the skills and interests of older adults enables this Centre to draw upon volunteers for not only clerical and related support but also for researching of briefs such as the recent presentation to the University's Academic Review Task Force. In that brief, the seniors called for, as resources become available, larger quarters, extended rural programming, and a coordinated approach to university and provincial gerontology resources.

The Centre has been involved in some of the following innovations:

- a world religions distance education program for seniors and others connecting Regina and Moose Jaw participants by video conferencing;
- the production of audio cassettes of course presentations;
- the cosponsoring in June 1987 with University of Saskatchewan Extension Division and the Saskatoon Seniors' Cultural and Creative Studies group, the first provincial conference on *Learning Opportunities for, with, and by the Older Adults in Saskatchewan*. Ten other senior organizations, government, and voluntary agencies were involved in this awareness-raising process; and
- the organizing and facilitating of the "Let's Talk About the News" program during the past five years together with several Regina nursing homes, utilizing university and community instructors and staff.

Our commitment is to lifelong learning and in a real sense preventive health care for all ages.

Why is the Senior Education Centre such a major drawing card to the seniors? A variety of reasons reflect the individual differences of the older adults:

1. It provides a second chance at learning for the cohort which experienced the Depression and the War and never had the opportunity to get or complete their education. For example, an 84-year-old woman travels two hours by car or bus with her friends to participate in a two-hour course, then travels back, taking another two hours.

2. It is a significant way of rebuilding one's life once a significant loss has occurred; for example, the loss of a spouse or moving into a strange city when one becomes too old to farm. Several have talked with me about the therapeutic effect that seniors' education provides: it enables them to find new friends and provides intellectual and emotional challenges (*resocialization,* in the literature).

3. Other seniors speak about the structure that the Centre's programs provide for their lives. "Something to get up for in the morning" is the way one senior puts it (*productivity of the retired and the nonretired,* in the literature).

4. The joy of learning.

5. The importance of physical activity and stimulation. Four courses each semester in the physical activity studies field are: Vitality Unlimited; Move to Music—peer taught; Basic Yoga; and T'ai Chi. The importance of physical activity in the aging adult has been well documented.

6. In a homogeneous setting open to other adults, seniors role-model positive healthy alternatives to the usual endless round of unimaginative drop-in center activities. The Centre, in short, is an integral part of the University's research, teaching, and community service purposes. In its pioneering efforts of meeting Saskatchewan's older adult learning needs, the Centre is a force to reckon with from a preventive health and aging perspective.

PANELIST QUESTIONS

I polled about a dozen Seniors' University Group Board and other members. Seven responded to the following questions:

1. What do older people think about being used as research subjects?

The research has to have a sense of mission, i.e., must improve the conditions of older adults. It has to be "tasteful," done in moderation, and the research subjects must not be used as objects for personal gain or used as guinea pigs.

I sense some latent skepticism in the seniors about the usefulness of a lot of research—perceptions of research being unrelated to reality and not improving society. At the Centre and within our university setting we are gradually trying to overcome some of those negative perceptions.

Critical to health and education research is the process of involvement of older adults. We need to take a leaf out of the adult educators' and community developers' book which constantly involves all the stakeholders in a trustworthy way.

2. **By and large, the health system for the elderly is planned and governed by those who do not use it. Would a health system for the aged run by older people be different from the one we currently have? If so, how?**

An overwhelming yes from the seniors and me. Yes, the health system would be different if seniors were involved in the planning and governance. It would change from a system of health care *for* to a system that emphasized *with and by*. The prepositions must change. Self-reliance and self-direction: mutuality and cooperation would be the outcomes.

According to the older adults polled, there would be a clearer focus on preventive health care needs. Seniors would stay in their own homes longer and maintain their self-esteem longer. There would be more emphasis on "staving off" old age instead of giving medication to keep people quiet. There would be a more effective pinpointing of needs if older people were asked to be involved with the planners. Older adults could also share their own experience and learnings gained from their illnesses and certain health practices.

A change in fiscal priorities would ensue. As one senior stated: "Less suffering by people means more money for dams and parks." Even the 1987 Canadian Medical Association "Health Care for the Elderly" report calls for more input from the seniors and a greater focus on preventive care. It reads (on pages 48 & 51):

> *Principles:* The elderly must participate in planning services that affect them. . . . Volunteers must be encouraged and supported but not stifled by bureaucracy.

> *Recommendations:* #12—the health and well-being of the elderly must be actively promoted, the emphasis on increasing their role in our society. #15—the use of appropriate incentives to expand programs that use the experience and skills of retired citizens.

3. Is the research agenda set by the scientific community and policymakers appropriate to the issues and dilemmas encountered by the elderly? If not, how might it change?

A buckshot response from the seniors polled. Generally, seniors are not aware of what the research agenda is, although two seniors indicated: "The elderly need to be consulted more" and "I feel enough research is being done—now we mainly need some action on what is already known."

The responses to question #2 can again be applied here. I believe that the research agenda is too focused upon the problematic, geriatrics, the institutionalized, and the medical model. The research and policy agenda needs to be shifted—especially in Saskatchewan—to gerontology, the 90% relatively well elderly, and a preventive/self-help focus in health, education, and social services. The Saskatchewan Gerontology Association annual meeting agenda is a case in point—there are very few topics on learning and the older adult or on the well elderly.

4. Are older people generally in favor of the directions the health system is pursuing? Is change occurring fast enough? Are there new directions which have not properly been considered up to now?

A variety of verbatim responses:

"I think the efforts to keep people in their own homes as long as possible and making available the help required to do this is the direction to go."

"Older people are fast becoming a larger segment of society. Senior housing and senior care centers are always less than the need. These items need to be more in balance."

"I believe older people think increased attention to their needs is a step in the right direction, but it must progress more in the direction of nursing home care."

"The new provincial policy on payments for prescription drugs [shifting from an almost completely insured service to a system of consumer charges] is very shortsighted. Agree that something must be worked out and keep health costs from rising faster than inflation."

"Everything is too complicated. [My desire is to stay healthy, but] if I should someday need lifesaving drugs of $100, I would perhaps have to go without them."

There is a lot of fear and stress regarding health and well-being, especially among single older women. One senior's statement sums up my response to this question:

"John—sorry, but I really don't know enough about the research that is being done. I do feel strongly that people should stay in their own homes as long as they possibly can, and that the resources needed in the community should be available. The situation is much better now than it was only a few years ago, but continuing work needs to be done. I suspect rural areas are in much greater need than are urban. I'm sure the emphasis on keeping people active mentally and physically as long as possible and with a good diet is very positive and needs to be extended. I'm also sure that medication should be kept to a minimum and that people should be encouraged to ask questions and find out what the medication is. As for illness itself, I'm sure more research is needed into Alzheimer's, Parkinson's, you name it!"

5. Are older people sufficiently consulted in the planning and administration of health services? If not, what mechanisms might be put in place to enhance the extent and influence of such consultation?

Generally, not enough consultation with the stakeholders occurs. "No, they are not consulted" is one response. "I have never been consulted" is another one. "More use could be made of [seniors'] experience and advice, possibly through their use on an advisory board"; "Boards of Health should have representation from the elderly"; "The elderly should organize and study their health needs, so they could have a means of dealing with the health officials"; "Improve the literacy levels so seniors can read and be involved more effectively"; "Hold a symposium or conference and reverse positions of doctors and patient(s). Seniors can speak for juniors."

My response is: Ask them—involve them at all possible levels and use a variety of problem-solving approaches; strengthen the community development and problem-solving skills and processes used by health officials and workers; experiment with stimulation, role reversals, and other adult learning techniques with and for health workers and seniors; and finally, build in the assumption at all levels that not all the health problems will be solved or alleviated in one generation.

PART IV

Applying Gerontological Research Effectively

32. Diffusion Across a Semipermeable Membrane, or the Process Through Which Research Influences Policy Development

DOROTHY PRINGLE

INTRODUCTION

I was asked to address the topic of how research gets used in the development of public policy as it relates to program development, within the context of aging and health in Canada. At the time, a number of colleagues from McMaster University and I (Mohide, Pringle, Streiner, Gilbert, & Roe, 1986) were in the data-gathering phase of a randomized trial of an in-home respite and support program for family caregivers of people with Alzheimer's disease. The various aspects of this experience stimulated my curiosity to investigate the process of how research affects the policy development process at a relatively micro level, i.e., policy that leads to program funding. In this chapter, on the basis of a reexamination of research on community support services for informal caregivers of disabled and impaired older people, I will (1) propose a model of the process as I think it works now; (2) review the approach of the task force on the periodic health exam and the implications for policy revision if it were adopted; and (3) summarize the pros and cons of our present system.

Aging and Health: Linking Research and Public Policy, © 1989 Lewis Publishers, Inc., Chelsea, Michigan 48118. Printed in U.S.A.

POLICY AND VALUES

MacPherson (1987) describes public policies as institutionalized political values and beliefs about what is right and good for society. In turn, public policies create and limit opportunities (Milio, 1986) for program development and, subsequently, for the services available to individuals within society.

Given this perspective, at a national level we have institutionalized the belief that all Canadians should be protected from the financial consequences of illness as long as that illness requires treatment in an acute care hospital or by a physician. Furthermore, we believe that this protection should be portable, so regardless of where illness strikes, access to hospital and physician care without financial penalty is guaranteed.

Apparently we do not have any national beliefs or values about it being good for society to protect individuals from the financial consequences of an illness that could be managed by another type of health professional, for example, a nurse, or if it could be managed at home. Some provincial governments have decided that it is right and good for residents of their provinces to be protected from the costs of community care. Manitoba decided it was right and good for Manitobans back in 1975, but Nova Scotia decided that it would not be right and good for residents of that province to be financially protected until the 1988–89 fiscal year. Nor is portability of community services an institutionalized belief at the national level. Waiting periods for new residents and visitors ranging from three months to a year are part of provincial policies.

Clearly, there are beliefs and values that do not get translated into public policies for a variety of reasons and you are as able to speculate on these as I: competing political agendas, economics, and history all play a role. The real question may be what role research has in influencing the political perception of what is right and good. Or, to put it another way, what role does research play in determining political values and beliefs?

REVIEW OF RESEARCH ON SUPPORT SERVICES FOR FAMILY CAREGIVERS

The area of informal or family caregiving has received a great deal of research attention, particularly since 1978. However, interest in this population goes back many years. In the first article I located on family caregivers' need for respite from the responsibilities of caregiving—in The Lancet, 1960—Macmillan noted that the policy of moving psychogeriatric patients to the community could backfire if family caregivers were burdened too long without relief. Resentment and rejection of the older person could set in, and once that happened no amount of hospital relief could change or reverse the situation. No one in this country apparently heard this warning. In the same year, Isaacs and Thompson (1960), physicians in a geriatric hospital in Scotland, reported on 46 men and women admitted for holiday relief and the circumstances of the caregivers, including the number of years they had gone without a break. They advocated holiday admissions and outlined very useful guidelines for caregivers to use in order to get the most out of their respite.

The next study did not show up until 1969. Golodetz, a social worker in a Boston hospital, and his colleagues examined the position of 50 family members who assumed responsibility for patients discharged home. Most patients were elderly and the caregivers were not young. He coined the term *responsor* and gave what I think is a classic description of a family caregiver (Golodetz et al., 1969, p. 390):

> She is not trained for her job, a priori. She may have little choice about doing the job. She belongs to no union or guild, works no fixed maximum of hours. She lacks formal compensation, job advancement and even the possibility of being fired. She has no job mobility. In her work situation, she bears a heavy emotional load, but has no colleagues or supervisor or education to help her handle this. Her own life and its needs compete constantly with her work requirements. She may be limited in her performance by her own ailments.

On the basis of the findings from these 50 caregivers, these authors proposed that both the patients and their caregivers should be treated as clients (Golodetz et al., 1969). Throughout the 1960s and 1970s Ethel Shanas (1971, 1979), an American sociologist, undertook a series of studies on the health and functional independence of random population samples of elderly community residents in a number of countries including Britain, Poland, Israel, Denmark and the United States but not Canada. Although she did not study the family caregivers, she described the amount of disability and impairment experienced by these individuals and what assistance they received from their families. She concluded that the vast amount of care that permitted these older people to remain in the community was delivered by family members. Shanas's work was by far the most comprehensive available on the extent of care provided by families.

Studies in the early 1970s began to document caregiver 'burden.' The majority were British, reflecting their early experience with the increasing proportion of people over 65. In 1971, Isaacs, from his position as geriatrician at the Queen Elizabeth Hospital in Birmingham, documented the characteristics of 280 patients referred to a geriatric unit from their homes. The reason for 63% of the admissions was "intolerable strain" on the caregiver. He reported that situations causing strain involved patients who were immobile, incontinent, or suffered from mental abnormality. In 1975, Sanford, another British geriatrician, offered the first quantitative measure of burden in the form of a tolerance factor. Based on interviews with the family caregivers of 50 patients admitted to a geriatric unit of a hospital in London, England, he found that the behaviors with the lowest tolerance factors were (1) immobility, (2) behaviors that disturbed sleep, and (3) behaviors that required constant supervision such as daytime wandering. Incontinence was not among the poorly tolerated group of behaviors.

The first Canadian study in the area did not appear until 1978. Ross and Kedward (1978) evaluated 100 elderly psychiatric patients admitted to a Toronto hospital, including the burden they caused for the family. One third of the family reported feeling burdened and half of them were assessed as severely burdened.

Summaries of Selected Characteristics of Frequently Cited Papers

From 1979 on, the volume of published studies accelerated considerably. Blythe (1987) states, "Judging from the library shelves, old age drives its explainers and managers to ink. A vast literature has emerged, most of it unfit for the elderly" (p. 41). My paraphrase suggests that the phenomenon of family caregiving drives the caregivers to drink and the investigators to describe. A vast literature has emerged, much of it unfit for policy development. American investigators took over from the British as the most prolific in publishing studies. Between 1979 and 1987, dozens of studies, descriptive papers, and a few review articles were published on family caregiving. The 45 articles whose selected characteristics are summarized below include the most frequently referenced articles in the area, but this list is by no means exhaustive.

Country of Origin

The country of origin of the 45 papers is as follows: Canada, 4; Britain, 7; United States, 33; and New Zealand, 1. Of the Canadian studies, 1 was done in Saskatchewan, 1 in Quebec, and 2 in Ontario.

Type of Study

The type of study gives an indication of the development of knowledge in a field. The types of study are identified as follows:

Descriptive survey	13
Correlational/Explanatory	20
Noncontrolled intervention	8
Randomized control trial	1
Review article	3

For the most part the descriptive surveys were the earlier ones, of which the majority (10) were published in or before 1983. The correlational or explanatory studies are still common as different facets of the experience of family caregivers are examined and related to such things as plans for institutionalizing the patient, their well-being, their use of support services, and so on. Three good review articles have appeared, a good indication of the complexity of the field.

Size of Sample of the Studies

If this research is to have policy implications, the size of the sample on which the findings and conclusions are based is important. In this group of papers, size of sample breaks down as follows:

10	2
11–25	6
26–50	9
51–100	6
100–500	11
>500	5
Not specified	6

As one would expect, the trend has been for the samples to get larger in the later studies, but this is by no means an absolute trend. The Canadian studies had samples ranging from 10 to 119. Three of the studies in the "not specified" category were the review articles. None of the intervention studies had a sample size of more than 50.

Use of Measurement Devices

Another indication of developing sophistication in an area is the appearance of scales and other measurement instruments. Examples from the literature are as follows:

- Tolerance Factor—Sanford, 1975 (Britain)
- Burden Scale—Zarit, Zarit, & Reever, 1982 (USA)
- Relative Stress Scale (RSS)—Greene et al., 1982 (Britain)
- Caregiver Strain Questionnaire—Robinson, 1983 (USA)
- Cost of Care Index (CCI)—Kosberg & Cairl, 1986 (USA)
- Caregiver Quality of Life Instrument (CQLI)—Mohide, Pringle, Streiner, & Gilbert, 1986 (Canada)

A valid and reliable measure of caregiver burden is critical to the assessment of interventions designed to reduce it. The instruments by Zarit et al. (1982); Greene et al., (1982); Robinson (1983); and Kosberg and Cairl (1986) are valid and reliable, but there is no evidence that they are responsive to true decreases in burden. In fact, there is evidence that the instrument by Greene et al. is not (Mohide, Pringle, Streiner, & Gilbert, 1986). Mohide et al. (1988) have designed an instrument to measure caregiver well-being rather than burden, and it is known to be responsive. The relation between burden and well-being and whether one is the converse of the other is not clear conceptually.

The literature is not entirely consistent in explaining what variables in the caregiver-patient environment contribute to burden and what ones reduce it. Correlates of burden according to the literature are:

- *age*—Older or younger caregivers are more burdened
- *sex*—Women are more burdened than men
- *kinship*—Daughters may or may not be more burdened than spouses; female spouses more burdened than male
- *length of caregiving*—Longer and shorter are more stressful
- *type of disorder*—Cognitive impairment more burdensome than other
- *type of behavior*—Immobility, incontinence, or sleep-disturbing, dangerous, or hostile behavior may or may not be burdensome
- *relationship*—Positive precaregiving relationship decreases burden

The role of age, length of caregiving, and types of behavior are particularly unclear, as is the relation between burden and the decision to institutionalize the patient. Burden certainly plays a role, but so do deteriorating caregiver or patient health, amount of assistance available, availability of acceptable institutional space, and recommendations from physicians. Although there are many conflicting findings, the literature is clear that upwards of 80% of family caregivers report feeling burdened and needing assistance.

There are many suggestions of what family caregivers require to reduce the strain of caring for an older person at home, whether that person is cognitively impaired, physically disabled, or both. The most common needs of caregivers are:

1. knowledge of the disease and clinical course
2. knowledge of health and social support services for patient
3. assistance with problem solving
4. supervision of and attention to their health
5. strategies to manage difficult patient behaviors
6. social support
7. assistance with the physical care of the patient
8. access to health and social support services for self
9. physical relief both through in-home and institutional respite
10. support from professional—either nurse or social worker
11. increased acknowledgement of the importance of meeting their own needs

Of the five studies that described and to some extent evaluated in-home respite programs, three were specifically for caregivers of patients with Alzheimer's disease or other types of cognitive disabilities and two were for caregivers of any older person. A variety of models were involved. One used a registered nurse exclusively, one used nurses and trained respite workers, two used only respite workers, and one used volunteers. None of the studies was a randomized trial nor used an analytic cohort design. The two studies that carried out pre- and post-measures of some version of caregiver burden showed few positive effects. One study showed no positive effects (Middleton et al., 1987). The other demonstrated that with respite, caregivers have more leisure time, which they appreciate and which they can devote to activities that interest them. They begin to use other relevant community services (George et al., 1986). In all the studies the caregivers reported that they found the respite helpful, satisfactory in terms of quality, and they were grateful for it.

Summary of the State of the Literature

This overview of a large proportion of the studies on family caregiving carried out since 1979 provides some sense of what information is available on which to base policy. The work is largely descriptive and explanatory, but when it is reviewed in total, it provides a comprehensive picture of the situation of caregivers of older people, who present a wide variety of health and social problems. The distress many of these people experience is obvious. That no government could afford to replace the care these family members are providing is also evident. What is helpful to them is less evident. The literature leaves many questions unanswered:

1. What is the relation between caregiver burden and institutionalization of the patient?
2. What is the aim of respite programs: to reduce burden on the caregiver or to reduce the likelihood of institutionalization of the patient?
3. How will we know what reduces burden, given the state of measurement?
4. How much of the work done in Britain and the United States can be generalized to Canada or to particular jurisdictions in Canada?
5. Should respite be targeted to only certain caregivers of particular types of patients or should it be available to all caregivers?
6. What model of respite is most helpful for what caregivers?
7. How much respite is needed to reduce burden and at what point in a caregiving career should it be introduced?

The dilemma is: should we wait until the answers to all these questions are known before developing policies, or should we act on the basis of what we know and, using our best judgment, construct policy alternatives?

Policy Initiatives and Research Available at the Time

Given these questions, it is interesting to track the record of funding of respite programs by provincial governments and to match this with research that was available at the time the policy was introduced—notwithstanding the fact that policy decisions do not occur overnight and it is likely that the decision to move toward funding was taken some time before the announced decision.

In 1975, Manitoba began funding in-home respite for family caregivers of older people as part of the home care program. At the time, there was little research on caregiver stress or burden on which to build policy—three British and one American study on caregiver stress; Shanas's work (1971) on caregiver tasks and time commitments, and no intervention studies. Clearly, other sources of knowledge formed the basis for policy and program development.

Ontario, in 1986, announced increased community support services for patients with Alzheimer's disease, and the policy to fund 70% of in-home respite services and program criteria was announced in 1987. There were no restrictions on the models that could be used, but only patients with Alzheimer's disease were eligible. Essentially all the research reviewed in this chapter was available, and this, combined with the pressure from special interest groups—particularly the Alzheimer's Society—resulted in the policy initiatives.

By contrast, the governments of New Brunswick and Prince Edward Island have no policy for funding or providing respite services to caregivers of older residents. Other provinces provide some funded respite when homemakers or respite workers are available. They are not, however, mandated services.

THE SEMIPERMEABLE MEMBRANE MODEL

This overview of research and the policy initiatives of some of the provincial governments makes it difficult to picture just what role, if any, research has in program funding policies. But I think research does play a role so let me speculate on how this occurs.

Descriptive Research

Research that ultimately influences public service policy development originates in a problem or need first noticed in the delivery system. Perhaps no service is available to meet a need, or the service that exists is overwhelmed. Sometimes the professionals in the system notice it first, sometimes the consumers. It seems each group responds to the problem differently: the consumers respond by forming a special interest group to pressure the system and/or the government for change. For example, in response to perceived poor care in Ontario nursing homes, the Friends of Residents of Ontario Nursing Homes, a Toronto-based group, formed to improve the quality of resident care and, ultimately, to augment community services so nursing home placement would not be needed. In contrast, the delivery system responds by doing descriptive research on the problem. If the caregiver research is at all typical, these initial studies are unsophisticated, with small samples drawn from the caseloads of the agency or institution involved and fairly crude measurement instruments usually generated for that study. Not until 20 years after the problem of caregiver stress was first described were the first true scales of burden published.

Emergence of Experts

These small studies get into the literature and others get reported at conferences, and if it is a widespread problem—frankly, only widespread problems get policy attention—research activity escalates. The research begins to explain as well as to describe the phenomenon. Two processes seem to follow: (1) the special interest groups become aware of some of this research and use it selectively to substantiate their demands that something be done, that is, in their lobbying, and (2) "experts" in the area emerge. These experts-cum-consultants, who are usually part of the research community, play a critical role in transmitting research to the policymakers. They are familiar with what research is being done, who is doing it, and where it is occurring; they are in a position to critique it and may have been involved in reviewing it for funding. Bureaucracies have their favorite experts called upon to inform the policymakers on the needs or problems and the perceived solutions. I think these experts are the major conduit for research into the policymaking process. They find their way onto commissions appointed by governments and are the ones who are phoned to check out possible alternatives or approaches. I find the bibliographies at the end of government working papers and discussion documents disappointing, if they exist at all, but then I find that the lists of consultants involved in producing the documents contain the experts in the field. They are the conveyors of research, and the research they convey and interpret is descriptive. Most descriptive research does not include policy implications, and it is left to the experts to formulate them.

Filtering of Research

I have labeled the process through which research influences policy development as *diffusion across a semipermeable membrane*—semipermeable, because there are filters that influence what information penetrates or, if it penetrates, gets acted upon. I expect that you are all familiar with these filters: overall government policy, the influence of competing special interest groups, the pressure exerted by the press, and the overall state of the economy. A jurisdiction perceived by the electorate as doing well economically is vulnerable to more pressure and cannot filter out as many demands as one perceived to have no money for new initiatives.

The Nonimpact of Demonstration Models

I have not mentioned demonstration models or program development as part of the process that influences policy because I do not think they play a role. They occur too late in the process to be useful. It is difficult to develop, submit, mount, and analyze a demonstration project in under four to five years. Demonstration models are driven by the compelling nature of the problem and they test potential solutions, but by the time these projects have results, the special interest groups have applied considerable pressure, the experts have been called in, and an election is on the horizon.

Program evaluation occurs too late to influence the policy that confines itself to whether, not how, a program will be established. The evaluation may affect the way the program is delivered in the agency conducting the evaluation (and that is its most useful role), and it may affect some aspects of programs that are developed in other agencies. But it will not affect policy in the general sense described above. Furthermore, the size of samples in most program evaluations, the biases involved in their selection, and the local conditions that affect the program delivery limit their representativeness and their ability to be generalized to policy that will affect large sectors of the public. Our study of a caregiver support program in Hamilton, with a sample size of 60 and a program tailored to the local delivery system, should not form the basis of a policy regardless of how effective it may be. I have tried to diagram this model of research influence on policy development in Figure 1.

Cousins and Leithwood (1986) do not support this position, and they identified 12 factors that they believe determine whether the evaluation of a program will have an impact on policy, 6 of which they claim are under the control of the researcher. These include (1) the quality of the evaluation; (2) the credibility of the researcher; (3) and (4) the nature of the findings and the way they are communicated; (5) the timeliness of the results relative to the policy development process; and (6) their relevance to the needs of the policymakers at that point in the process. Most researchers have only tenuous control over some of these factors, such as nature of the findings and the timeliness relative to the decisionmaking process. The vagaries of the political process can alter the timing of policy development regardless of the original schedule. In recent years, we have seen political dynasties with long-standing commitments to particular policies come to an end in several Canadian provinces.

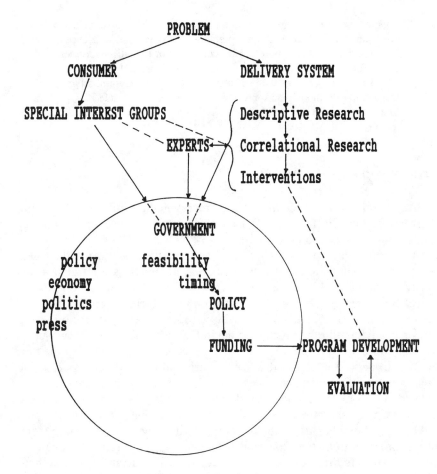

Figure 1. Model of research influence on policy development.

The other six factors (Cousins & Leithwood, 1986) are completely beyond the control of the researcher. These are: (1) the information needs of the policymakers; (2) how the policy developers make decisions; (3) the political climate at any time; (4) information that becomes available from competing sources; (5) the personal inclinations of the policymakers; and (6) their receptiveness to the information made available to them. These two lists provide support for my and many others' contention, that program evaluation has no impact on policy.

To summarize the main tenets of this model:

1. The descriptive research responds to and confirms the perceived need and affects policy.

2. This research reaches government through experts who have the ear of the government and through the interpretation of special interest groups.
3. The research must penetrate a filter consisting of overall government policy, influence of competing special interest groups, and the perception of the financial capacity of the jurisdiction to undertake new initiatives.
4. Demonstration models and evaluations of programs mounted in response to and funded through policy initiatives have no impact on policy development or revision.

THE FERTILIZATION MODEL

An alternate way of looking at the process is the fertilization model of research and policy (Figure 2). This analogy has some severe limitations so it cannot be pushed too far.

The sperm represent researchers, and the egg is the government, the maker of policy. When there is interest in an area, it stimulates a lot of research activity. Although this research goes on, it may have no impact on government (i.e., the egg), because the egg is only available at certain times and only receptive to influence for limited periods. A variety of factors affect this receptivity, all of them beyond the influence of the sperm. However, at certain times it is possible for a sperm to penetrate the egg. Most of the time only one sperm does it, but that sperm carries all the information needed to make policy. Depending on the orientation of the sperm, some policies would come out looking like a girl and some like a boy. It is unclear just why any given sperm gets selected to penetrate the egg. It may be a matter of being in the right place at the right time, swimming faster, wiggling more, being prepared to go the extra mile to find the egg. Penetrating the egg does not guarantee fertilization, and fertilization does not guarantee a viable fetus at the end of a predetermined period of time. Even though a sperm may penetrate the egg, the egg may not be able to become implanted in the wall of the uterus, so it cannot develop. Even if fertilization and implantation occur, a miscarriage can take place, or the whole process can be aborted. If a viable pregnancy occurs, it is subjected to all sorts of influences that can affect its development: smoking, nutritional limitations, drugs, accidents. The actual birth can also be smooth or stormy, and you may or may not like what the kid looks like when it's born but, regardless, you are stuck with it pretty much the way it is for the rest of your life.

I used only one area of research to illustrate the model, but with policy development and research in the areas of home care, day care, and palliative care a similar process occurred. Program evaluation has had no impact on the policy developments or revisions.

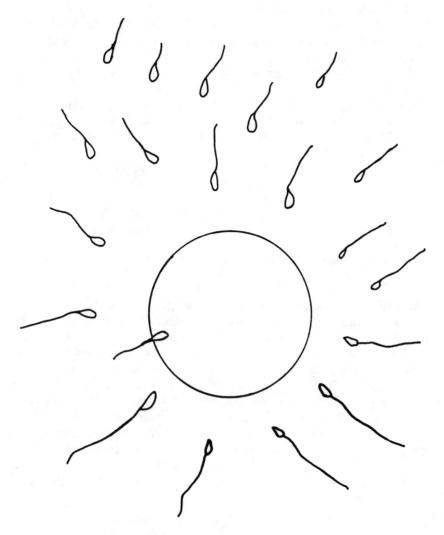

Figure 2. The fertilization model of research and policy. The sperm are researchers; the egg is the government.

ALTERNATE APPROACH: SYSTEMATIC REVIEW OF POLICY INITIATIVES

New policy initiatives will continue to be based on descriptive research and public perceptions of need, but the adequacy or inadequacy of those initiatives perhaps could be examined more systematically. In turn, this could result in policy changes.

The Canadian Task Force on the Periodic Health Examination under the leadership of Dr. Walter Spitzer (1984) has developed "a standardized method for evaluating and weighing scientific evidence on the effectiveness of preventive interventions" (p. 2). Based on a grading scheme, a recommendation is made about whether this intervention should continue to be part of a regular medical examination. This methodology has had considerable effect on the practice of many physicians, and it has the potential to affect policies about what provincial health insurance schemes will pay physicians to do. I wondered if there were any lessons from this approach for revisions in the area of public policy.

Evaluations of interventions are graded on a 4-point scale (Spitzer, 1984):

Grade 1—Evidence from at least one randomized trial

Grade 2.1—Evidence from case-control or cohort analytic studies

Grade 2.2—Evidence from comparisons between times or places with or without the intervention

Grade 3—Opinions of respected authorities, based on experience, descriptive studies, or reports of expert committees

This grading scheme and some other relevant factors lead the task force to recommend that either (1) the intervention should absolutely or possibly be included in a regular exam, or (2) it should absolutely or possibly be excluded. The question is whether a similar type of systematic review of evidence of program effectiveness would contribute anything to the policymaking process. At the very least, it would provide information to government about how well the policy was reaching its objectives. This information could be useful in pointing out when policy revisions were needed.

Service providers are encouraged to evaluate their programs and are frequently funded by government to do so. However, the results of only one evaluation tell about as much about policy effectiveness as one descriptive study tells you about need: it is the aggregate systematically reviewed that provides direction.

THE PROS AND CONS OF OUR PRESENT SYSTEM

The way research seems now to influence public policy has both advantages and disadvantages. Probably the major disadvantage is its unpredictability. What experts are consulted, the research they know, how they interpret the policy implications, the way that assessment gets added into all the competing forces is unpredictable. It is also fairly invisible, so it is difficult to scrutinize. However, it is a relatively open system. Most governments utilize a fairly broad spectrum of scientific opinion, so potentially they have access to most of the research that is carried out. When they do not consult widely and only a chosen one or two experts have the ear of government, the research community must decide either to try and influence the expert or to persuade the government to expand its horizons. A system in which only one or two studies could have a profound effect on public policy has potentially more limitations than the one that we have now. Although I value what research can contribute to knowledge, I value all the other ways of knowing as well.

One of the ways to increase the impact of research is to discuss the policy implications of findings in descriptive and explanatory research whenever it is appropriate to do so. Someone is going to draw these conclusions regardless, and the researcher is frequently the best person to do it. Also, as a research community, we do not always use the influence of the special interest groups to our advantage. If these special interest groups are kept informed of research in their area of concern and its implications, they can be a powerful ally—or if they are not well informed, a terrible liability.

It is hard to feel satisfied with the way things work now, but it is even harder to identify concrete ways of changing the current pattern. In Canada, there are several positive signs of government commitment to health research: six provincial governments now support extramural research programs in their provinces. This research can only enhance the amount of information on the identification and management of health care problems. If these developments are matched by systematic reviews of the research findings in each of the provinces, incorporation of research into policy may be enhanced. But, a systematic review may already be carried out by the experts and conveyed to government in one of the many channels in existence: commissions, telephone calls, consultations. I'm just glad that the topic assigned to me was not how to *improve* the way research affects public policy.

REFERENCES

Blythe, R. (1987, August). Reviews: In the long, late afternoon of life. *Hastings Center Report,* 41–43.

Cousins, B., & Leithwood, K. (1986). Current empirical research on evaluation utilization. *Review of Education Research, 56*(3), 331–365.

George, L. K., Gwyther, L. P., Fillenbaum, G. G., & Palmore, E. (1986). *Respite care: A strategy for easing caregiver burden?* Paper presented at the Gerontological Society of America Annual Meeting, Chicago, IL.

Golodetz, A., Evans, R., Heinritz, G., & Gibson, C. D. (1969). The care of chronic illness: The 'responsor' role. *Medical Care, 7,* 385–394.

Greene, G., Smith, R., Gardiner, M., & Timbury, G. C. (1982). Measuring behavioural disturbances of elderly demented patients in the community and its effects on relatives: A factor analytic study. *Age and Ageing, 11,* 121–126.

Isaacs, B., & Thompson, J. (1960). Holiday admissions to a geriatric unit. *Lancet,* April 30, 969–972.

Kosberg, J. I., & Cairl, R. E. (1986). The Cost of Care Index: A case management tool for screening informal care providers. *Gerontologist, 26*(3), 273–285.

MacPherson, K. I. (1987). Health care policy, values, and nursing. *Advances in Nursing Science, 9*(3), 1–11.

Middleton, L., Cairl, R., Miller, L., Keller, D., & Doblas, R. (1987). *The impact of Alzheimer's in-home respite care on patients and family caregivers.* Tampa: University of South Florida Medical Center, Suncoast Gerontology Center.

Milio, N. (1986). *Promoting Health Through Public Policy,* Ottawa: Canadian Public Health Association.

Mohide, E. A., Pringle, D. M., Streiner, D. L., & Gilbert, R. (1986). *Progress report for the feasibility study for the evaluation of a caregiver support program #01657.* Ontario Ministry of Health Grant.

Mohide, E. A., Pringle, D. M., Streiner, D. L., Gilbert, R., & Roe, D. J. (1986). *An evaluation of a family caregiver support program in the home management of demented elderly.* Ontario Ministry of Health Grant.

Mohide, E. A., Torrance, G. W., Streiner, D. L., Pringle, D. M., & Gilbert, R. (1988). Measuring the well-being of family caregivers using the time trade-off technique. *Journal of Clinical Epidemiology, 41*(5), 475–482.

Robinson, B. C. (1983). Validation of a caregiver strain index. *Journal of Gerontology, 38*(3), 344–348.

Ross, H. E., & Kedward, H. B. (1978). Social functioning and self care in hospitalized psychogeriatric patients. *Journal of Nervous and Mental Disease, 166,* 25–33.

Sanford, J. R. A. (1975). Tolerance of debility in elderly dependents by supporters at home: Its significance for hospital practice. *British Medical Journal,* August 23, 471–473.

Shanas, E. (1971). Measuring the home health needs of the aged in five countries. *Gerontologist, 11,* 37–40.

Shanas, E. (1979). The family as a social support system in old age. *Gerontologist, 19,*(2), 169–174.

Spitzer, W. O. (1984). A periodic health examination: 1. Introduction. *Canadian Medical Association Journal, 130*(10), 1276–1278.

Zarit, S. H., Zarit, J. M., & Reever, K. F. (1982). Memory training for severe memory loss: Effects on senile dementia patients and their families. *Gerontologist, 22*(4), 373–377.

SUGGESTED READING

Anderson, M., Pringle, D. M., Buzzell, E. M., Roe, D. J., & Eybel-Misch, B. (1985). Family caregivers' self-assessed stress and need for respite and the relationship to assessments by nurses and gatekeepers-to-services. In K. King et al. (Eds.), *Nursing research: Science for quality care.* Toronto: University of Toronto.

Archbold, P. G. (1980). Impact of parent caring on middle-aged offspring. *Journal of Gerontological Nursing, 6*(2), 78–85.

Argyle, N., Jestice, S., & Brock, C. P. B. (1985). Psychogeriatric patients: Their supporters' problems. *Age and Ageing, 14*, 355–360.

Arling, G., & McAuley, W. J. (1983). The feasibility of public payments for family caregiving. *Gerontologist, 23*(3), 300–306.

Barnes, R. F., Raskind, M. A., Scott, M., & Murphy, C. (1981). Problems of families caring for Alzheimer patients: Use of a support group. *Journal of the American Geriatrics Society, 23*(2), 80–85.

Bowers, B. J. (1987). Intergenerational caregiving: Adult caregivers and their aging parents. *Advances in Nursing Science, 9*(2), 20–31.

Cantor, M. H. (1983). Strain among caregivers: A study of experience in the United States. *Gerontologist, 23*, 597–604.

Casserta, M. S., Lund, D. A., Wright, S. D., & Redburn, D. E. (1987). Caregivers to dementia patients: The utilization of community services. *Gerontologist, 27*(2), 209–214.

Chenoweth, B., & Spencer, B. (1986). Dementia: The experience of family caregivers. *Gerontologist, 26*(3), 267–272.

Clark, N. M., & Rakowski, W. (1983). Family caregivers of older adults: Improving helping skills. *Gerontologist, 23*(6), 637-642.

Crossman, L., London, C., & Barry, C. (1981). Older women caring for disabled spouses: A model for supportive services. *Gerontologist, 21*(5), 464–470.

Doty, P. (1986). Family care of the elderly: The role of public policy. *Milbank Quarterly, 64*(1), 34–75.

Drinka, T. J., Smith, J. C., & Drinka, P. J. (1987). Correlates of depression burden for informal caregivers of patients in a geriatrics referral clinic. *Journal of the American Geriatrics Society, 36*(6), 522–525.

Fengler, A. P., & Goodrich, N. (1979). Wives of elderly disabled men: The hidden patients. *Gerontologist, 19*(2), 175–183.

Fitting, M., Rabbins, P., Lucas, M. J., & Eastham, J. (1986). Caregivers for dementia patients: A comparison of husbands and wives. *Gerontologist, 26*(3), 248–252.

Gallagher, D. E. (1985). Intervention strategies to assist caregivers of frail elders: Current research status and future research directions. In M. P. Lawton & G. Maddox (Eds.), *Annual review of gerontology and geriatrics.* Chicago: Springer Press.

George, L. K., & Gwyther, L. P. (1984). *Family caregivers of Alzheimer's patients: Correlates of burden and the impact of self-help groups* (pp. 1–17). Durham, NC: Duke University Center for the Study of Aging and Human Development.

George, L. K., & Gwyther, L. P. (1986). Caregiver well-being: A multidimensional examination of family caregivers of demented adults. *Gerontologist, 26*(3), 253–259.

Gilhooly, M. L. M. (1984). The impact of care-giving on care-givers: Factors associated with the psychological well-being of people supporting a dementing relative in the community. *British Journal of Medical Psychology, 57*, 35–44.

Gilleard, C. J., Belford, H., Gilleard, E., Whittick, J. E., & Gledhill, K. (1984). Emotional distress amongst the supporters of the elderly mentally infirm. *British Journal of Psychiatry, 145,* 172–177.

Goodman, C. (1986). Research on the informal carer: A selected literature review. *Journal of Advanced Nursing, 11,* 705–712.

Hildebrandt, E. D. (1983). Respite care in the home. *American Journal of Nursing, 83*(10), 1428–1431.

Isaacs, B. (1971). Geriatric patients: Do their families care? *British Medical Journal,* Oct. 30, 282–286.

Johnson, C. L., & Catalano, D. J. (1983). A longitudinal study of family supports to impaired elderly. *Gerontologist, 23*(6), 612–618.

Jones, D. A., & Vetter, N. J. (1984). A survey of those who care for the elderly at home: Their problems and their needs. *Social Science and Medicine, 19*(5), 511–514.

Kahan, J., Kemp, B., Staples, F. R., & Brummel-Smith, K. (1985). Decreasing the burden in families caring for a relative with a dementing illness. *Journal of the American Geriatrics Society, 33*(10), 664–670.

Koopman-Boyden, P. G., & Wells, L. F. (1979). The problems arising from supporting the elderly at home. *New Zealand Medical Journal, 89,* 265–268.

Kraus, A. S. (1984). The burden of care for families of elderly persons with dementia. *Canadian Journal on Aging, 3*(1), 45–50.

Levine, N. B., Dastoor, D. P., & Gendron, C. E. (1983). Coping with dementia: A pilot study. *Journal of the American Geriatrics Society, 31*(1), 12–18.

Macmillan, D. (1960, December). Preventive geriatrics. Opportunities of a community mental health service. *Lancet,* 1439–1441.

Netting, F. E., & Kennedy, L. N. (1985). Project RENEW: Development of a volunteer respite care program. *The Gerontological Society of America, 25*(6), 573–576.

Niederehe, G., Fruge, E., Scott, J. C., Neilson-Collins, K. E., & Woods, A. M. (1982). *Measuring family system characteristics in families caring for dementia patients.* Paper presented at the Gerontological Society of America Annual Meeting, Boston, MA.

Niederehe, G., Fruge, E., Woods, A. M., Scott, J. C., Volpendesta, D., Nielsen-Collins, K. E., Moye, G., Gibbs, H., & Wiegand, G. (1983). *Caregiver stress in dementia: Clinical outcomes and family considerations.* Paper presented at the Gerontology Society of America Annual Meeting, San Francisco, CA.

Poulshock, S. W. & Diemling, G. (1984). Families caring for elders in residence. Issues in the measurement of burden. *Journal of Gerontology, 39,* 230–239.

Rabins, P. R., Mace, N., & Lucas, J. G. (1982). The impact of dementia on the family. *JAMA: Journal of the American Medical Association, 248,* 333–335.

Robertson, D., & Reisner, D. (1982, September). Management of dementia in the elderly at home: Stress and the supporter. *Canada's Mental Health,* 36–38.

Robinson, B. C., & Thurnher, M. (1979). Taking care of aged parents: A family cycle transition. *Gerontologist, 19*(6), 586-593.

Sheldon, F. (1982). Supporting the supporters: Working with relatives of patients with dementia. *Age and Ageing, 11,* 184-188.

Smallegan, M. (1985). There was nothing else to do: Needs for care before nursing home admission. *Gerontologist, 25*(4), 364-369.

Soldo, B. J., & Myllyluoma, J. (1983). Caregivers who live with dependent elderly. *Gerontologist, 23*(6), 605–611.

Spence, D. L., & Miller, D. B. (1986). Family respite for the elderly Alzheimer's patient. *Social Work and Alzheimer's Disease,* 101–112.

Ware, L. A., & Carper, M. (1982). Living with Alzheimer disease patients: Family stresses and coping mechanisms. *Psychotherapy: Theory, Research and Practice, 19*(4), 472–481.

Winogrond, I. R., Fisk, A. A., Kirsling, R. A., & Keyes, B. (1987). The relationship of caregiver burden and morale to Alzheimer's disease patient function in a therapeutic setting. *Gerontologist, 27*(3), 336–339.

Worcester, M. I., & Quayhagen, M. P. (1983). Correlates of caregiving satisfaction: Prerequisites to elder home care. *Research in Nursing & Health, 6,* 61–67.

Zarit, S. H., Reever, K. E., & Bach-Peterson, J. (1980). Relatives of the impaired elderly: Correlates of feelings of burden. *Gerontologist, 20*(6), 649–655.

Zarit, S. H., Todd, P. A., & Zarit, J. M. (1986). Subjective burden of husbands and wives as caregivers: A longitudinal study. *Gerontologist, 26*(3), 260–266.

Zarit, S. H., & Zarit, J. M. (1982). Families under stress: Interventions for caregivers of senile dementia patients. *Psychotherapy: Theory, Research and*

33. Profession Without Practice: An Administrator's Perspective on Barriers That Restrict the Use of Research in Public Policy

RICK ROGER

INTRODUCTION

This chapter identifies and examines barriers to the use of research findings in the development and evaluation of policies and programs directed at aging populations. Potentially limiting aspects of the health service environment are considered from the administrative perspective. System elements that hinder management participation in research are appraised with a review of restrictions to the use of available research conclusions. Proposals intended to extend the future applicability and use of gerontological research are put forward in a final section of the chapter. The views of 15 senior health sector managers, assembled by questionnaire, are incorporated at various stages in the analysis. It is acknowledged, however, that the central arguments identified have not been recycled through the reference group of managers, many of whom may disagree with some of the opinions expressed.

Aging and Health: Linking Research and Public Policy, © 1989 Lewis Publishers, Inc., Chelsea, Michigan 48118. Printed in U.S.A.

BACKGROUND: THE HEALTH SERVICE ENVIRONMENT

Unique Aspects of the Service Environment

Acute care and continuing care policymakers, managers, and practitioners analyze problems and administer responses in an environment that is increasingly turbulent and challenging. Well-known factors—technological and demographic imperatives, increasing cost consciousness at all levels of the system, professional and interest group rivalries, and an overlay of conflicting ideologies—intermix with a forceful impact on the care delivery structure. Health system outputs are difficult to measure. Moreover, inputs are complex, specialized, and interdependent in some respects, but "loosely coupled" in others (Howell & Wall, 1983). It is further recorded that the dominant profession in acute care delivery has an exceptional organizational status, controlling the utilization of services and generating expenditures outside the traditional boundaries of organizational control. This is hardly new information, but it supports the contention that "the political, legal, and financial environments that confront health care organizations are extremely complex and pluralistic requiring the development and maintenance of complicated intra- and inter-system linkages" (Fottler, 1987, p. 369). The research community is only one of several constituencies health care administrators must address, just as the policy development audience is only one of several destinations for the research effort.

Future Organizational and Research Needs

The managerial and care delivery practices of past decades should not be expected to define or delimit the future for health care providers and organizations. This condition is particularly clear to researchers, practitioners, and policymakers when the materializing needs of increasing populations of dependent elders are assembled as a challenge to program development. Just as the past successes of medicine are converted into the next decade's dilemmas (Wildavsky, 1977), service delivery models of past decades are unlikely to furnish a fully effective response to future demands for an integrated, but diverse, range of care and service options (Robertson, 1986).

Health care delivery for seniors has been based on institutional-dominant models and methods, which in turn create a public demand from (and later for) health care providers (Mechanic, 1979; Miller & Miller, 1981). Noting the inconsistency between sound rehabilitative principles and institutional models for care of the elderly, Mechanic (1979) argued that current health policies, which engender dependence and reliance on medical authority, will be displaced through the lobbying efforts of seniors seeking a wider range of programs and benefits in a social climate that encourages deinstitutionalization. Research evidence continues to accumulate on the specific cost impact of population aging, with a concurrent identification of factors that propel cost increases. It would be unwise to assume, however, that the resources of the next century will be sufficient to finance a growing infrastructure of community programs coincident with the high institutional utilization levels that have characterized the past. Creative, informed policymaking must be part of a strategy for future system effectiveness.

Innovative modes of service delivery will be developed with difficulty. It is, for example, a much simpler matter to establish nursing home beds than to link existing beds with community support care services in an integrated system. The development of discharge planning beds to displace long-stay patients from the acute care system is a less exacting task than the development of early intervention systems to obviate or delay the need for acute care admission. Implications for research will follow from organizational futures characterized by increasingly complex system interactions and accelerating conditions of change.

Davis (1985) maintained that research can influence public policy by identifying problems that require intervention and by identifying appropriate solutions. Adopting the relative simplicity of the argument, we need to know what works and what does not as new programs are developed and transferred to different delivery settings. At the patient care level, we must learn how to fit specific services to individual client needs (Mechanic, 1979), recognizing that successful intervention must be directed at changing the rate of chronic disease progression (Fries & Crapo, 1982). Finally, we must learn how to maintain flexibility and build in capacities for organizational self-evaluation and renewal from the front-line care level to the executive office. As Wildavsky (1979) reminds us, evaluation and organization are somewhat contradictory terms. The self-evaluating organization is easy to conceptualize, but difficult to sustain.

Role of Policy Analysis

Under prevailing circumstances, Canadian society must place an increased premium on constructive policy analysis with a concurrent reinforcement of the role of research in policy formation. Paralleling the increasingly sophisticated policy formulation process reported in the United States (Davis, 1985), there should be additional opportunities for decisionmakers at all levels to apportion greater emphasis to good analytical research, statistical evidence, and evaluation of existing programs. Indeed, a growing accumulation of health care literature testifies to the active research interest in emerging policy choices, but contemporary issues associated with the provision of human services to an aging population have not been examined to the universal satisfaction of managers or researchers.

Paradoxically, competent and well-presented research has not always found a receptive audience of policymakers. The former Deputy Assistant

Secretary of Planning and Evaluation for the U.S. Department of Health and Human Services notes "many gaps remain to be bridged. . . . The research community is rarely familiar with specific questions for which policy officials want answers, the types of information, or method of presentation that could be helpful in assisting policymakers in making choices among alternatives" (Davis, 1985, p. 2). Policymakers and administrators surveyed for this chapter disclosed similar views about their affiliations with the Canadian research community. These reservations notwithstanding, all respondents were optimistic about the potential contribution of research to public policy development.

Differential Accountabilities

Practitioners attempting to apply and disseminate acquired knowledge respond to demands for accountability from patients, from professional bodies, from society in a general sense, and from the organizations in which they practice. The health care manager/policymaker, on the other hand, is primarily accountable to a single employing organization. Professional and patient accountabilities may not be well served by the bureaucratic-to-political-to-electorate accountability linkage. Surely this is the underlying allegation behind occasional charges of "squelched research," which, in the Canadian context, originate primarily with interest groups aligned against governing parties at the federal or provincial levels.

Accountability issues shape the research results interpretation and dissemination process in the form of public discernment of issues. Policy is developed in an environment made up of political ideologies, interest group lobbying, media attention, public opinion, and broad economic and social forces (Davis, 1985). Research is only one factor that shapes policy.

Acceptance of the argument that perceived needs of populations change over time—requiring the periodic restriking of balance points between needs, resources, and system utilization (White et al., 1977)—forces consideration of those factors that change public perception. The prevalent American cultural outlook, which distrusts the political system and places greater faith in the "nonpolitical" judgments of professional experts (Bjorkman & Altenstetter, 1979), has gained evident momentum in Canada in recent years. If professional peer accountability has indeed been substituted for government accountability in the public mind, the effective introduction of research findings into policy is at least somewhat dependent on the degree of concurrence between professional and public interests.

The accountability issue was introduced here for two reasons: (1) to emphasize the importance, in a pluralistic society, not only of research, but also of the dissemination and dispensation of research results; and (2) to confirm the setting of health care policy development, providing a background to the opinions solicited from a small survey of officials in positions to influence health care policy.

SURVEY OF HEALTH ADMINISTRATORS

Process

The organizing committee for CONNECTIONS '88 asked for a presentation of views from the "field" concerning barriers to the use of research augmented by a review of mechanisms and procedures by which these barriers could be overcome. As a representative "policymaker/administrator" with a background in the government and service delivery flanks of the health care sector, I have firm opinions on the efficacy of contemporary research and decisionmaking processes. Portraying the views of more than 15,000 managers in the Canadian health care system is not, on the other hand, an easy task. As the various organizational segments are only mildly responsive to one another (Howell & Wall, 1983), there is limited reason to suspect that a homogeneous body of opinion exists. Moreover, if the "differentiated accountability" assertion presented previously is valid, viewpoints will differ among practicing managers (e.g., head nurses), client advocates, and executive managers.

Input was sought from executive level officials involved or influential in health care policymaking. A group of senior administrators, selected from a range of backgrounds, was commissioned as an informal panel and surveyed by mail. A brief three-page questionnaire was used to extract and distill opinions. Questions were structured about an elementary conceptual model incorporating a "researcher" sending an encoded message (research results) to a "policymaker" with requisite decoding skills. Survey responses were interpreted from the systems perspective with specific reference to three areas that received extensive comment in the survey returns: the research environment; researcher/policymaker interaction; and administrative acceptance of research products and findings.

Twenty-two mailed questionnaires drew 15 responses from three groups of equivalent size: 5 respondents with present or previous positions at the assistant deputy minister level in provincial government health or social service departments; 5 senior health care administrators located at facilities in five different provinces; and 5 respondents with specific policy-forming roles in provincial government planning units, health care interested advocacy associations, or research funding agencies. The distinct culture of Quebec was not represented in the responses received.

The survey was developed without scientific pretense. The extent to which findings can be generalized to a larger Canadian community of Canadian health service administrators and policymakers is not a function of population or survey instrument validity, but of a commonsense interpretation of the consistent themes identified in the returns. The questionnaire was intended to encourage a very busy group of officials to take time to respond. Structuring opinions into a predetermined format was a secondary consideration. Input from the panel was not intended to be tabulated or quantified. Respondents were promised anonymity.

Administrative Views: The Research Environment

The pervasive reaction of respondents to an unasked question is noteworthy. The single overriding issue of concern centered on the actual extent to which provincial governments are prepared to provide a role for research in decisionmaking. Responses were permeated with references to hospitals and extended care facilities built in the "wrong" locations, "wrong-headed" reactions to task force and commission recommendations, "ill-advised" cutting of community programs during periods of restraint, and "uninformed" intersectoral policy initiatives as, for example, when hospitals are encouraged to expedite patient discharge without consideration of implications for home support programs. These developments were attributed universally, and perhaps somewhat unfairly, to the obligations of the political process. Many respondents acknowledged their own cynicism in this regard. Research has a limited future according to administrators convinced that the policy development process will continue to address political motivations and to discount "rational" analysis.

Economic influences were cited almost as frequently as political motivations in the responses dealing with the research environment. There is a general perception that funding for "program delivery" and "organizational" research has been limited in recent years. Several respondents reported the discontinuation of "evaluation" funding for new initiatives, noting that this type of support was probable a decade ago, but less likely in the resource-restricted 1980s. The "lack of incentives" rallying cry of contemporary administrators was also prevalent, usually as part of a larger argument that a system without spurs to innovation will not present well as a target for research.

Administrative Views: Researcher/Policymaker Interaction

Respondents observed that more and more policy-oriented jobs in government are filled by people with graduate level education, providing the potential for a growing research perspective in policy development. Computer technology and data base accessibility were identified as supporting elements, enabling more research and policy analysis activity. Communication of research results and subsequent researcher/policymaker dialogue was thought to be facilitated with computer graphics and interactive data presentation technologies.

Many asserted that, when under pressure to establish a firm policy direction on a contentious issue, the typical decisionmaker in government is likely to prefer contracted research to general academic studies. Researchers under contract are perceived to be more responsive to administrative direction. Contracted research offers the joint advantages of design and publication control. Academic research was not, however, distrusted or found consistently deficient by the responding group of managers.

Respondents frequently mentioned communication difficulties. A portion of the problem was attributed to a relatively unsophisticated audience receiving the research results, whereas others referred to poor communication skills of the researcher. It was argued that researchers and policymakers can be suspicious of each others' motives and methods. Policymakers funding research wish to avoid uninformed or questionable findings and recommendations at the conclusion of the investigative process. Those involved in research could be troubled, on the other hand, by an acknowledged tendency on the part of managers and policymakers to oversimplify and generalize results inappropriately.

Respondents describing their own involvement in the implementation of research conclusions pointed to (1) deficiencies in data bases which have gone unnoticed in research and (2) limitations in research design which have not been recorded in published literature. Problems arising from "lack of expertise" at the receiving end of the research process were also conceded.

One respondent, a senior policy advisor in a provincial health department, provided an excellent summary of the differences in orientation between researchers and policymakers. Research, Pallan argues in a paper delivered to an audience of research-oriented dieticians (personal communication, January 13, 1988), is directed at achieving a better understanding of issues; policy development seeks out facts in support of decisionmaking. Researchers must attempt to simplify reality, minimizing the number of variables under investigation; policymaking is obligated to deal with a larger encompassing system of contributing elements. Research focuses on hypothesis testing and controlled experimentation; policy development often must act from limited information and imperfect science. Research results are qualified and cautious; policy communication is optimistic with an orientation towards marketing.

One respondent noted a further barrier to researcher/policymaker interaction: the limited movement of personnel among the academic environment, government, and service delivery organizations. The academic reward system was considered by many of the surveyed administrators to encourage researchers to avoid policy-orientated studies in favor of academic research directed at the requirements of review journals.

Administrative Acceptance of Research Findings

Respondents recognized the need for research findings to be condensed and interpreted for senior officials and politicians. In this regard, the potential role of policy units of government health departments across Canada was identified. Many respondents expressed reservations about the effectiveness of these units when dealing with other parts of the provincial health bureaucracies. One respondent suggested that group lobbying efforts, on behalf of seniors, had more impact on policy development for geriatric care than decades of "in-house" demographic analysis pointing to emerging problems. Several respondents speculated that Provincial Health Ministers simply do not have time to read anything longer than one page, and questioned how complex research findings could be communicated in such a condensed format.

Respondents stressed the need for senior officials comfortable and confident with research data interpretation. The benefit of contemplative and self-evaluating organizational modes was recognized. Organizational fragmentation and specialization at the provincial government level, and high policy development staff turnover rates in some jurisdictions, were cited as concerns.

Synthesis of Survey Returns

The survey returns are not, as a package, encouraging. Administrators and policymakers believe that political and economic constraints have overpowered past research efforts, limiting potential contributions of research to policy development. Moreover, communications problems and competing objectives are considered to have compromised researcher/administrator interaction to the detriment of the research product. Respondents acknowledged and supported the role of research, but offered only cautious optimism with regard to future prospects.

PROFESSION WITHOUT PRACTICE

Canadian administrators, tracking the introduction of prospective payment under the American Medicare system, witnessed a policy development process quite distinct from the Canadian experience. The underlying diagnosis-related-group method of patient classification was research based, with a stream of published literature dating to the mid-1970s. Virtually every interest group commissioned research in support of its particular cause. Policy options were debated in several forums with frequent references to research findings. An entire field of study, institutional policy analysis, is dedicated to the study of government reform and its consequences (Gormley, 1987).

Contrast this American background with the Canadian tradition of restricted federal/provincial dialogue on funding issues, unaided by research or interest group involvement. Both health administrators and researchers in Canada have been insufficiently vigilant in pursuit of their potential roles in the policy formation process.

Health Administrators

Health administrators profess interest in enhancing the contribution of research to policy development. In practice, however, only a very limited number of administrators have invested significantly in this option. Allocating time to the proper interpretation and generalization of research findings requires a diversion of management attention from other day-to-day activities. Few managers have accomplished this transition, although most would note the importance of an executive vision inspired by new ideas and methodologies. Many health administrators professing a conviction that policy should be further influenced by research findings have not yet become actively involved in the presentation and dissemination of research findings. Professed interest in self-evaluating organizational models often translates into active management interest in research that buttresses previously held opinions and preserves the status quo.

Research Community

Researchers profess interest in the applied use of research findings. In practice, however, academics often appear unprepared or unwilling to contribute to public dialogue on health issues that would raise the profile of research. Moreover, researchers have not always understood or accepted the need to keep pace with the mechanisms and timing of the policy-development process. Researchers are not universally comfortable with the view that good policy decisions often derive from more than one discipline and that multidisciplinary research enhances the policy-development process. Researchers have not spent significant time with policy developers investigating those factors that would strengthen research as an input to policy formation. Professed academic interest is not matched consistently with contributions in practice.

WHERE TO NOW: OVERCOMING BARRIERS

Challenging the Policy Development Environment

System improvement is dependent upon the stimulus to research associated with informed interest group participation and open dialogue. A new threshold of research influence on policy can be achieved only if there is acceptance that research can actually influence policy. Researchers and managers must be prepared to integrate research findings more extensively in public discussions of health care issues.

Framework for Future Health Priorities

Many of the predominant barriers to immediate gains in research effectiveness as a policy determinant can be removed without funding infusions. At the federal government level, for example, the National Health Research and Development Program (NHRDP), the policy-oriented research funding arm of Health and Welfare Canada, has made strong efforts to better signal priorities and to improve the project review process. Relevance screening is more applicable than in the past. There is more involvement by health administrators and planners at the project review stage and priorities are shifting toward a problem-solving focus. Nevertheless, research still tends to cluster around clinical planning and health status determination issues, as noted in an earlier review (Sutherland, 1984). As administrators, we have not achieved great success in the communication of our real research needs, and frustrated individual researchers continue to be unable to secure NHRDP funding for worthy administrative projects. Administrators must become proactive communicators of research priorities, working through governments, interest groups, and professional bodies.

At the provincial level, in-house planning efforts, which were perhaps more characteristic of the 1960s and early 1970s, have been augmented by or replaced with provincial funding for health research bodies. On the whole, there have been positive developments that have encouraged promising research in new areas of interest. However, the existence of several provincial funding agencies in itself complicates the funding process, obligating administrators to question if the true potential effectiveness of current research is being achieved on a national scale.

A published five-year plan for federal financing of research on national health issues, similar to that of the 1985 report of the Social Science and Humanities Research Council of Canada, would assist provinces in the development of their own research funding program. A published plan for NHRDP would also serve as a focal point for reaction from scholars and managers.

Bridging Gaps

Administrators and researchers must learn to interact more effectively. When new initiatives are contemplated at the facility or program level, researchers should be consulted at an early stage to ensure that appropriate evaluation protocols are developed and that the data base is manageable from the research perspective.

The enabling role of policy development units in provincial government must be strengthened. These units have the potential of bringing research closer to policymaking and serving as vital linkages between the research, funding, and program delivery systems.

Affiliation arrangements between government policy planning units and individual university research units have started to emerge. These are yet to be evaluated but offer several advantages. Cross appointments between policy planning units and universities should also be further promoted.

We must be prepared as administrators to encourage new researchers in their roles. We must recognize that the natural tendency of the research funding system, left to its own momentum, is to continue in established directions, using established researchers and established funding arrangements.

A newsletter sanctioned or produced by NHRDP is an absolute necessity. We cannot trigger responses from administrators and policy developers without better forums to engender interest.

Data Base Development

As Canadians, we know too little about the health status of our population. We must reexamine prospects for an upgraded and comprehensive national health survey, ensuring that all provinces have a reasonable chance of achieving statistically valid results within their area of program jurisdiction. We have also done too little to document the utilization of our health institutions, to record admission and discharge severity within clinically meaningful groups, and to trace patients through the community and institutional networks. Our national data banks tell us far more about system inputs than outputs, a situation that must be challenged.

CONCLUSION

I have attempted to present the case for more effective researcher involvement in policy development. A conforming attitude prevalent among health administrators and policy developers has been identified as one fundamental barrier to increased use of research findings. In our collective efforts to design, fund, implement, and evaluate more effective health care strategies, we have been too often discouraged by the failures of the past. We must avoid the temptation to portray population aging itself as the cause of current delivery system deficiencies, recognizing that policy challenges deriving from aging will require a reevaluation and reassessment of the entire spectrum of health services for seniors (McDaniel, 1987). Researchers, managers, and policymakers must envisage and encourage a future more influenced by good research and analysis and less influenced by the constraints of political and professional accountability.

REFERENCES

Bjorkman, J. W., & Altenstetter, C. A. (1979). Accountability in health care: An essay on mechanisms, muddles, and mires. *Journal of Health Politics, Policy and Law, 4*(3), 360–381.

Davis, K. (1985). Using research in policy formulation. (Prepublication Draft). Prepared for L. H. Aiken, & D. Mechanic (Eds.), *Applications of social science to clinical medicine and health policy*. Revised February 6, 1985.

Fottler, M. D. (1987). Health care organizational performance: Present and future research. *Journal of Management, 13*(2), 367–391.

Fries, J. F., & Crapo, L. M. (1982). Physiologic aging and the compression of morbidity. In *Proceedings of the Conference on Health in the '80s and '90s and its Impact on Health Sciences Education* (pp. 87–114). Toronto: Council of Ontario Universities.

Gormley, W. T. (1987). Institutional policy analysis: A critical review. *Journal of Policy Analysis and Management, 6*(2), 153–169.

Howell, J. P., & Wall, L. C. (1983). Executive leadership in an organized anarchy: The case of HSO's. *Health Care Management Review, 8,* 17–26.

McDaniel, S. A. (1987). Demographic aging and the welfare state. *Canadian Public Policy, 13*(3), 330–336.

Mechanic, D. (1979). *Future issues in health care: Social policy and the rationing of medical services*. New York: The Free Press.

Miller, A. E., & Miller, M. G. (1981). *Options for health and health care: The coming of post clinical medicine*. Toronto: John Wiley and Sons.

Robertson, D. (1986). *Alternative methods of health care delivery for Canada's aging population*. Paper presented at the Colloquium on Aging with Limited Health Resources, Winnipeg. (Sponsored by Economic Council of Canada)

Sutherland, R. W. (1984, Spring). Federally funded health administration research— A new era? *Health Management Forum,* 43–51.

White, K. L., Anderson, D. O., Kalmo, E., Kleczkowski, B. M., Purola, T., & Vakmanovic, C. (1977). *Health Services: Concepts and information for national planning and management*. Geneva: World Health Organization.

Wildavsky, A. (1977). Doing better and feeling worse: The political pathology of health policy. In J. M. Knowles (Ed.), *Doing better and feeling worse: Health in the United States* (pp. 105–123). New York: W. W. Norton and Company.

Wildavsky, A. (1979). *Speaking trust to power*. Toronto: Little, Brown and Company.

34. Overcoming Barriers to Using Research in the Policymaking Process: A Researcher's Perspective

PETER R. GRANT

INTRODUCTION

This chapter is divided into two parts: First, the literature on the factors that influence whether policymakers will utilize social science research findings will be reviewed in the context of three general propositions. Arising from these propositions are actions both the researcher and the policymaker can take to maximize the chances of the latter obtaining important and relevant information from a research project.

During the 1970s, a number of prominent social scientists expressed concern that policymakers were not using the results from large scale evaluation research projects available to them (Beyer & Trice, 1982; Leviton & Hughes, 1981; Weiss, 1972). This concern led to a number of investigations into the factors that influence *research utilization* (defined as "serious consideration of the results of a research project in the decisionmaking process"). Usually this research involved identifying a number of well-known research projects in a particular field and then interviewing the evaluators, policymakers, and project officers associated with these projects.

For example, Patton et al. (1977) selected a stratified random sample of 20 national health program evaluations conducted in the United States between 1971 and 1973. Using in-depth, open-ended interviews, the evaluator, the decisionmaker (usually a director or division head in the Federal civil service), and the project officer were asked whether the results were utilized and, if so, to describe the nature of the utilization. The results showed that two factors were considered very important if research is to be utilized:

Aging and Health: Linking Research and Public Policy, © 1989 Lewis Publishers, Inc., Chelsea, Michigan 48118. Printed in U.S.A.

(1) someone within the organization needs to be a consistent and strong supporter of the research and (2) the political climate must be favorable. As is typically the case in this kind of study, both the evaluators and decision-makers were very experienced people (on average, members of both categories had worked 14 years in their field).

Thus, the strength of this kind of research is that it reflects the opinions of people who have considered the implications of research results for program and policy change over a long period of time. Its weakness is that causal links between the identified factors and research utilization are never directly tested and remain informed speculation. Although simulations have been used to manipulate variables and observe their impact in an experimental design (Braskamp, Brown, & Newman, 1982), they are of limited utility, and the in-depth interview remains the dominant procedure used to investigate research utilization.

The literature review that follows will express the relation between three broad, related factors and research utilization in the form of general propositions.

- *Proposition 1*—The more research results enlighten and inform policymakers about a social program or problem, the more these results will be used in the program and policy development process.
- *Proposition 2*—Factors that increase the credence that policymakers place in research findings are likely to increase the use of these findings in the program and policy development process.
- *Proposition 3*—Involvement by policymakers in the research process is likely to increase the use of research results in the program and policy development process.

Aspects of these propositions will be elaborated upon in the context of specific research findings. Consistent with Leviton and Hughes (1981), *utilization* is defined as "serious consideration of research findings in the decisionmaking process (conceptual utilization) or the use of this information to make specific policy decisions (instrumental utilization)."

FACTORS THAT INCREASE RESEARCH UTILIZATION: THREE PROPOSITIONS

1. The more research results enlighten and inform policymakers about a social program or problem, the more these results will be used in the program and policy development process.

There seems to be general agreement that *utilization* means "using research results when discussing program and policy formation and change." Research can enlighten and inform policymakers about the parameters of a social program or problem as they engage in this decisionmaking process (Cook, Levinson-Rose, & Pollard, 1981; Knorr, 1977; Patton et al., 1977; Thomas & Tymon, 1982; Weiss & Bucuvalas, 1977; Weiss, 1979). From this perspective, the results of outcome evaluations are not all that useful, because often they are not directly relevant to this decisionmaking process. Information on how a program is implemented and which describes its components is at least as desirable. According to Leviton and Boruch (1983), research that documents how education programs are implemented (process evaluations) has more impact on the decisions of middle management than research that demonstrates the effects of these programs (outcome evaluations). These authors suggest that, ideally, evaluation research should provide both implementation and outcome information for maximum impact on program and policy decisions. In the same vein, Bickman (1985) argued that program *components* need to be described and evaluated rather than *entire* programs to facilitate program change and development. As well, Siegel and Tuckel (1985) used two case studies to argue that research findings that suggest small incremental changes to programs and policies rather than their wholesale adoption or abandonment are of more use to administrators and managers.

2. *Factors that increase the credence that policymakers place in research findings are likely to increase the use of these findings in the program and policy development process.*

At the heart of this proposition is the notion that researchers and policymakers live in two different communities with different practices, values, and priorities and that these differences partially prevent researchers from communicating the program- and policy-related implications of the research findings to policymakers (Caplan, 1977; Shrivastava & Mitroff, 1984). Indeed, the evidence suggests that sophisticated methodological and analysis strategies used by researchers to ensure that their results have scientific validity are not always appreciated by research consumers (Cohen & Weiss, 1977; Patton et al., 1977; Van de Vall & Bolas, 1981). Rather, communication of research results in frequent, informal conversations, short nontechnical reports, and ad hoc policy-related meetings seems to be of importance (Rich, 1979; Sproull & Larkey, 1979; Stevens & Tornatsky, 1980; Van de Vall & Bolas, 1981, 1982). Further, qualitative information often has more impact than quantitative information because it more clearly confirms or contradicts a policymaker's daily experience (Dawson & D'Amico, 1985; Beyer & Trice, 1982; Oman & Chitwood, 1984; Patton et al., 1977).

In this regard, the research also shows that surprising findings often do not have much impact because, it is suggested, they do not fit with other information (including past research findings) that policymakers bring to bear in the decisionmaking process. Results that have impact are those that clarify and extend the issues involved and help build a consensus among key decisionmakers on the direction that changes to programs and policies should take (Patton et al., 1977; Rich, 1977; Weiss & Bucuvalas, 1977; Van de Vall & Bolas, 1982).

3. *Involvement by policymakers in the research process is likely to increase the use of research results in the program and policy development process.*

The industrial-organizational area has shown that participative decision-making is conducive to organization change (Beyer & Trice, 1982). Thus, it is not surprising to find that staff involvement in the research process leads to greater utilization of research results in the decisionmaking process (Dawson & D'Amico, 1985; Stevens & Tornatsky, 1980). To facilitate staff involvement, steering committees and interdepartmental policymaking units can be formed (Oman & Chitwood, 1984; Polivka & Steg, 1978; Van de Vall & Bolas, 1981, 1982). Although these units can be coopted for political purposes (Peck & Rubin, 1983), they can be very effective if their function is to integrate relevant research findings into the program and policy development process. For example, Polivka and Steg (1978) discuss an evaluation unit set up by the Florida Department of Health and Rehabilitation Services. This unit set up a formal mechanism in which, over a two- to three-month period, evaluation results were reviewed in meetings among administrators, program managers, and evaluators of the program with the goal of developing policy recommendations. In this review process, the program director was responsible for presenting the evaluation results—thus ensuring his/her commitment to the research project. Recommendations were passed on up the government hierarchy for approval. This process worked very well and the authors report that major policy changes in the areas of retardation, mental health, and youth services had been effected based, in part, upon the research conducted by the evaluation unit. As well, a European study has shown that even in the absence of a formal mechanism, in-house evaluators appear to spend more time on ad hoc, policy-related conferences, and the degree to which this activity occurs is associated with utilization (Van de Vall & Bolas, 1981).

Commitment to the research project by an influential person in the organization is a key factor that affects whether the project's results are utilized (Caplan, 1977; Johnson, Frazier, & Riddick, 1983; Oman & Chitwood, 1984; Patton et al., 1977; Van de Vall & Bolas, 1982; Webber, 1987). Essentially, this person acts as an advocate for the project within his/her organization and builds support for inclusion of the results in the decisionmaking process. This is often a linking role, because the person maintains a link between the research team and management and facilitates consensus building at all stages of the research project.

Several studies suggest that the degree to which research findings meet user needs and expectations is related to utilization of these findings (Bedell et al., 1985; Johnson et al., 1983; Rich, 1979; Weiss & Bucuvalas, 1977; Van de Vall & Bolas, 1982). That is, for a policymaker to be involved in a research project, he or she must feel that it addresses important information needs.

Additionally, it has been argued that utilization occurs when research results are compatible with organizational needs. For example, how decisions are made within the organization, its communication network, its organizational structure (hierarchy), and its past history all will influence the way research results are received (Beyer & Trice, 1982; Shapiro, 1984; Weiss, 1979). However, it appears that no research has been done to test these ideas.

In summary, research utilization is increased when research results are felt to be both informative and credible by policymakers who have been involved with the research from its beginning. These factors are related and together suggest strategies that researchers and policymakers can adopt in order to maximize research utilization—the focus of the remainder of this chapter.

STRATEGIES FOR INCREASING RESEARCH UTILIZATION

Increasing the research consumer's involvement in the research process and ensuring that the research results are communicated effectively are part of a very political process (Posavac & Carey, 1985; Weiss, 1975). However, it is my experience that although political considerations are of obvious importance, policymakers primarily support research projects because they are very interested in obtaining useful and valid information on the social program or policy with which they are concerned. Thus, it is useful to consider how the researcher and the policymaker might act in order to ensure that the utilization of research findings is maximized in the context of the propositions discussed earlier.

Before doing so, it should be noted that directives for the policy *researcher* are common throughout the literature, whereas, parallel directives for *policymakers* are made conspicuous by their absence. This is understandable in that often the policymaker commissions the research or, at least, proposes to sponsors that such research needs to be funded. Further, if the research is conducted in-house, the researcher may report directly to this policymaker. Obviously, it behooves the in-house researcher to ensure that the results of his/her project are communicated accurately and completely and to convince his/her boss that the research project was worthwhile, whereas the policymaker experiences no such pressure. Indeed, while in-house evaluators usually have more impact on policymakers (Van de Vall & Bolas, 1982), they are also subject to pressures to produce the "expected" results. That is, their research may be more suspect because they may be perceived as having a conflict of interest. At any rate, it has been estimated that 75% of program evaluations and policy studies in North America are conducted by external consultants on a contractual basis (Van de Vall & Bolas, 1981). Therefore, for this reason alone, policymakers might find it productive to pay more attention to this issue.

Strategies for the Policy Researcher

First, consider advice given to the policy researcher:

1. Consult with the policymaker to ensure that relevant descriptive information on the social program or problem is collected.
2. If an evaluation is required, explore the usefulness of describing and evaluating key program components.
3. Clarify that program evaluation is an important part of program planning and development.
4. Communicate research results through informal conversations, short nontechnical reports, and ad hoc policy meetings.
5. Spend time discussing the research project with the organization's staff.
6. Contract for management's continual involvement in the research process through a steering committee or other policymaking unit, or regular meetings with representatives of the organization committed to the research project.
7. Try to ensure that the research addresses the needs of key policymakers.
8. Try to ensure that the policy implications of the research results are extensively discussed in a series of post final report meetings between researchers and policymakers.

Such a person is exhorted to explore a proposed research project with representatives of the "client" consumer groups. This process ensures that the research is relevant to the issues considered to be of critical importance by the consumer. In the evaluation research literature, this is called the utilization-focused approach to program evaluation (Patton, 1978). Obviously the chances of the research findings having an enlightenment function (Proposition 1) is increased using such a strategy. Further, it is an attempt to ensure consumer involvement and commitment right from the beginning of the project (Proposition 3).

Contracting is also considered to be very important (Gallessich, 1982; Posavac & Carey, 1985). In the contract (whether formal or informal), mechanisms can be set in place which facilitate continuing commitment and involvement in the research process (Proposition 3). For example, a steering committee could be established to allow the researcher to discuss the research with decisionmakers or their representatives. Also, informal reports to this body allow the researcher to discuss the findings and to gear them toward questions of particular interest (Proposition 2). If this is not possible or desirable, the contract can clearly state to whom the researcher should report.

In negotiating the contract, the researcher needs to try and obtain the commitment of at least one key decisionmaker to the project in order to ensure its success (Proposition 3). Indeed, it is well known that if all key players are not consulted at this time, there is a real danger that the project will either be sabotaged or, upon completion, shelved (Posavac & Carey, 1985).

Contracting can be viewed as helpful in increasing the chances that research results will be utilized, because it tries to ensure that the research is answering policy or program relevant questions in consultation with management (all propositions). That is, it is directed toward clarifying policy or program development issues, maintaining management's involvement, and creating a mechanism to ensure frequent communication between the researcher and administrative personnel.

Often evaluators talk of overcoming the resistance of the staff of the organization to the evaluation (Weiss, 1975; Posavac & Carey, 1985). Research, particularly evaluation research, can have negative consequences, and research as a tool to facilitate program and policy development is an idea that needs to be sold. In the field of program evaluation, this direction has led researchers to focus more on program planning and development. Thus, evaluability assessment—a procedure that documents a program's components and their intended effects—is becoming more widespread as a management tool for joint discussions between the researcher and administrative staff on the direction of evaluation efforts (Proposition 3). Further, process evaluation, which describes the activities of program staff and the client characteristics, has become popular for establishing accountability. Fisher and Peters (1985) argued that program evaluation should follow a certain sequence to be maximally effective in terms of program planning and development: (1) evaluability assessment, (2) process evaluation, (3) outcome evaluation. Part of the effectiveness of this approach lies in the continual involvement of management in the research process (Proposition 3).

At a different level, research consultants such as the PhD students trained in the Applied Social Division of the Psychology Department at the University of Saskatchewan use a process-oriented consulting model, which advocates the continuous involvement in the research process by policymakers and program managers (Proposition 3). Students are trained to develop and maintain relations with key decisionmakers in the organization so that this happens (Lippitt & Lippitt, 1978). For example, when investigating policy issues, the consultant may suggest that management commission a needs assessment to provide useful information on important policy-related questions, or a process evaluation to obtain an accurate and complete description of a program. Then the consultant works on establishing an internal mechanism to ensure that this information is fed into the policymaking/program development process (all propositions).

Finally, a number of authors have suggested that the researcher become an advocate of his/her research findings and their policy implications follow-ing completion of the final report (Stevens & Tornatsky, 1980; Van de Vall & Bolas, 1981). Such post-report activity is likely to increase the utilization of research findings, because they focus on the link between the research results and possible program and policy change (Proposition 2).

Strategies for the Policymaker

Possible strategies of a policymaker to maximize research utilization in the program and policy development process include:

1. Make sure the information needs of the organization are discussed thor-oughly with the research team and that these needs form the basis of the research project.
2. Ask for short, nontechnical, interim reports and discuss them with members of the research team.
3. Create a steering committee or policy unit to monitor the research.
4. Identify a contact person (project officer) to meet regularly with the re-search team.
5. Arrange for post–final report discussions between policymakers and re-searchers to discuss the policy implications of the research findings.
6. Arrange for staff to attend workshops on basic research design and program evaluation.

First, it is important to create a mechanism to encourage staff involvement in the research process. For in-house research projects, this may mean the establishment of a permanent interdepartmental unit that routinely discusses the policy and program development implications of each research project (Polivka & Steg, 1978). For an externally conducted project, regular meet-ings between the researcher and a steering committee or key individual in the organization should be arranged. If these actions lead to staff becoming more involved with the research project, Proposition 3 would suggest that the use of research findings in discussions of possible program and policy changes is more likely to occur. Leviton and Hughes (1981) indicate that one reason for lack of involvement by government staff in a research project is due to staff turnover. Often transfers occur during the period when the research project is being conducted. The establishment of an interdepartmental unit or steering committee should help maintain staff involvement under these circumstances, because there is a formal mechanism for acquainting new employees with the history and objectives of the research project, as well as with key members of the research team.

Second, it can be very helpful if the administrator/manager with whom the researcher has the most contact has some insight into the research process. There is nothing so frustrating to a researcher as the continual lack of appreciation for basic research design issues. For example, the reasons for pilot-testing the measures used in a study, for a no-treatment control group, and for the random assignment to different treatments are not hard to grasp. Nevertheless, as an applied researcher, I know that I am probably going to have to work hard to convince administrative personnel of their importance whenever I start a new research project. Policymakers will likely benefit from efforts to close the gap between their world and the world of the researcher—for example, by attending workshops on the basics of research design or evaluation research. The assumption is that the program and policy implications of research findings will be more apparent to policymakers with this knowledge (Proposition 1) and whether credence can be placed in the research findings will be more congruent with methodological criteria (Proposition 2). Note I am not suggesting that a policymaker abandon common sense, nor am I suggesting that methodological rigor should be given greater weight than other factors in the decisionmaking process. But understanding a little about the research process will allow a policymaker to hold more in-depth discussions with the researcher on the program and policy implications of the results. Because the policymaker is likely to be much more familiar with the issues than the researcher, such discussions are likely to maximize the usefulness of these results in ensuing meetings concerned with program and policy change. Post–final report discussions are likely to be more productive if policymakers are familiar with the research process.

In summary, the literature suggests that informative and credible research results communicated to a policymaker who has been closely involved in the research process are most likely to be utilized.

REFERENCES

Bedell, J. R., Ward, J. C., Archer, R. P., & Stokes, M. K. (1985). An empirical evaluation of a model of knowledge utilization. *Evaluation Review, 9,* 109–126.

Beyer, J. M., & Trice, H. M. (1982). The utilization process: A conceptual framework and synthesis of empirical findings. *Administrative Science Quarterly, 27,* 591–622.

Bickman, L. (1985). Improving established statewide programs: A component theory of evaluation. *Evaluation Review, 9,* 189–208.

Braskamp, L. A., Brown, R. D., & Newman, D. L. (1982). Studying evaluation utilization through simulations. *Evaluation Review, 6,* 114–126.

Caplan, N. (1977). A minimal set of conditions necessary for the utilization of social science knowledge in policy formulation at the national level. In C. H. Weiss (Ed.), *Using social research in public policymaking* (pp. 183–197). Lexington, MA: Lexington Books.

Cohen, D. K., & Weiss, J. A. (1977). Social science and social policy: Schools and race. In C. H. Weiss (Ed.), *Using social research in public policymaking* (pp. 67–83). Lexington, MA: Lexington Books.

Cook, T. D., Levinson-Rose, J., & Pollard, W. E. (1981). The misutilization of evaluation research: Some pitfalls of definition. In H. E. Freeman & M. A. Soloman (Eds.), *Evaluation studies review annual* (Vol. 6, pp. 727–748). Beverly Hills: Sage.

Dawson, J. A., & D'Amico, J. J. (1985). Involving program staff in evaluation studies: A strategy for increasing information use and enriching the data base. *Evaluation Review, 9,* 173–188.

Fisher, R. J., & Peters, L. (1985). The role of evaluability assessment in mental health program evaluation. *Canadian Journal of Community Mental Health, 4,* 25–34.

Gallessich, J. (1982). *The profession and practice of consultation.* San Francisco: Jossey-Bass.

Johnson, K. W., Frazier, W. D., & Riddick, M. F. (1983). A change strategy for linking the worlds of academia and practice. *The Journal of Applied Behavioral Science, 19,* 439–460.

Knorr, K. D. (1977). Policymakers' use of social science knowledge: Symbolic or instrumental. In C. H. Weiss (Ed.), *Using social research in public policymaking* (pp. 165–182). Lexington, MA: Lexington Books.

Leviton, L. C., & Boruch, R. F. (1983). Contributions of evaluation to education programs and policy. *Evaluation Review, 7,* 563–598.

Leviton, L. C., & Hughes, E. F. X. (1981). Research on the utilization of evaluations: A review and synthesis. *Evaluation Review, 5,* 525–547.

Lippitt, G. & Lippitt, R. (1978). *The consulting process in action.* San Diego: University Associates.

Oman, R. C., & Chitwood, S. R. (1984). Management evaluation studies: Factors affecting the acceptance of recommendations. *Evaluation Review, 8,* 283–305.

Patton, M. Q. (1978). *Utilization-focused evaluation.* Beverly Hills: Sage.

Patton, M. Q., Grimes, P. S., Guthrie, K. M., Brennan, N. J., French, B. D., & Blyth, D. A. (1977). In search of impact: An analysis of the utilization of federal health evaluation research. In C. H. Weiss (Ed.), *Using social research in public policymaking* (pp. 141–163). Lexington, MA: Lexington Books.

Peck, D. L., & Rubin, H. J. (1983). Bureaucratic needs and evaluation research: A case study of the Department of Housing and Urban Development. *Evaluation Review, 7,* 685–703.

Polivka, L., & Steg, E. (1978). Program evaluation and policy development: Bridging the gap. *Evaluation Quarterly, 2,* 696–707.

Posavac, E. J., & Carey, R. G. (1985). *Program evaluation: Methods and case studies* (2nd ed.). Englewood Cliffs, NJ: Prentice-Hall.

Rich, R. F. (1977). Use of social science information by federal bureaucrats: Knowledge for action versus knowledge for understanding. In C. H. Weiss (Ed.), *Using social research in public policymaking* (pp. 199–211). Lexington, MA: Lexington Books.

Rich, R. F. (1979). Problem-solving and evaluation research: Unemployment insurance policy. In R. F. Rich (Eds.), *Translating evaluation into policy* (pp. 87–110). Beverly Hills: Sage.

Shapiro, J. Z. (1984). Conceptualizing evaluation use: Implications of alternative models of organizational decision making. In R. F. Conner, D. G. Altman, & C. Jackson (Eds.). *Evaluation studies review annual* (Vol. 9, pp. 633–645). Beverly Hills: Sage.

Shrivastava, P., & Mitroff, I. I. (1984). Enhancing organizational research utilization: The role of decision-makers' assumptions. *Academy of Management Review, 9*, 18–26.

Siegel, K., & Tuckel, P. (1985). The utilization of evaluation research: A case analysis. *Evaluation Review, 9*, 307–328.

Sproull, L., & Larkey, P. (1979). Managerial behavior and evaluator effectiveness. In H. C. Schulberg & J. M. Jerrell (Eds.), *The evaluator and management* (pp. 89–104). Beverly Hills: Sage.

Stevens, W. F., & Tornatsky, L. G. (1980). The dissemination of evaluation: An experiment. *Evaluation Review, 4*, 339–354.

Thomas, K. W., & Tymon, W. G. (1982). Necessary properties of relevant research: Lessons from recent criticisms of the organizational sciences. *Academy of Management Review, 7*, 345–352.

Van de Vall, M., & Bolas, C. A. (1981). External versus internal social policy researchers. *Knowledge, Creation, Diffusion, Utilization, 2*, 461–481.

Van de Vall, M., & Bolas, C. A. (1982). Using social policy research for reducing social problems: An empirical analysis of structure and functions. *Journal of Applied Behavioral Science, 18*, 49–67.

Webber, D. J. (1987). Factors influencing legislators' use of policy information and implications for promoting greater use. *Policy Studies Review, 6*, 666–676.

Weiss, C. H. (1972). *Evaluation research: Methods of assessing program effectiveness*. Englewood Cliffs, NJ: Prentice-Hall.

Weiss, C. H. (1975). Evaluation research in the political context. In E. L. Struening & M. Guttentag (Eds.). *Handbook of evaluation research* (Vol. 1, pp. 13–26). Beverly Hills: Sage.

Weiss, C. H., & Bucuvalas, M. J. (1977). The challenge of social research to decision making. In C. H. Weiss (Ed.), *Using social research in public policymaking* (pp. 213–233). Lexington, MA: Lexington Books.

Weiss, J. A. (1979). Access to influence: Some effects of policy sector on the use of social science. *American Behavioral Scientist, 22*, 437–458.

35. Research and Public Policy on Urinary Incontinence: Can We Afford Not to Evaluate?

LARRY W. CHAMBERS
GRAHAM WORRALL

THE NEED FOR KNOWLEDGE ABOUT EFFECTIVENESS AND EFFICIENCY

It is exceedingly important to ensure that scarce resources are used to deliver care that is not only efficient (that is, costs are small in relation to effects) but also meets an adequate standard of effectiveness in delivery of care (that is, how well are we doing in alleviating or preventing the health problem?). As the absolute amount of societal resources used for health care of seniors increases, the proportion of resources devoted to evaluation should increase at the same rate. Non–health care industries use approximately 6% of their operating expenditures on quality assurance activities (Chambers, 1986). Similarly, governmental and nongovernmental agencies responsible for financing health care for seniors should view investment in health care evaluation activities as extremely important and devote adequate resources to this.

Editor's Note: Dr. Chambers' original paper used two examples to illustrate his program evaluation perspective: urinary incontinence and dementia. Due to space limitations we reluctantly restricted the discussion to the case of urinary incontinence. In so doing we hope we have preserved the theoretical and analytical integrity of the paper while undeniably reducing the fullness of the illustrations.

Aging and Health: Linking Research and Public Policy, © 1989 Lewis Publishers, Inc., Chelsea, Michigan 48118. Printed in U.S.A.

TYPES OF HEALTH CARE EVALUATION—THE MEASUREMENT ITERATIVE LOOP

The Department of Clinical Epidemiology and Biostatistics at McMaster University has produced an evaluation approach called the *measurement iterative loop* (Tugwell et al., 1985). The loop consists of seven steps:

1. measuring the burden of illness

2. determining the cause of the health problem(s)

3. community effectiveness

4. efficiency (economic evaluation)

5. synthesis and implementation of an intervention/program

6. monitoring the intervention/program

7. reassessing the burden of illness

The iterative loop is a framework which provides for logical and functional organization of health-related information. Once organized, this information can be examined to determine how the burden of illness (both morbidity and mortality) of a given population can be reduced. It can be used to identify

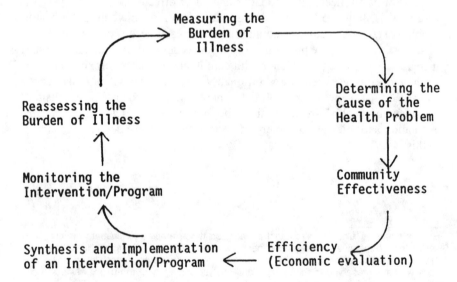

Figure 1. The measurement iterative loop. (From Tugwell et al., Copyright 1985 by Pergamon Press, Inc. Reprinted by permission.)

areas in which health care evaluation research is lacking or of poor quality. It can also be useful to the health policymaker in determining health care policy priorities.

THE ITERATIVE LOOP APPLIED TO URINARY INCONTINENCE

To illustrate the application of the loop to health problems among elderly persons, this chapter will focus on the problem of urinary incontinence, that is, involuntary loss of urine that is objectively demonstrable (Bates et al., 1979), which frequently precipitates institutionalization. The remainder of this chapter will describe the use of the loop in assessing how well we are doing (1) in meeting community health needs of elderly persons with this health problem, (2) in setting community health policy priorities for this health problem, and (3) in identifying areas in which research is lacking or of poor quality—research that will be essential in order to make informed and intelligent decisions in providing health care to persons with urinary incontinence.

Step 1—Measuring the Burden of Illness

What is the impact of the health problem on the individual, family, and the community? The consequences of a health problem can be defined in terms of the *nine D's:*

- disease activity—clinical presentation, asymptomatic process
- distress—symptoms
- death—mortality rate
- disability—impairment, handicap
- dysfunction—physical, social, and emotional function
- disadvantages—increased risk for another health problem
- disharmony—family, work, friends
- dissatisfaction—patient satisfaction
- debt—money problems

Taken together, delineation of these problems constitute Step 1—measuring the burden of illness.

Studies (Kirshen, 1983; Mohide, 1986; Milne, 1976) have indicated that between 5% and 10% of persons 65 and over living independently in the community have incontinence, as do 10–20% receiving home care and 50% of persons in long term care institutions. It appears that the prevalence of incontinence increases with age and is more common in women than men.

The available information reveals that in the 65-and-over age group, urinary incontinence exists in epidemic proportions, especially among the institutionalized seniors.

Step 2—Causation

What are the known or suspected causes of the health problem? In searching for putative causal factors, four broad categories of factors should be considered: genetic (e.g., biological marker); behavioral (e.g., sociocultural); environmental (e.g., physical and chemical environment); and other (e.g., including access to health services). A variety of epidemiological study designs and "diagnostic tests" for causation must be employed to tease out these factors (Sackett, Haynes, & Tugwell, 1985).

Bates et al. (1979) outline five types of urinary incontinence, and Williams and Pannill (1982) suggest different causes for each type. For example, detrusor instability and overflow incontinence may be due to central nervous system problems such as dementia (Yarnell & St. Leger, 1979; Campbell, Reinken, & McCosh, 1985) or stroke. Sphincter insufficiency may be due to estrogen imbalance, muscle weakness, urologic surgery, severe neuropathy, and urinary infections. Functional incontinence may be due to psychological factors, impaired mobility (Isaacs & Walkey, 1964), inconvenient facilities, and inflexible staff schedules. Finally, iatrogenic incontinence may be due to various drugs, especially diuretics, sedatives, and autonomic nervous system agents, or due to physical restraints. Little information is available on the frequency with which these different types of urinary incontinence occur in institutionalized and community populations of seniors.

Step 3—Community Effectiveness

How well are we doing in alleviating or preventing the health problem? This step considers information about whether an intervention or health program is available with the potential to reduce or prevent the health problem, and thus the burden of illness, when applied in the community. If an intervention is available, information is needed about five components of community effectiveness: diagnostic accuracy, health provider compliance, patient compliance, efficacy, and coverage. The more each component achieves a targeted level, the more an intervention or program will increase its community effectiveness. Each component is now discussed in relation to urinary incontinence.

Diagnostic Accuracy

How well can we identify the problem? Urinary complaints of all types are common in elderly persons, and symptoms are often not specific. True stress incontinence as an isolated complaint (incontinence only on physical activity) has a high positive predictive value for sphincter weakness (Drutz & Mandel, 1979; Farrar et al., 1975) (that is, the proportion reporting stress incontinence that are subsequently confirmed to have sphincter weakness—96% to 98%). Although frequently recommended (Fossberg, Sanders, & Beisland, 1981; Castleden, Duffin, & Asher, 1981), the predictive value (see Sackett et al., 1985) of urodynamic, neurologic, cognitive, and functional status assessments are not available. In fact, there is a dispute regarding whether a patient history alone is sufficient to diagnose detrusor instability or overflow incontinence (Wein, 1981; Kirshen, 1983; Williams & Pannill, 1982; Hilton, 1987) or whether urodynamic studies are also needed.

Health Provider Compliance

Will health care personnel provide the intervention or health program? Many health professionals are unaware of the most recent treatment of urinary incontinence, and therefore do not deliver the most effective care (Mohide et al., forthcoming). With urinary incontinence, there are obvious risk factors that can be eliminated, such as access to toilets, but this is often overlooked.

Greater amounts of evidence are being produced demonstrating that health professionals do not always comply with present recommendations for optimal management of a variety of health problems. Battista (1983) studied the behavior of Quebec family physicians; he found that their behavior fell far short of the recommendations of the Canadian Cancer Society in regard to preventive and early screening procedures. Evans (1984) examined financial factors that may influence practitioner behavior. He found that where preventive interventions are concerned, there is a need for the fee schedule to reward a procedure that is simple and quick and which can be repeated at regular intervals. Detection of high blood pressure by blood pressure measurement is an example of a success story (with the subsequent reduction in stroke and cardiovascular disease in North America), but no simple, quick, and repetitive procedure exists for detection of urinary incontinence.

Patient Compliance

Will a person's behavior, in terms of taking medications, following diets, or executing lifestyle changes, coincide with medical or health advice (Haynes, Taylor, & Sackett, 1979)? Drug compliance in elderly patients is notoriously poor (Haynes et al., 1979). Studies of treatments for urinary incontinence have not separately assessed level of compliance (Williams & Pannill, 1982).

Efficacy

Under ideal conditions of making an accurate diagnosis, and patient and provider compliance, will the intervention/program work? Some cases of urinary incontinence can be completely cured and other cases improved with careful investigation and treatment of their condition (Overstall, Rounce, & Palmer, 1980; Fossberg et al., 1981). A variety of bladder training techniques (a behavioral intervention in which the interval between voluntary voidings is gradually extended) have been shown to achieve cure rates of 44–97% for some types of urinary incontinence (Hadley, 1986). These studies have included only a small number of patients, either in institutions or attending university research centers, and their generalizability to patients at home has yet to be demonstrated. These efficacy studies have attempted to show that bladder training does more good than harm to patients under ideal conditions of diagnostic accuracy, patient compliance, and provider compliance. Methodological criteria for critically appraising the quality of evidence from efficacy studies have been reported by Sackett et al. (1985).

Usually clinicians have no difficulty in detecting incontinence of urine, but to diagnose its cause in the majority of patients who do not have major neurological problems is more difficult. Some claim that urodynamic studies are cheap and feasible (Fossberg et al., 1981; Castleden et al., 1981) and are a necessity before rational and effective treatment can begin. Others claim that such studies are not without risk (Sabanathan, Duffin, & Castleden, 1985), expensive, and impracticable in a frail elderly population based mostly in the community; an algorithmic approach at the patient's home or bedside is claimed to be at least as sensitive as urodynamic studies (Hilton, 1987). To date no controlled trial comparing the two approaches exists.

Coverage

Does the intervention (health program) reach those who need it? Even when treatment is relatively efficacious, as can justifiably be claimed for urinary incontinence, there is still the problem of delivering care to the population in need. With 11% of those over 65 and 21% of those over 80 years of age being incontinent (Campbell et al., 1985), it is unlikely that many of the incontinent have received professional treatment. In a survey of home care program patients with incontinence, incontinence pads and protective garments (palliative rather than remedial forms of treatment) were used in 56% of patients (Mohide et al., forthcoming). This level of community coverage may be viewed as inadequate coverage (below the targeted level), given our knowledge of the efficaciousness of such remedial actions as bladder training.

The assessment of community effectiveness may also be conducted through the execution of community trials (Cadman et al., 1984). In such trials, all five components (diagnostic accuracy, provider compliance, patient compliance, efficacy, and coverage) are examined together, but one has the problem of teasing out the relative contributions of each component. Their use in decisions about specific health problems is enhanced if they provide information on one or more of the following: (1) the selection of subjects for study (so that the reader may determine both the internal and external validity of the study); (2) the program's mix of services (so that replication may be facilitated); (3) the manner of execution of the study (so that bias, the cause of incorrect conclusions, may be minimized); and (4) the health outcomes and how they are measured (so that one may determine their relevance and validity) (Vogel & Pelman, 1982).

Step 4—Efficiency (Economic Analysis)

How can we put our limited resources where they will do the most good? Health care consumes vast amounts of societal resources (personnel and equipment) and costs are increasing, including care directed at seniors (Barer et al., 1987). If the marginal (extra) costs of enhancing a program/intervention exceed the marginal (extra) benefits of the enhanced program/intervention, then the enhancements (for example, a two-hour as opposed to a ten-minute assessment) will not be justified. The social value that seniors place on maintaining their quality of life and the cost of health programs/interventions from their point of view should be considered. Increased resources for health care of seniors must be weighed against how these same resources might be used for other age groups and/or for other services, for example, transportation for seniors.

A number of pitfalls in determining costs of care are outlined elsewhere (Drummond, 1980; Sackett et al., 1985). For example, chronically ill or elderly patients in acute care facilities have been referred to as bed-blockers—which implicitly suggests that if they could be housed elsewhere (anywhere), new acute admissions would be generated to use the freed space. A study claiming cost savings to society of a new program to provide alternative housing for bed-blockers would have to demonstrate that the freed acute care facility beds had been closed. That is, efficiency studies compare two or more programs in terms of their costs and benefits.

Economic analyses force the decisionmaker to consider all the alternatives for support of persons with urinary incontinence. For example, efficiency analyses should compare health provider interventions directed at seniors with alternative interventions such as tax breaks for home conversions for the disabled, more homemaker services, perhaps more chronic care beds, or income supports for the chronically ill or their informal caregivers (Doty, 1986).

Determination of the efficiency of a program is particularly important when making decisions about whether to support curative as opposed to preventive/rehabilitative interventions (programs) for elderly persons. Indeed, advocates of preventive interventions for seniors use the argument that such actions will prevent many seniors from ending their lives in institutionalized care. Whereas the provision of adequate housing does help to keep seniors out of institutions (Schwenger & Gross, 1980), as does the status of being married and having children (Shanas et al., 1968), keeping seniors at home with a wide range of health problems, including urinary incontinence, does not reduce the cost of care to society. For example, Weissert, Cready, and Pawelak (in press), in a review of 30 community care programs with control groups, found that costs increased in all but four programs. In addition, most of the studies found no significant differences in health status between the experimental and control groups. Increases in community care, therefore, will have to be justified on the value society places on staying at home to receive health care even though it might cost at least as much as institutional care.

Similarly, in a recent review of day hospital cost effectiveness, Eagle et al. (1987) found a large number of enthusiastic descriptive studies and four randomized control studies. One of the four studies demonstrated credible improvement in physical and emotional function in the day hospital versus a conventional care control group. The three randomized studies in which costs were examined revealed, however, substantially greater costs in the day hospital group. Cost-effectiveness analyses are thus forcing providers and policymakers to be much more explicit in defining the mix of care provided in a day hospital and the objectives of these programs.

No studies of the efficiency of programs for seniors have focused on specific interventions for patients with specific health problems such as urinary incontinence. One exception is a report by Hopper et al. (1984) in which specific interventions for patients with a specific health problem (diabetes) were compared. Such research would be useful for decisionmaking about who should be eligible for programs. That is, eligibility should be based on evidence that there is an effective and efficient intervention for patients with urinary incontinence. Present efficiency research does not exist to permit such fine-tuning of eligibility criteria or selection of the type of interventions to be included in health programs for seniors.

Step 5—Synthesis and Implementation of an Intervention/Program

Will I, as health provider or program manager be able to use the intervention (health program) with my patients and my resources? This step involves analyzing the information from all the other loop steps along with identifying constraints (social, cultural, political, and ethical). The synthesizing of findings of studies from other communities as well as from one's own community and deciding whether to implement or continue a program locally should be based on applicability, resource availability, and leverage.

Applicability

The intervention or program must (1) be within the mission of the organization; (2) conform with existing practices, regulations, and standards (for example, in Ontario, the Hospital Act or the Health Promotion and Protection Act); (3) be compatible with existing programs; and (4) be consistent with the goals and objectives of the health agency/facility) as stated in its strategic plan.

Resource Availability

Resource availability does not refer to the matching of budget dollars to program costs. Rather, it is intended to take into account the broad mandate and scope of a health agency or facility. Any single intervention or program should not dominate the activities of a health agency or facility. Programs for urinary incontinence could be built onto existing home care programs providing nursing, Meals On Wheels, and other services.

Leverage

This factor involves judging whether a intervention is (1) politically feasible and (2) beneficial to the stature of the organization. A white paper on health and social services for seniors in Ontario (Van Horne, 1986) had focused on "providing a broader and more innovative range of community support services." The board of the community home services agency would obviously benefit from supporting the new program as the agency strives to demonstrate its ability to provide a range of home services for seniors.

Step 6—Monitoring the Intervention/Program

How well is the intervention (program) doing? If we are to learn whether a health care intervention reduces the burden of illness on the individual, family, community, or society, we must have mechanisms for ongoing review of the impact of a program/intervention. Ongoing assessment of quality of the care provided is conducted by comparing what an individual health professional or group of professionals agree should be done with what is actually done. Methodological issues in quality of care assessment are outlined in Tugwell (1979) and Chambers et al. (1981). The monitoring methods usually focus on one or more of the following categories: (1) structure—for example, buildings built and equipped, and qualifications of health workers; (2) health care administrative and clinical process—the actions of the personnel; and (3) patient-resident health outcomes—changes in symptoms, disability, and mortality.

In a recently completed study in Ontario (Mohide et al., in press), 60 nursing homes were randomly allocated to receive or not to receive a quality assurance intervention that consisted of (1) use of predeveloped quality assurance packages; (2) the services of a quality assurance consultant; and (3) the process of working through the quality assurance cycle (Chambers, 1986) with criteria established for care of residents with the specific health problems of hazardous mobility and constipation. The care for 1525 residents was examined before and after the intervention using a retrospective record review initiated for the study purposes. Improvement in management of the principal conditions, hazardous mobility and constipation, was greater in the experimental group.

This trial demonstrates how behavior change of the caregivers, that is, improved provider compliance, was achieved using quality assurance within a facility. One of two hidden conditions reviewed in this trial was the management of urinary incontinence. No corresponding differences were found in this health problem and the other hidden problem (potential skin breakdown), suggesting that the observed changes resulted from the quality assurance intervention rather than from some other possible interventions. Monitoring, supplemented with the strategies used in this trial, might not only provide information but also improve care provided. When monitoring, it is important to involve the providers of care in carrying out the quality assurance cycle in order to maximize their ownership in any changes that are recommended and subsequently implemented.

These examples of monitoring programs demonstrate both what might be done and the early stage of introduction of such monitoring for all seniors with urinary incontinence.

Step 7—Reassessment of Burden of Illness

Have we changed the burden of illness? In the example of urinary incontinence, did the introduction of the bladder training program reduce the incidence of urinary incontinence in long term care facilities? This step represents the closing of the measurement loop, by returning to the burden of illness, which should continue to provide the anchor for decisions about programs targeted at seniors with urinary incontinence.

Few Canadian studies of elderly persons have been attempted to examine the burden of illness of different conditions over time. In addition, health surveys such as the Canada Health Survey (Health and Welfare Canada, 1981), the Nutrition Canada National Survey (Health and Welfare Canada, 1973), and the Canadian Health and Disability Survey (Statistics Canada, 1986) have lacked this basic descriptive information, because they considered everyone aged 65 and older to be "old," with few or no distinctions made between those aged 65 and 95. There are two exceptions: the Manitoba Longitudinal Study of Aging (Mossey et al., 1981) and the Ontario Longitudinal Study of Aging (Hirdes et al., 1986). However, these studies have produced little information that will permit evaluation of the impact of programs/interventions specifically aimed at urinary incontinence. As this is such a common affliction of seniors, attempts should be made to introduce information about these patients both in routinely collected health information (for example, hospital vital statistics) and in special studies (for example, future national health surveys of seniors by Statistics Canada).

CONCLUSION

Decisionmakers in a variety of health care settings need to improve their skills at critically digesting and evaluating health care evaluation results. Increased pressure to constrain health care expenditures for seniors has led to the need for detailed review of the quality of new and established health care programs. Devolution of responsibility for planning and priority setting to the local level in some jurisdictions has greatly increased the number of individuals who must use health care evaluation results obtained by proceeding through the seven steps of the measurement iterative loop. Health care providers and administrators require the skills necessary to use information from each step in developing health policies.

The distinction between users and doers of research is important, though often overlooked. Doers of research may conduct one or more studies focusing on one or more steps of the measurement iterative loop. Users not doing studies may not require the design and analysis skills of doers. On the other hand, they must be able to interpret and assess the usefulness of research results (health care evaluation). In particular, they must be able to determine and judge whether the evidence supports the specific policy or health care evaluation recommendations based on it. In addition, they must be able to determine what health care evaluation (research) will be useful for policy development. Therefore, physicians, government planners, local planning authority directors, hospital administrators, clinical program directors, and such others need some general guides for interpreting and setting priorities for such studies. The measurement iterative loop provides such guidelines.

Only rarely (or never) will ideal information (for example, health statistics, effectiveness research, and efficiency research) be available to address each step of the loop. However, the amount of evidence available to decisionmakers can be substantial. Because there are gaps in the evidence, it is all the more important to systematically organize available information and explicitly identify gaps so that an informed decision can be made—whether it be a recommendation for further interventions to reduce the burden of illness, policymaking, funding, or further study to fill the information gaps.

This review of our application of the seven steps of the loop to urinary incontinence has highlighted the need for information about the cause, about patient and caregiver compliance, the efficiency of programs, and the need for community surveys to reassess the burden of illness over time.

The review has also emphasized the epidemic nature of urinary incontinence. Also, although the causes, detection, and efficacy of interventions is well established for urinary incontinence, the community effectiveness of programs targeted at this health problem is unknown because of the lack of information about patient compliance with the interventions and the lack of information about the extent to which patients are actually receiving these efficacious interventions.

In summary, we cannot afford *not* to conduct health care evaluation. This is especially so as the amount of health resources devoted to care of seniors increases. With the geriatric imperative upon us, the potential for support of ineffective and inefficient programs is great. The measurement iterative loop provides a useful framework for both providers and researchers to gauge the deficits in our knowledge and to base our health program policy decisions.

REFERENCES

Barer, M. L., Evans, R. G., Hertzman, C., & Lomas, J. (1987). Aging and health care utilization: New evidence on old fallacies. *Social Science and Medicine, 24*(10), 851–862.

Bates, P., Bradley, W. E., Glen E., et al. (1979). The standardization of terminology of lower urinary tract function. *Journal of Urology, 121,* 551–554.

Battista, R. N. (1983). Adult cancer prevention in primary care: Patterns of practice in Quebec. *American Journal of Public Health, 73,* 1036–1039.

Cadman, D., Chambers, L. W., Feldman, W., & Sackett, D. L.. (1984). Assessing the effectiveness of community screening programmes. *JAMA: Journal of the American Medical Association, 251*(1), 1580–1585.

Campbell, A. J., Reinken, J., & McCosh, L. (1985). Incontinence in the elderly: Prevalence and prognosis. *Age and Ageing, 14,* 65–70.

Castleden, C. M., Duffin, H. M., & Asher, M. J. (1981). Clinical and urodynamic studies in 100 elderly incontinent patients. *British Medical Journal, 282,* 1103–1105.

Chambers, L. W. (1986). *Quality assurance in long term care: Policy, research and measurement.* Paris: World Health Organization and the International Center on Social Gerontology.

Chambers, L. W., Sibley, J. C., Spitzer, W. O., et al. (1981). Quality of care assessment: How to set up and use an indicator condition. *Clinical and investigative Medicine, 4*(1), 41–50.

Doty, P. (1986). Family care of the elderly: The role of public policy. *Milbank Quarterly, 64*(1), 34–75.

Drummond, M. F. (1980). *Principles of economic appraisal in health care.* Toronto: Oxford University Press.

Drutz, H. P., & Mandel, F. (1979). Urodynamic analysis of urinary incontinence symptoms in women. *American Journal of Obstetrics and Gynecology, 134,* 879–892.

Eagle, E. J., Guyatt, G., Patterson, C., & Turple, I. (1987). Day hospitals: Cost and effectiveness. *Gerontologist, 27*(6), 735–740.

Evans, R. G. (1984). *Strained mercy: The economics of Canadian health care.* Toronto: Butterworths.

Farrar, D. J., Whiteside, C. G., Osborne, F. L., et al. (1975). A urodynamic analysis of micturition symptoms in the female. *Surgical Gynecology and Obstetrics, 141,* 875–881.

Fossberg, E., Sanders, S., & Beisland, H. O. (1981). Urinary incontinence in the elderly (Pilot Study). *Scandinavian Journal of Urology and Nephrology* (Suppl. 60), 51–53.

Hadley, E. (1986). Bladder training and related therapies of urinary incontinence in older people. *JAMA: Journal of the American Medical Association, 256,*(3), 372–379.

Haynes, R. B., Taylor, D. W., & Sackett, D. L. (1979). *Compliance in health care.* Baltimore: The Johns Hopkins University Press.

Health and Welfare Canada. (1973). *Nutrition Canada: National Survey.* Ottawa: Bureau of Nutritional Sciences, Health Protection Branch.

Health and Welfare Canada. (1981). *Health of Canadians: Report of the Canada Health Survey.* Ottawa: Statistics Canada.

Hilton, P. (1987). Urinary incontinence in women. *British Medical Journal, 295,* 426–432.

Hirdes, J. P., Brown, K. S., Forbes, W. F., et al. (1986). The association between self-reported income and perceived health based on the Ontario longitudinal study of aging. *Canadian Journal on Aging, 5,*(3), 189–204.

Hopper, S. V., Miller, D., Birge, C., & Swift, J. (1984). A randomized study of the impact of home health aides on diabetic control and utilization patterns. *American Journal of Public Health, 74,* 600–602.

Isaacs, B., & Walkey, F. A. (1964). A survey of incontinence in elderly hospital patients. *Gerontology Clinic, 6,* 367–376.

Kirshen, A. J. (1983). Urinary incontinence in the elderly: A review. *Clinical and Investigative Medicine, 6*(4), 364–369.

Milne, J. S. (1976). Prevalence of incontinence in the elderly age groups. In F. L. Willington (Ed.), *Incontinence in elderly.* London: Academic Press.

Mohide, E. A. (1986). The prevalence and scope of urinary incontinence. *Clinics in Geriatric Medicine, 2*(4), 639–655.

Mohide, E. A., Pringle, D. M., Robertson, D., & Chambers, L. (forthcoming). Prevalence and implications of urinary incontinence in home care programs. *Canadian Medical Association Journal.*

Mohide, E. A., Tugwell, P., Caulfield, P., et al. (in press). A randomized trial of quality assurance in nursing homes. *Medical Care.*

Mossey, J. M., Havens, B., Roos, N. P., & Shapiro, E. (1981). The Manitoba longitudinal study on aging: Description and methods. *Gerontologist, 21*(5), 551–558.

Overstall, P. W., Rounce, K., & Palmer, J. H. (1980). Experience with an incontinence clinic. *Journal of American Geriatrics Society, 28,* 535–538.

Sabanathan, K., Duffin, H. M., & Castleden, C. M. (1985). Urinary tract infection after cystometry. *Age and Ageing, 14,* 291–295.

Sackett, D. L., Haynes, R. B., & Tugwell, P. (1985). *Clinical epidemiology: A basic science for clinical medicine.* Toronto: Little, Brown and Company.

Schwenger, C., & Gross, J. (1980). Institutional care and institutionalization of the elderly in Canada. In J. V. Marshall (Ed.), *Aging in Canada: Social perspectives.* Toronto: Fitzhenry and Whiteside.

Shanas, E., Townsend, P., Wedderburn, D., et al. (1968). *Old people in three industrial societies.* New York: Atherton Press.

Statistics Canada. (1986). *Report of the Canadian Health and Disability Survey 1983–1984* (Catalogue No. 82–55E). Ottawa: Ministry of Supply and Services.

Tugwell, P. (1979). A methodological perspective in process measures of the quality of medical care. *Clinical and Investigative Medicine, 2,* 113–121.

Tugwell, P., Bennett, K., Haynes, R. B., et al. (1985). The measurement iterative loop: A framework for the critical assessment of the need, benefits and costs of health interventions. *Journal of Chronic Diseases, 38*(4), 339–351.

Van Horne, R. (1986). *A new agenda: Health and social service strategies for Ontario's seniors.* Toronto: Office on Seniors' Affairs, Queen's Park.

Vogel, R. J., & Pelman, H. C. (1982). *Long term care: Perspectives from research and demonstrations.* Washington, DC: Health Case Financing Administration, U.S. Department of Health and Human Services.

Wein, A. J. (1981). Urodynamics: Promises, promises, promises (editorial). *Journal of Urology, 126,* 218.

Weissert, W. E., Cready, C. M., & Pawelak, I. E. (in press). Net costs of home and community care: Three decades of findings. *Milbank Quarterly.*

Williams M. E., & Pannill, F. C. (1982). Urinary incontinence in older persons. *Annals of Internal Medicine, 97,* 895–907.

Yarnell, J. W. G., & St. Leger, A. S. (1979). The prevalence, severity and factors associated with urinary incontinence in a random sample of elderly. *Age and Ageing, 8,* 81–85.

Commentary

CARL D'ARCY

INTRODUCTION

There is a well established and honorable debating tradition in which participants are arbitrarily assigned to defend a particular side of an argument, e.g., titling my comments "What Can We Afford to Evaluate?" or "How Much Evaluation is Really Needed and in How Much Detail?" You are then required to marshall the facts to support your side of the debate irrespective of how much or how fervently you believe in the rightness of the position you have been assigned. Although intimidating to one's belief system, such a tactic stimulates debate. It also trains one to 'think on your feet' and dispassionately and logically muster an argument. Though such a tactic also exposes one to flim-flam tools for convincing an audience, it trains one to be less caught in the rhetoric of an argument and evaluate its merits on more objective grounds.

In some respect, in being asked to comment on the chapter by Chambers and Worrall on "Research and Public Policy on Urinary Incontinence: Can We Afford Not to Evaluate?," I feel that I am being asked to argue for the sake of arguing. How can one be opposed to rationality? After all, as a researcher whose livelihood and career is intimately tied to research and evaluation, how can I be opposed to doing more research and evaluation, in having more impact on public policy, in having things done the way I think they should be done?

However, drawing upon my 15 years of experience as a contributor of information to governments, programs, and agencies as well as conducting independent grant-funded research, I wish to comment on the process of translating research into policy and program decisions. That process is at the nub of Chambers and Worall's chapter. I am not sure that the method proposed in the chapter will solve the problem(s). In essence, I wish to comment on the model of decisionmaking implied in this chapter. I leave the specifics of the argument about urinary incontinence to others.

DISCUSSION

We all get blamed for not making more and better use of research findings in developing policy and programs. In the health field, it can be legitimately argued that we accept and continue to use too many procedures on the basis of precedence without subjecting them to evaluation (MRC, 1980).

Failure to use research and evaluation findings is usually seen as a failure of:

- the politician and/or bureaucrat/manager to respond to and use data and information that are being proffered to them;
- the researchers to provide useful and timely information in a format and language understandable by decisionmakers; and
- technique—we need better methods and techniques that provide better information.

Chambers and Worrall's chapter is premised on the notion that in order to make better public policy we need to make better use of the research findings, and that the failure to make better use of existing research findings is one of technique. We need better metamethods for collating and evaluating research findings.

Chambers and Worrall note that in light of the "geriatric imperative" facing our nation we cannot afford not to conduct health care evaluation. The potential cost of supporting ineffective and inefficient programs is too great. It is "important to ensure that scarce resources are used to deliver care that is not only efficient (that is, costs are small in relation to effects) but also meets an adequate standard of effectiveness in delivery of care (that is, how well are we doing in alleviating or preventing the health problem?)." Finally, Dr. Chambers reminds us that we must have the tools to provide information about decisions that we must take regardless of our role—provider, manager, bureaucrat.

The authors promote the "measurement iterative loop" (Tugwell et al., 1985) as the tool for more effectively translating research findings into public policy. The loop is composed of seven steps: (1) measuring the burden of illness; (2) determining the cause of the health problem; (3) community effectiveness; (4) efficiency; (5) synthesis and implementation of an intervention program; (6) monitoring; and (7) reassessment. The measurement iterative loop is touted as a tool that provides both health administrators and researchers with a method for evaluation of existing programs, identifying gaps in knowledge, and a rational basis for evaluation of existing programs. The use of the method will, it is suggested, deliver us from evil (that is, the nonuse of research findings).

The cartoon that is Figure 1 typifies a common sort of organizational cynicism about research and its application. I found it circulating around the health office of a Canadian provincial health agency.

The cartoon serves to emphasize that the use(s) of research is a precarious exercise:

- what is recommended by the research study is not what gets approved by administration and/or politicians;
- what gets ordered may be a further modification;
- what gets delivered may even further deviate from the original plan;
- what gets implemented may again be more divergent; and, of course, as a final kicker,
- what was "really needed" was not even recommended by the research study in the first place.

Researchers have long felt that the application of their knowledge and research findings would improve societal, government, and bureaucratic functioning. However, despite this desire for application, they generally

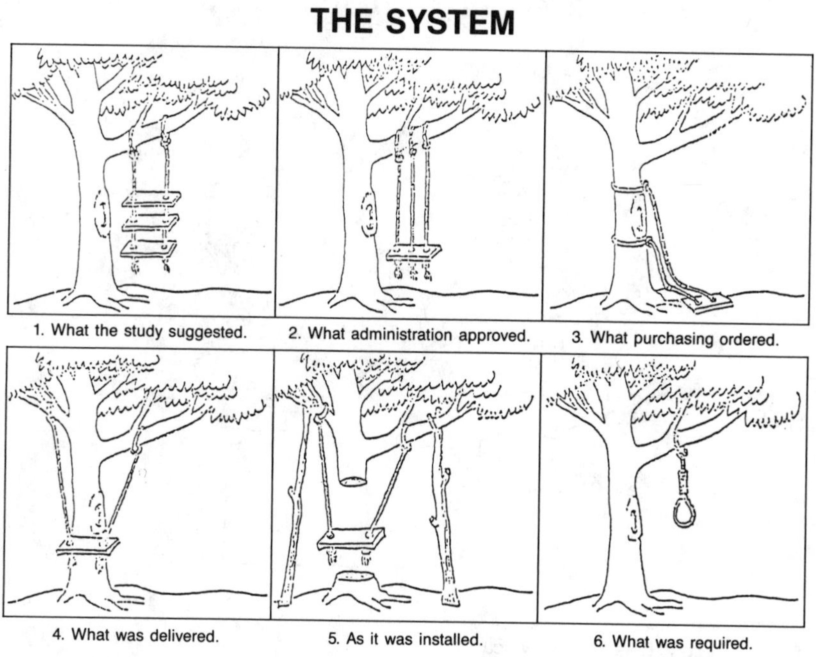

THE SYSTEM

1. What the study suggested.   2. What administration approved.   3. What purchasing ordered.

4. What was delivered.   5. As it was installed.   6. What was required.

Figure 1. It's hard not to be cynical about research and its application.

doubt that their research is used, or used where its application would be most effective. We have our own cynicism and cartoons (Figure 2).

I am reminded of an experience I had when consulting for a senior level bureaucrat about program and policy issues in the mental health field. As indicated in Figure 2, I was icily informed that he "didn't want to know about how to drain the swamp," all he really wanted to do was keep the "alligators" from chomping on his legs. I presume that the alligators were pressure groups, more senior bureaucrats, politicians, and the like. I, of course, informed him that if he didn't drain the swamp, although he might bash down one alligator, it and possibly others would be there again to chomp on him.

This experience illustrates an important issue: bureaucrats, administrators, and politicians have relatively limited time horizons. The yearly budget cycle, length of tenure, the electoral process, and the fickleness of media and interest groups necessitate a concern for immediate solutions. Implementors may not be around five years down the road; the actors and issues may also have changed. Should you as an implementor be interested in a research

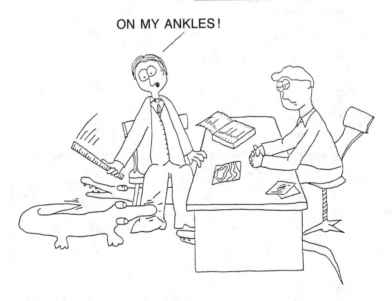

Figure 2. Researchers can be cynical, too.

solution that may be more expensive and debatable in the short term but is both therapeutic and cost-effective in the long term? It is hardly surprising that some research is criticized by potential users "for being esoteric and irrelevant; for not contributing to the public good, for providing research that is often contradictory, imprecise, late and impractical, and perhaps worst of all, for not being a source of creative ideas" (Trent, 1982). Researchers in general look for long-term solutions rather than the "quick fix."

There are other concerns about being enlisted in the cause of decisionmaking, particularly government decisionmaking. What happens then to priorities? Do we lose an essential detached focus needed for scientific inquiry? Is it worse to have your research not used or to have it used inappropriately or taken out of context?

Is the lack of use of scientific research in health care solely a failure of technique in terms of summarizing that information and communicating it? We all should know how to do good research, e.g., Campbell and Stanley (1963), Cook and Campbell (1979), and others. In addition, there is ample evaluative technique, e.g., Cronbach et al. (1981). The metaanalysis techniques of Glass, McCaw, and Smith (1981), Light and Pillemer (1984), Rosenthal (1984), and others enable us to summarize findings and estimate effects from a large number of studies. (I am puzzled by the lack of reference to this literature by Chambers and Worrall.)

I suggest that the failure to utilize research findings is not a failure of technique but rather a failure to understand the dimensions of the process of translating research into policy, a failure to understand the roles and interests of the various actors involved.

We should recognize translating research into policy as a social process. We need to understand that process so that we are not surprised by it, so that we can influence it more. And, of course, we need to recognize that we as researchers have our own self-interests.

Scientists tend to feel that information is a good thing per se, and more would be better. It is assumed that there is one clear and single truth; scientists have it by the tail; decisionmakers will heed this truth; and this truth is independent of the clash of vested interests and political stakes. It would seem, by their intrinsic nature, scientists only give "good" never "bad" advice. Experience tells otherwise.

In reality, no matter how we as scientists like it, research findings are used, but they may not be used as we would like. At the same time, although we can and do make a significant contribution to policy debate, there are areas in which we may have little to offer that is important. These are areas in which more research and more methodologically sophisticated research does not provide a firmer basis for policy choice and action. The world is revealed as having greater complexity than anticipated.

Most discussions on knowledge utilization assume that at some specific place and time policy decisions are made by "decisionmakers" who arrange to solve a "problem." In truth, it is difficult to know when "a decision" is made, how it was made, and who was responsible for making it. Not surprisingly, upon reflection one discovers that "decisionmaking" is a diffuse and complex social process.

We need to know more about the policy and decisionmaking process. How are problems defined and given priority? Who makes decisions? How concentrated or diffuse is the process? How can the process be influenced?

Research information enters this complex process in a variety of ways. According to Weiss (1977, pp. 11–16), it may enter the decisionmaking process:

1. *instrumentally*—with its direct application to solve a given policy problem;
2. *as knowledge*—in which as the fruit of basic research applications new policies emerge;
3. *interactively*—in which research information is one part of a complicated process involving experience, political insight, pressure politics, social technologies, and judgment;
4. *as political ammunition*—in which research information becomes ammunition for the side that finds its conclusions most congenial and supportive. Research is used to neutralize opponents, convince waverers, and bolster supporters;
5. *miscellaneously*—as research is used to delay action or avoid taking responsibility for a decision; and
6. *as conceptualization*—in which social research is used in recognizing the character of a problem and its attendant policy issues. Research information can sensitize decisionmakers to new issues and revise thoughts concerning "old issues."

THE MESSAGES

For Knowledge Utilizers

I am reminded of three laws of information:

1. The information you have is not that which you want.
2. The information you want is not that which you need.
3. The information you need is not that which you can obtain.

There are two corollaries that should go with these three laws.

a) You have to make the most of the information that is available.
b) You have an obligation to make decisions and take actions that are in the long-term interests of the clients or population which you serve, even if that means short-term heat and discomfort.

At some point action is required. The decision(s) cannot be put off. The information is rarely complete.

For Researchers

Data and information will be used in making, and in justifying, decisions and policy choices. It is your (our) obligation to see that it is used to its best advantage. Scientists need and have to have a greater input into the implementation, evaluation, and decisionmaking processes. Decisionmaking is a process. Input, therefore, has to be an educative process rather than a "take it or leave it," one-shot presentation of data and information.

It is legitimate to ask what can we afford to evaluate, at what cost, and in what detail? We cannot evaluate everything; everything does not need rigorous evaluation.

We, as scientists, need to rise above our own self-interest and participate as partners in the decisionmaking process.

Research and policymaking should be collaborative processes involving researchers not just as scientists but also as utilizers involved in the social and political life of the community.

REFERENCES

Campbell, D. T., & Stanley, J. C. (1963). *Experimental and quasi-experimental designs for research.* Chicago: Rand McNally.

Cook, T. D., & Campbell, D. T. (1979). *Quasi-experimentation: Design and analysis issues for field settings.* Chicago: Rand McNally.

Cronbach, L. J., Ambion, S. R., Dornbusch, S. M., et al. (1981). *Toward reform of program evaluation.* San Francisco: Jossey-Bass.

Glass, C. V., McCaw, B., & Smith, M. L. (1981). *Meta-analysis in social research.* Beverly Hills: Sage Publications.

Light, R. J., & Pillemer, D. B. (1984). *Summing up: The science of reviewing research.* Cambridge, MA: Harvard University Press.

Medical Research Council of Canada (MRC). (1980). *The application of biomedical research to health care* (Report of the MRC Sub-Committee on the Improved Clinical Application of Existing Knowledge). Ottawa: Ministry of Supply and Services, Canada.

Rosenthal, R. (1984). *Meta-analytic procedures for social research.* Beverly Hills: Sage Publications.

Trent, J. E. (1982, December). Promoting the social sciences: Lessons for four years. *Social Sciences in Canada, 10*(3), 2–4.

Tugwell, P., Bennett, K., Haynes, R. B., & Sackett, D. L. (1985). The measurement iterative loop. A framework for the critical assessment of the need, benefits and costs of health interventions. *Journal of Chronic Diseases, 38*(4), 339–351.

Weiss, C. H. (Ed.). (1977). *Using social research in public policy making*. Lexington, MA: D. C. Heath & Company.

36. Integrating Research into the Delivery Environment: One Community-Based Agency's Struggle

PHIL GAUDET

INTRODUCTION

There exists a "pecking order" in the health care system, and community-based health delivery programs tend to glean resources left after the more powerful institutions have had their fill. The problems outlined by my colleagues—insufficient resources, lack of trained staff, lack of time—all contribute to great difficulties in integrating research into the delivery environment. We in the community have them all—in spades! The only perceived advantage we have is that the pain and suffering of those we minister to is generally thought not as acute and, consequently, we might ignore them with relative impunity in order to find time for research.

Let there be no doubt—the time and resources required for research could always be used in the delivery of care. Whether it is in a teaching hospital, a long term care facility, or home care, someone will argue that is where all scarce time and resources should go. In my view, the commitment to research must be solid and recognized first at the highest level, with a full understanding that those nearest the suffering patient will rightly hesitate to make time for it. It is consequently with new and additional resources that research is most palatably introduced into a tight delivery environment. Government has a role to play in such resource allocation.

This chapter will describe some of our agency's methods of integrating research into our operations. These methods are not presented as an ideal model but rather a description of our own travails.

Aging and Health: Linking Research and Public Policy, © 1989 Lewis Publishers, Inc., Chelsea, Michigan 48118. Printed in U.S.A.

OUR AGENCY—SASKATOON HOME CARE

Ours may be the largest home care program in Saskatchewan, but it is still a relatively small program in the system. We have a budget of $4.3 million (1988) and responsibility to provide and coordinate home nursing; personal care; homemaking; Meals On Wheels; home maintenance; security calls; friendly visitors; and transportation to the elderly, disabled, or those convalescing in Saskatoon and district (population 200,000). We employ approximately 130 professional staff and 200 paraprofessionals. We operate as a nonprofit society with a locally elected Board, and most of our revenue is from the provincial Department of Health in the form of per capita and other grants.

INTEGRATING RESEARCH—TWO BROAD AVENUES

From its inception in 1981, the Board has had membership from the University of Saskatchewan who insisted on research in the organization. Consequently, they incorporated the goal "to initiate and support research" in their original mission statements. Subsequent Board members from the University, though few in number, have continued to be strong advocates for research. Although we may seem not to be doing very much, without a strong commitment at this level, I wonder if we would be doing anything at all.

We pursue this part of our mission partially as a component of quality assurance. Quality assurance programs in the delivery environment must be fundamentally concerned with integrating research. The very idea of establishing standards (whether process, structure, or outcome) and evaluation measures, forces an organization to consider whether accepted professional judgments about what is good and desirable ought not be tested for demonstrated efficacy.

Formal Link to the University

A small agency in the community cannot hope to have the time, knowledge, and skill in-house to respond to research inquiries, let alone initiate them. Recognizing this, we developed a joint Research and Development Committee with the University of Saskatchewan College of Medicine, administered through the Department of Community Health and Epidemiology. This structure, though not unique, requires a small amount of funding to ensure its stability; our Board committed the interest earned on operating funds. On this committee sit representatives of several colleges, and it is the University's responsibility to provide them. Senior staff and a Board member round out the committee, whose primary functions are:

1. to review and advise the Board on all research inquiries to the agency;
2. to encourage students in various colleges to investigate particular problems in our agency and to provide them access to field data or research ideas;
3. to initiate research, including obtaining external funding where possible;
4. to provide access to library and expert resources of the University where required.

From 1985 to 1988, five projects (three MA theses, two special reports) were completed, on subjects ranging from palliative care and self-help groups to resource allocation and management information systems.

The committee turned down a few student requests for a variety of reasons, thereby making the agency's response to inquiries more thoughtful and easier than it would otherwise have been. We have found that this form of commitment and structure has provided us with a strong and economical link to a research community. In the future, we will seek membership on the committee from Engineering and Physical Therapy.

Students will always be a major contributor to formal research in all fields, and it is important to facilitate their choosing our field for investigation. We also hope that the areas they will choose to investigate are realistic and have practical relevance to our operations. Too often, their proposals are of marginal relevance or so overambitious that the probability of providing any useful answers is slim. Through our Research and Development Committee, we encourage staff in all departments to contribute lists of projects and research questions developed in the course of their work. If adopted as a research project, some of these staff-generated ideas will receive additional resources from the Board.

The results of these investigations find their way into the field very quickly. Sometimes research findings alter staff behavior before publication. For example, Remus (1987) found that staff assigned to relieve a dying client's family were insufficiently experienced; staff took remedial steps immediately.

Staff Development

The other avenue for integrating research into the delivery environment is a commitment to staff training and development. The three traditional cornerstones of staff development continue to be (1) enrollment in further education that has a research component; (2) access to information in journals, books, and other publications; and (3) travel to centers of excellence.

Although there are remarkable exceptions to the rule, typically research and internal evaluation do not become part of the professional's daily bread without exposure to university education. There are many innovative ways in which agencies can promote and support the desire of staff for further education: fully or partially paid leaves, tuition reimbursement, and so forth. In our opinion these are sound investments.

We challenge staff to learn what others have done in a certain area through literature reviews and visits to other programs. These have proved important in introducing and developing protocols for such new home treatment modalities as hypodermoclysis drips and the computerized ambulatory drug delivery system, or in firming up guidelines for staff in treatment of AIDS victims. There is always more to read and an exciting place to visit; time and resources limit what is possible.

Taking what you read and knowing whether to try it is also not always straightforward. Roberts and Burke (1986) suggest a three-step approach: (1) validation—subjecting the article to a vigorous critique of its scientific merit; (2) comparative evaluation of the article with any other published studies; and (3) decisionmaking and continued evaluation—pilot-project the implementation and evaluate its outcome.

Reading circles, where individuals take responsibility for reading certain journals and distributing relevant articles to the group, are a useful and practical way to get material read in the first place.

CONCLUSION

There is no magic to integrating research in the delivery environment— only thoughtful hard work, many problems, and insufficient resources. But for us, there is no question that the process is essential to quality assurance, and we will continue to protect some research capacity. I hope government departments that fund operations like ours will not only permit a small portion of funds to be dedicated to research and development, but in the future will actually encourage it. Also, a government that funds entire systems of care should facilitate research that requires either (1) samples larger than a small agency like ours can generate or (2) the tracking of a population across different sectors of care from one agency to another. Such research is not within our scope but is necessary to the sound evolution of health care. Otherwise, research will continue to meet the needs of "professionals," "sectors," or other "partisans" and not necessarily the people they intend to serve.

REFERENCES

Remus, G. (1987). *Dying at home: The experience of family care givers.* Unpublished master's thesis, University of Manitoba.

Roberts, C. A., & Burke, S. O. (1986, May). Applying nursing research: Getting started. *Canadian Nurse, 82*(5), 20–22.

37. Integrating Research into the Long Term Care Setting

SUELLEN ARCHIBALD

INTRODUCTION

In this chapter I will (1) discuss the difficulties one encounters in conducting research while employed in the service area; (2) examine some of the barriers to integrating research findings into the long term care setting; and (3) provide a specific example of applying some of the principles of environmental design for the elderly to the long term care setting.

OUR FACILITY

I am fortunate to be employed at a large long term care facility that has many resources not enjoyed by some of the smaller and rural homes. As Director of Resident Care Services, I oversee the operations of the departments of Nursing, Occupational Therapy, Physical Therapy, Social Work, Recreation, Adult Day Care, and Volunteers. We believe that education and research are important priorities in our facility. This focus was one of the features that attracted me to this facility and in turn, my research background was important to the facility.

OBSTACLES TO CONDUCTING RESEARCH

In my naïveté, I believed that research would receive high priority in my work, but I encountered several obstacles to carrying out active research projects. One of the first difficulties was finding the time to plan, organize,

Aging and Health: Linking Research and Public Policy, © 1989 Lewis Publishers, Inc., Chelsea, Michigan 48118. Printed in U.S.A.

and implement a project. As an administrator, I spend a great deal of time overseeing the general operations of the departments I supervise. It is easy to identify research questions but difficult to set aside time for investigation.

It is alarming how quickly the time passes from the point at which one identifies a problem to the time at which the opportunity for studying it has passed. Several opportunities have come and gone in the past year. An example is a relocation project undertaken to create a ward for the cognitively impaired. A perfect opportunity to perform before and after measures with a comparison group passed before we could formulate a well thought out plan to evaluate the effects of the moves on our residents. The administrator-researcher faces the dilemma of wanting to complete a project quickly and also wanting to measure the impact of an intervention which is so time consuming.

Another difficulty, experienced perhaps more so in the institutional long term care environment, is the lack of coworkers who possess research backgrounds. The odds are that employees with research training (typically master's degree or beyond) are in administrative positions where access to researchable clinical areas is limited.

Another barrier to conducting research is the underutilization of the nursing home sector by graduate and baccalaureate students. Traditionally, care of the elderly has not attracted students, because they often prefer the more fast-paced and high technology environments. Community health and home care also appear to have more appeal to the students and universities. Fortunately, this is slowly changing as gerontology gains strength and popularity as a specialty in its own right. With this comes the emergence of master's-prepared practitioners who are beginning to take service positions in long term care. These practitioners can then act as preceptors to postgraduate students, which makes the long term care setting a more desirable place for students in the eyes of universities.

The slowly increasing number of students in long term care institutions brings with it two obvious benefits. The first is that researchers/professors have access to clinical areas in which to generate research findings that have more relevance to long term care. In addition, the opportunities to collaborate with faculty on research projects expand. The importance of research carried out by graduate students also merits recognition as a valuable contribution.

The second benefit is that students placed in clinical settings introduce new concepts, techniques, and research findings to the front line staff. I am making the assumption that new findings and techniques are introduced into university curricula faster than into the service areas. Joint appointments between universities and service agencies would further increase research in the service environment.

The lack of in-house resources earmarked to support research in service settings is a real problem. In times of fiscal restraint, we have difficulty acquiring sufficient resources to maintain a reasonable quality of care for residents. It is difficult, if not impossible, for an administrator to justify expenditures on research when direct line staff are overworked. This financial problem certainly underlies the other problems I identified. The obvious recourse is to apply for external research funding, for which competition is fierce. Social science research often loses out to the more exciting and rigorous biomedical projects when resources are scarce.

Compounding these barriers is the difficulty of carrying out rigorous research in the clinical setting. I believe this is one of the reasons that a lot of qualitative and nonexperimental research takes place in nursing. Researchers must compromise their desires for tight and clean methodologies due to the realities of the clinical world, which is not easily molded into experimental designs. Administrators, on the other hand, must often change the normal care routines in order to facilitate research design without compromising the quality of care, the rights of residents, and the efficiency of staff.

Given the barriers to carrying out research in the nursing home setting, the integration of available research findings is a logical compromise. Since the barriers characterize the whole field, however, it is hardly surprising that the research literature is scarce.

OBSTACLES TO INTEGRATION OF RESEARCH FINDINGS

Several problems confront the integration of research findings from the literature into the clinical setting. First, 90% of our staff have no health-related or postsecondary education, which means they are unlikely consumers of health care journals and, particularly, research journals. A further complication is that when resources are tight, the workloads of staff tend to increase; time for reading is not a priority or even possible for most direct line staff. Here again, the importance of students practicing in the care setting becomes apparent, because they can share their knowledge with front line staff.

Generally it is those who are not at the bedside who are reading the clinical journals and translating the literature into policy and procedure. Evaluating the integration and success of new policies and procedures can also be difficult, because access to the bedside is limited for those in administrative positions.

The next major difficulty is that the bulk of long term care literature is not research based. Most of the articles in long term care journals are based on the experience of service providers. For this reason, it is difficult to evaluate the reliability and validity of the content. Research articles that might be appropriate often appear in research journals, which are not the daily fare of practitioners or are full of disciplinary jargon far beyond the comprehension of the reader. To make this point clear, I will outline some of the difficulties I encountered while doing research on color vision in the elderly.

I first became interested in the use of color in environments for the elderly while taking a course in gerontological nursing. I learned about the sensory changes that occur as a result of normal aging and how these impair the elders' ability to perceive the environment accurately. One of the most interesting changes is the change in color vision. The literature is replete with articles describing the changes in vision and color vision that occur in the elderly. Very few articles are research based. Assuming that this information had not merely been contrived to capture the interest of practitioners, I set about to find its source. After frustrating hours spent trying to locate these data, I found myself in the ophthalmology literature, where I had to learn a whole new language in order to capture the essence of the information. I was appalled to realize how inaccessible this information was to me, considering how valuable I thought it was to the long term care community.

The second difficulty I experienced was that most of the research that had produced this knowledge was carried out under tightly controlled, artificial conditions. I was not convinced that the information could be generalized to the real world setting nor was I convinced that the information I had read in the non-research based gerontology articles had been interpreted correctly. These concerns led to the development of my research questions.

I designed a study that would examine the color vision abilities of the elderly under controlled laboratory conditions comparable to the everyday environments in which people function. Although my findings were not supported in the gerontological literature, they were reasonably consistent with the ophthalmological literature. My major finding was that illumination is the crucial variable in determining color perception abilities in the elderly.

The need for increased lighting by the elderly is well documented in the gerontological literature, but not in terms of its impact on color vision. As a result, the information on color vision has been presented and used in isolation from the information on illumination. Using the gerontological literature, practitioners concerned about altering the environments of the elderly to make them more functional created environments with meaningless stimuli that could be at times aesthetically offensive. The practitioners decorated the environments using bold yellow, oranges, and reds so that the elderly person could "experience" color, when all that was really necessary was to provide increased lighting and appropriate contrast to important landmarks.

Most elderly people in my study could distinguish the desaturated (pale) colors as easily as the highly saturated (bold) colors. There were two combinations of colors that posed problems for them whether they were pale or bold: oranges and reds, and blues and greens. Those who could be diagnosed as being color-vision anomalous, as opposed to those who simply had normal but aged eyes, had more difficulty with the desaturated colors when lighting was poor. Interpretation led to the principle that one can use most colors, whether pale or bold, in the environments for the elderly, when lighting levels are sufficient. Neither blue and green, nor orange and red should be used together if important landmarks are to be distinguished. An additional finding was that most persons in the sample preferred to have the walls in their rooms painted off-white so that their personal belongings would not clash with the room.

HOW OUR FACILITY APPLIED PRINCIPLES OF ENVIRONMENTAL DESIGN

One of the characteristics of my facility was that most of it needed refurbishing and renovation. Many of the original wallcoverings, floorcoverings, and window dressings were still in use, dating back to the '60s and '70s. The facility told the history of design in long term care—new ideas were tried as they appeared in the literature.

Our unit for the cognitively impaired has 85 beds that were divided into three subunits by three wings. The formation of the three wings is very much like a stubby T, the base of the T being shorter than the top. Each of the three wings has a lounge for the residents. The nursing desk is located where the wings meet in the center of the unit. This core area also includes the medication and service rooms. The hallways on the unit are long and poorly lit. Before renovation, the walls were papered in a variety of different patterns. The wallpaper formed archways on the walls, with pictures hung in the centers. The flooring was highly waxed. At the end of each of the three wings was a fire exit with an alarm system. Two additional exits into the core area of the facility were located on either side of the nursing station.

We had a limited budget for renovation and so options for major changes were limited. Our goal in renovating was to create a secure and safe environment that would allow freedom for the residents while on the unit, and to make the environment both as functional as possible and aesthetically pleasing.

The core area of the unit underwent the most major renovation. One of the exit doors into the core area was closed off, and the alcove in front of the door was modified to provide an office for the nursing manager. The high writing surface of the nursing desk was lowered to wheelchair height with a foot of Plexiglas mounted on the top to prevent the residents from removing charts and so forth while still allowing them clear visibility. The nursing desk was also covered in a seafoam-green arborite, which was quite a change from the previous dark wood. The medication room was expanded, and more functional writing and storage areas were created.

Floor space from the central core area of the building was converted to a dining room for 20 of the residents. A light, dull-finish floor was installed, and the lighting was upgraded to approximately 75 footcandles. Cork ceiling tiles were installed to absorb sound and reduce echo. A plain, small-patterned wallpaper was applied to the lower 80 centimeters of the wall. An oak chair rail, or wainscotting board, was installed above the wallpaper to prevent the chairs from damaging the walls. A variety of floral prints were hung above the chair rail at a height low enough to be enjoyed from a sitting position. The room has a very peaceful dining room atmosphere.

Another smaller dining room for eight people was created near the core area. The occupational therapist holds a self-care dining group with selected residents. A large picture window was installed which overlooks a small garden. The walls were painted a pale peach color, and the woodwork that marks the important landmarks of the door and window were painted a dark rust. Appropriate dining pictures were hung on the walls.

A third dining area, which included a wheelchair-accessible kitchen, was created in the core area. This room accommodates approximately 16 residents for meals at one sitting. The kitchen is well used by the residents in supervised cooking groups. All important landmarks are well contrasted with color distinguishable by the aged eye. Large posters of food reinforce the purpose of the room. The room also boasts an outside exit into a protected green space with a circular walking path and a patio where meals or coffee can be enjoyed in summer.

The concept behind the creation of the smaller dining room is that the cognitively impaired generally function better when confusing stimuli are reduced and many cues signal the same event. Ideally, the dining rooms should accommodate six to eight residents, which was the norm for many of these people in years past. Such an arrangement would have been very labor intensive.

The hallways were painted off-white to increase available light. Dark surfaces absorb light, whereas light surfaces reflect light. All paints were an eggshell finish to reduce glare. The hallways were adorned with pictures that differed in theme on each of the wings. This type of cueing is helpful only if the staff use the cues in giving directions: "Your room is the one next to the picture of the barn." The important landmarks for residents to observe in the hallway were contrasted with a dark seafoam-green paint. All other doorframes and doors where resident access was not desired (e.g., linen closet) were painted in the off-white so they were not easily distinguished from the walls. We installed a light-colored, nonglare sheet floor.

The three lounges in the wings were all decorated slightly differently with different-colored blinds and different pictures. We designed both a lounge and dining chair using the appropriate anthropometrics and ensured that there was ample lumbar support. The covers of the chairs, removable for laundering, were upholstered in a variety of fabrics to provide contrast and color.

All windows, including those in the resident rooms, were covered with vertical fabric blinds. This allowed us to provide variable lighting and avoid glare from the sun.

The fire exit doors on the unit posed our most challenging problem. For fire safety, the doors had to be barrier free to allow easy escape, but residents continually opened the doors to wander off the unit. The doors were alarmed, which led to constant buzzing noise. Our solution to this problem was very simple and very effective. We taped a 1-meter-by-3-meter strip of black crepe paper horizontally over the push handles of the door. It is now very rare for a resident to exit through the doors, because it no longer looks like a traditional exit. Many residents examine it, then turn around and walk away. Our plan is to make a more permanent arrangement using black cloth applied to the doorway with Velcro, which will easily strip away in the event of a fire.

The exit/entrance into the core area of the building also posed a problem. This door was not alarmed because it was in frequent use by families and staff. On evenings and nights, when staff numbers were fewer, a resident could leave the unit without staff being aware. This problem was solved by mounting on the door two knobs that had to be turned at the same time to open the door. Most cognitively impaired residents have difficulty figuring this out. Initially, some of the staff had a problem with it as well.

The renovations created an environment that was more functional, secure, and aesthetically pleasing than the original. Our modifications were relatively simple and inexpensive. To substitute for upgraded illumination that we were unable to afford, we used light-colored paint with an eggshell finish to reduce the severity of the problem.

The renovation of our ward for the cognitively impaired should have been carried out as a research project. Fortunately, I am able to make some measurements using archival data. In retrospect, it is apparent that much of what we did was through trial and error and common sense. There was little research-based information available upon which to rely. The long term care community needs to test the knowledge we glean through trial and error through rigorous research designs. Finally, some of the principles of environmental design used in this example were research based and successfully implemented. It is important that experiences like this are documented for other health practitioners to evaluate and test.

38. Integration of Research in Clinical Practice

LINDA KESSLER

INTRODUCTION

Few would question the need to utilize, integrate, and generate research at the practice level; the realities of converting need into operation, however, are far more complex. This chapter will address the issues of utilization, integration, and generation of research from a nursing perspective in a Geriatric Assessment Unit in University Hospital, Saskatoon, Saskatchewan, Canada.

On our 18-bed Geriatric Assessment Unit, there has not been, to date, any clinical nursing research. As in many hospital units, however, there has been "coincidental" research, in which nurses note that something has happened a certain way in certain circumstances and then draw a conclusion. It could be compared to an episode of the television show "Three's Company" in which Chrissie, "the dumb blond," was reading the obituary column in the local newspaper. She exclaims, "Oh my God, it's happening again! People are dying in alphabetical order." Chrissie and her roommates thought of appropriate interventions such as changing their names to something that starts with Z (Norbeck, 1987). Although this example exaggerates, it does illustrate what can happen and the pitfalls of procedures established from observations and assumptions without adequate examination.

UTILIZATION OF RESEARCH

How existing research is used in the practice setting is best illustrated by reviewing the most basic nursing care procedures and noting the changes that have evolved based on rigorous investigation.

Aging and Health: Linking Research and Public Policy, © 1989 Lewis Publishers, Inc., Chelsea, Michigan 48118. Printed in U.S.A.

Examples

Good skin care, for many years was taught as having three basic components: reposition the person every two hours, vigorously rub bony prominences, and apply liberal amounts of moisturizing lotion at each turn. Looking back to my early years as a medical staff nurse, I do not know what prevented patients from slipping right out of bed—they were so well lubricated by 6 A.M.! Now we know that rigorous rubbing was actually increasing the skin breakdown by grinding already fragile skin directly over a hard object, and that the temporary increase in circulation—the rationale for the procedure—was of little consequence. The ritualistic lathering of skin with lotion created excessive moisturizing, again leading to the possibility of increased skin damage. Even the perfect schedule of every two hours has had to be reevaluated, and the time frame adjusted downward in accordance to the length of time the skin remains reddened after each turn. These changes in clinical management would not be considered "high tech," yet can do much to increase patient comfort and decrease hospitalization time by preventing decubitus ulcers.

A second component of nursing care, which has been changing, but perhaps more slowly, is that of bowel management and treatment of constipation, particularly among the elderly. Brocklehurst (1985, p. 539) states: "The use of laxatives, suppositories, and enemas among elderly people, particularly those in hospital, often has no more rational basis than the experience and prejudices of the nurse or relatives in charge." One should be less than eager to focus the cause of irrational decisions solely on nurses and relatives, considering the physician frequently decides on the order for a patient's bowel management by saying, "So, what do you want?" suggesting a no more rational basis for the treatment plan. Although this has been a well-researched component of patient care, translation into practice has been less than encouraging. As in skin care, not enough consideration is given to the consequences of inadequate management.

Barriers

The examples cited raise the important question of how do research findings become part of patient care and what are the barriers that might prevent this from happening? The first that comes to mind is the power of tradition. How does one rid oneself of a practice that was part of both the educational process and practical application for so many years? What will be the institution's reception of the individual who questions a particular clinical practice? There are practices so entrenched in the system they are like breathing. How many of us must, even now, hold back our hand to prevent our rubbing of a patient's red, bony hip!

The second hurdle to utilizing research findings in practice is the whole process of finding the appropriate literature and then evaluating those research findings for application to practice based on their scientific merit and their significance and usefulness to the practice setting (Luckenhill, 1987). This assumes access to an individual who has both skills in critical appraisal and the time designated for the task. When it is available, does dissemination of the appropriate research information translate into changes in practice? Again, this is dependent on the power of tradition, the climate of the care setting to new ideas, and the receptiveness of the institution itself to new innovations.

INTEGRATION OF RESEARCH

In spite of the various barriers, utilization of research in the clinical setting occurs more readily than integration and generation of research. Both imply that research and evaluation are integral parts of the unit's function. On the Geriatric Assessment Unit, although integration of research and evaluation is a goal, it is a goal for the future. Hospitals are task-oriented institutions. To change this orientation means an alteration of an entire thought process, which takes time. This change can happen only if all levels of nursing management acknowledge its value and the institution supports it as a priority. Though it sounds easy, the reality is, particularly in times of economic restraint, that administrative support must be contingent upon not increasing costs and ensuring direct patient care is not compromised.

Equally important as the administrative support for the research process is the support of the staff nurse. This support does not just happen because we want it to, and without it integration and generation will never be a reality. In the times of staff cutbacks, the staff nurse is not likely to consider research a priority. It is only through direct support, encouragement, and education that the staff nurse will know that her contribution is not only valued, but essential.

GENERATION OF RESEARCH

There are even more practical barriers to the generation of research at a unit level. One of the most obvious is that of obtaining an adequate sample size from one small study site. On a geriatric assessment unit, only a more general clinical problem would be seen frequently enough to generate adequate numbers. A second issue is the need for at least master's-prepared nurses working directly in or in conjunction with the clinical setting. As more nurses are obtaining graduate degrees, will the priority be their placement at a clinical level, and will research and evaluation be recognized as part of their work?

The next step is to see if any existing mechanism in hospitals could be used to "hurry along" the research process. The introduction of quality assurance programs has had a positive impact within hospitals, particularly on documentation. Because these programs are mandatory to meet accreditation standards, hospitals have had to spend the monies required to institute and maintain them. Because the quality assurance program is mandatory and evidence of research is not, can the first be used to enhance the second? At present, there is a lack of established validity of quality assurance measures. It is suggested that quality assurance studies are similar to exploratory research studies in nonexperimental field settings, in which most variables are outside the investigator's control and the investigator is left observing what is happening (Brink, 1984). Quality assurance studies are needed in nursing. Assuring that the measurement criteria are both reliable and valid would allow the data to also be used for scientific evaluation.

Even university hospitals, which tend to be viewed as "having it all," face restraints and realities encountered elsewhere in the health care delivery system. In times of economic restraint, the first priority must always be delivery of patient care services. The review of appropriate literature, its critical appraisal, and its dissemination assumes the availability of individuals trained for the task and a receptive audience for the information. All of these factors suggest well-developed research programs; reality dictates that they do not exist.

How can the gap between reality and the ideal be decreased? One approach is the further integration of the clinical practitioner and the academic. Each has a specialized talent and should complement the other in the research process. Essential to these changes is the need to change the thought process in the clinical setting to look beyond the task and to begin questioning what we are doing and why. This change does not happen quickly, but is a realistic goal. A questioning attitude produces fertile ground for implementation and evaluation of new ideas.

What does the future hold? Nurses will become an integral part of the process of developing data bases on the clientele we serve, and rational interventions will be formulated based on that information. The staff nurse will be encouraged to continue looking for patterns emerging from practice and circumstance—the coincidental research—then this information needs to be taken one step further to a quantitative level from which predictive models may be developed. Research would then be an integral part of the clinical practice. The goal is not unrealistic, but is a future outcome of the process of change.

REFERENCES

Brink, P. J. (1984). Are quality assurance studies really research? *Western Journal of Nursing Research, 6,* 365–366.

Brocklehurst, J. C. (1985). The gastrointestinal system—the large bowel. In J. C. Brocklehurst (Ed.), *Textbook of geriatric medicine and gerontology* (pp. 534–556). Edinburgh: Churchill Livingstone.

Luckenhill, J. L. (1987). Use of nursing practice research findings. *Nursing Research, 36,* 344–349.

Norbeck, J. S. (1987). In defense of empiricism. *Image, 19,* 28-30.

PART V

Cementing Research and Policy Connections

39. Research and Policy: Cementing the Connections

A. ROD DOBELL

INTRODUCTION

In this chapter I will address (1) fundamental as well as practical questions of research-policy interactions, (2) the importance of using good research in policy development, and (3) some practical problems of building links from research to policy, and in the words of Steven Lewis, finish with a "cerebral call to arms to bridge the vast research-policy gulf."

There is a vast literature dealing with this "vast research-policy gulf." In many ways, however, it all boils down to the recognition that we try to *think* (undertake research) within a finely-tuned framework of rigorous analysis and precise calculation, whereas we *act* (form policy) within a framework of very rough indicators and very broad values, attitudes, and beliefs. A now-classic statement of the dilemma is set out by David Cohen and Charles Lindblom in their discouraging but persuasive little book called *Usable Knowledge* (1979). They make the case that professional social inquiry (research) is usually far from conclusive, far from authoritative, and far from the action. Decisions are driven, they suggest, by ordinary knowledge, in a process of interaction and adjustment, not by a program of analysis and deduction designed to find the optimal solution to a well-posed policy problem. In the words of former Canadian Cabinet Minister Bud Drury (1979), "Some policy choices are not so much decisions that are taken as they are accidents that happen." A more basic concern about what we can know in fields like this was expressed in Oskar Morgenstern's monograph *On the Accuracy of Economic Observations* (1963), which reviewed some of the limitations of statistics and data gathering as means to understanding the economic or social world around us.

Aging and Health: Linking Research and Public Policy, © 1989 Lewis Publishers, Inc., Chelsea, Michigan 48118. Printed in U.S.A.

I plan to examine briefly a few illustrative policy issues in which my own Institute for Research on Public Policy has been involved and then examine why a large body of relevant research is so little used in their successful resolution. I will suggest possible directions for further work and orientations for policy, and briefly digress on the roles of think tanks.

In some ways, my conclusions amount to working out the consequences of a diagnosis that says: in research, the supply has been too much dictated and shaped by the supplier, and in health care, the provision is too much dictated and controlled by the provider. On various occasions I have been impressed by the arguments of Japanese executives that the source of their postwar success in sophisticated manufacturing and technologies is the obsessive concern of their industrialists with consumers' reactions. They design, we are told, for the consumer; the preferences of suppliers carry no great weight. We in the research industry might ponder that lesson. I will argue that you in the health industry should, too.

SOME ILLUSTRATIVE POLICY ISSUES IN SEARCH OF RESEARCH

Two definitions to begin: (1) a *patient* is a moving bundle of medical intervention opportunities; (2) *health* is a transitory state of inadequate or insufficiently detailed diagnosis. The following themes are drawn from this meeting:

The Survival Curve and Morbidity

The *rectangularization of the survival curve* (which *is* happening) does not necessarily mean the *compression of morbidity* (which may *not* be occurring). (I will come back to this point later.)

Fiscal Planning and the Age-Use Curve

The aging of the Canadian population does not, in itself, mean any inevitable fiscal crisis. Many studies exist to demonstrate that the growth of the proportion of old and very old people in the population entails, at current utilization rates, a gradual but continuing increase in the share of resources devoted to this age group—a reallocation eminently manageable.

Our history is one of increasing rates of utilization of medical and hospital services, and the results cited by Bob Evans (Chapter 14) suggest dramatic further twisting of the age-use curve. If that continues, with increasing numbers, something very like a pending fiscal crisis would seem to be very hard to rule out.

Barriers to Effective Allocation

The biggest single barrier to more effective allocation of health care resources is that we do not know until afterward which interventions will prove to be terminal. (It is not age that creates the spike in utilization, but treatment in the period immediately prior to death.) Obviously there is nothing we can do about that gap in our knowledge.

The next biggest barrier is dealing effectively with two powerful interest groups: the elderly themselves and the physicians for whom those elderly are (in Evans's words, Chapter 14) the solution to a grave economic problem.

Birth, Death, and Postponement of Disability

The key dilemmas we face in research relating to health policy are increasingly focused on the fuzzy boundaries at the two ends of the life cycle:

- when life *begins,* and how to apply our new-found technological powers and discretion in marginal cases of viability
- when life *ends,* and how to exercise our growing technological capacities and discretion to alter the point of "natural" death—whether to do, in Andrew Malcolm's phrase (Chapter 15), all that we obviously can do to prolong life

In both cases our problem is, in part, one of substitute judgment—taking action on behalf of an individual who is not or might not be competent to defend his or her own rights in the matter. In the case of the elderly, the consequence (again in Andrew Malcolm's words, Chapter 15) is that death often comes where the machinery is gathered, not where the family can gather.

For me, this is perhaps the most vivid impression I carry away from this meeting:

- the focus on a right to die at home with dignity, without being subject (quoting Evans) to the precept that no one can be allowed to leave this Earth with unbroken ribs;
- the concomitant focus on acceptance of natural death as natural; or, more generally,
- the need to ensure that decisions about treatment are based on an individual responsibility exercised through personal choice and a social responsibility exercised through a political process—not only through a patient, passive acceptance of professional judgment.

This emphasis on birth, death, and the postponement of the onset of disability or activity limitation suggests, from a research perspective, an emphasis on life cycle structures and a longitudinal microsimulation approach to health statistics. (I will return to this point later.)

Health Status as the Goal of Health Policy

At the level of the overall system as well as for the individual, the final theme I will discuss is the focus on *health status,* not treatment technologies, as the goal of health policy. For illustration, I will sketch a few examples of research that could be linked to policy processes, concentrating on work in which the Institute for Research on Public Policy or its associates have been involved.

1. Life technologies (or new reproductive technologies) and the issues of responsibility, accountability, or liability that they raise, and ethical dilemmas they create. The 1986 IRPP publication by David Roy and Maurice de Wachter *(The Life Technologies and Public Policy)* offers a path-breaking exploration of some of these questions.
2. Treatment technologies and their evaluation, in particular the ethical dilemmas generated by research designs based on randomized controlled trials. What is efficacious for the older patient—not just in increasing longevity (or extending the period of dying) but in promoting the quality of life—is not easy to determine without confronting some controversial ethical choices. These questions are examined in the 1986 IRPP publication edited by Feeny, Guyatt, and Tugwell *(Health Care Technology: Effectiveness, Efficiency, and Public Policy).*
3. Information technologies and their implications for medical practice, medical education, and (most important) assignment of responsibility for treatment outcomes, where decisions are a consequence of judgments by patient, health care professional, *and* software designer. Problems of risk perceptions and risk analysis arise along with further ethical dilemmas as the promises of artificial intelligence, expert systems, and information retrieval are realized in diagnosis and treatment. Proposals for collaborative research activities in this area are under development.
4. Health status indicators and healthfulness—healthful equivalent life expectancy (Wilkins-Adams, 1983). In particular, the link from socioeconomic status to life expectancy and health status demands examination. What is the mechanism? What are the intermediating processes? What factors explain this "wealthier is healthier" feature of our social structure or lifestyles?
5. Microsimulation frameworks for systems of health statistics (Wolfson, 1987) promise a statistical structure based on individual activities and health status in a way that promises a more positive attack on evaluation problems in the health policy arena.
6. Institutional or organizational evaluation and expenditure control; incentive systems and mechanisms for establishing geographically differentiated fee schedules and appraisal of practice profiles; and links from fee schedules

to utilization of health care resources and the twisting of the age-use profile. At the societal level, the balancing of statistical lives and aggregate outcomes against expenditures drawn from other purposes altogether introduces a different—but still urgent—set of ethical dilemmas.

The Institute has just released preliminary results suggesting that those Canadians in the top 1% of the income distribution are likely to benefit most from current proposals for income tax reform (Maslove, 1988). The consequences of income distribution are not only direct (on purchasing power and material well-being), but also indirect (for health and happiness). Aaron Wildavsky has circulated a paper called "richer is safer," which in part is actually about the proposition that "wealthier is healthier" (Wildavsky, 1987).

Let me quote from a seminal Institute publication by Russ Wilkins and Owen Adams (1983):

> The results of our analyses of income-related differences in healthfulness of life are shown in Table 5.4. In terms of life expectancy at birth, the estimated disparity between the wealthiest 20 per cent of the population (fifth quintile) and the poorest 20 per cent (first quintile) is approximately 6.0 years for men and 3.0 years for women. By comparison, the 1978 disparity in life expectancy among regions is but 1.9 years for males, and 1.3 for females.
>
> Taking into consideration degree of health enjoyed as well as overall length of life, we see that Canadian males from the highest income group can expect an additional fourteen years of life free of activity restriction, or eleven more years of quality-adjusted life compared to Canadian males from the lowest income group. For wealthier females, the corresponding advantages are an additional eight years of life free of activity restriction, or six more years of quality-adjusted life.
>
> In spite of their shorter life, low-income males must endure almost twice the number of years of disability, and low-income females, an additional 40 per cent, compared to their high-income counterparts. (The disability figures cited here exclude long term institutionalization, for which data cross-classified by income were not available.)
>
> Even at age 65, the disparity between males of the highest and lowest income levels is 2.0 years of remaining life expectancy in all states of health, 3.0 years of quality-adjusted life, and 4.0 years of disability-free life. For females, the disparity is 0.4 years for all states of health, 1.4 years for quality-adjusted life, and 2.0 years for disability-free life. In each case, the advantage is in favour of the highest income group.

In my view it is this issue—the link from socioeconomic status to health status—that will pose the greatest social policy problem of the coming decades. The age-use curve—utilization rates for health services—will have to be constrained. Will utilization rates be controlled by rationing through income and socioeconomic status? Will lifestyle choices be permitted to be decisive either directly or through links with socioeconomic status? Herein lies, without doubt, the crunch issue for social policy over the next couple of decades.

All these examples illustrate areas in which research might do much to inform public policy and illuminate public choices. Yet little seems to be used, and direct impacts are hard to document. Reasons for this state of affairs are the subject of the next section.

WHY IS ANALYSIS SO HARD TO USE FOR POLICY PURPOSES?

There is an extensive literature explaining why government responses to problems so often differ dramatically from the analytically "correct" choices; many barriers exist to using results of research.

Different Interpretations of Evidence

The first major barrier to using research results in the policy process is simply a lack of agreement or a lack of clarity about what these research results are and how they should be interpreted. Scientific evidence is interpreted very differently by different scientists. For example, Jim Fries (Chapter 1) suggested not only a very clear and persuasive objective in identifying the "compression of morbidity" as the target of policy, but also a very optimistic reading of evidence suggesting that such reduction of morbidity is occurring. Verbrugge and Evans suggested much less optimistic readings based on different evidence about changes in morbidity. How dramatic is the impression that the scientific evidence is confused and that the scientists cannot agree.

Note also how easily I have slipped into plausible but careless language: as Fries defined *compression of morbidity,* it is quite possible—indeed, perhaps even likely—to achieve it in a period of nondecreasing morbidity. There is no real contradiction. But the readings of the evidence sound very different and, in fact, they are, depending on the starting point adopted by the individual scientists and the datasets employed. Here, obviously, is one concrete candidate for our list of items for further research work.

There is surprising consensus among researchers about some broad general features. We agree, for example, on the value of universal health care while admitting the importance of organizational experimentation around the fringes. We seem to agree that if ways can be found to handle the needs of a small fraction of very elderly people consuming a disproportionate amount of health care funds, then even present demographic trends need not pose an insurmountable challenge to our fiscal capacity. We also agree on a general philosophy emphasizing health and prevention as opposed to illness and treatment. But what comes through more strongly than these broad agreements are the disputes and disagreements over the numbers and their interpretation. Disputes and disagreements in the process of interest group exchange and adjustment to determine policy are big barriers to use of research results.

Saskatchewan's Health Minister, the Honourable George McLeod, observed that in his experience, one finds the program people and caregivers, the policy development people, and the researchers to be three solitudes in Canada. The first two exchange ideas in occasional encounters; the last two pass as ships in the night. His suggestion that all three might try to come together in the same harbor once in a while provides the motivation and explanation underlying this meeting.

Failure to Consider the Political Setting

Policy analysts often overlook the need for consensus, or support or political will. They often neglect the setting of the agenda itself. They forget that facts and concerns are filtered—the problem is to explain which facts are selected, or which risks are registered as objects of concern. It is hard to bring analysis to bear on political decisions, where *costs* are subtle, uncertain, distant, diffuse, and possibly undetectable or even unknowable, but where *benefits* are immediate, concrete, concentrated, and visible (or the other way around). The asymmetries involved in balancing statistical lives against identifiable people, or statistical risks against budget dollars (or employment dollars) pose almost insurmountable problems. The difficulties of public choice and collective decisionmaking can be explored at either a theoretical or pragmatic level. Either way they add up to a litany sufficient to scare off the most ardent analyst. What then is to be done?

BETTER LINKS: SOME DIRECTIONS FOR FURTHER WORK

1. *Research and advocacy to pursue the general reorientation of objectives within the health system identified above in our selective review of policy issues.* This orientation argues for emphasis on (1) health status rather than health care; (2) a health environment and lifestyle rather than treatment technology; and (3) active individual responsibility for personal health and treatment strategies rather than passive acceptance of professional judgment.

2. *Continuing emphasis on our pluralist tradition in policy formation, particularly on getting research results and research capabilities (data, models, computational capacity, analytical power) out into the hands of all sorts of interest groups.* We must ensure that the participants in public policy formation have the power to contend effectively in processes of mutual adjustment and research-policy interaction. The biggest single step in most of these complex issues comes when one can demystify the problem and disperse the attacks upon it.

These two practical steps can be focused, joined, and supported through the work now going on within Statistics Canada and the Canadian Institute for Advanced Research on the development of a system of health statistics. This initiative to develop a new conceptual framework for health accounts (building on the concept of healthful equivalent of life expectancy [Wilkins & Adams, 1983]) is one of the most promising steps we will take to bring research more fully to bear on policy in an enlightened way. I encourage you to support as actively as possible Health and Welfare Canada's efforts to establish a uniform system of statistics and management information from the bottom up, working with institutional management information systems. Because these administrative data are oriented toward visits and resources, not patients, I urge you even more strongly to support efforts to establish a conceptual framework and data-gathering effort with federal and provincial involvement—perhaps in some quasi-independent continuing Centre of Health Statistics or within Statistics Canada itself.

3. *Development of a patient-centered life-cycle longitudinal microsimulation framework (Wolfson, 1987) so that one can correlate episodes of disability, treatment, and interactions with activity outside the health system.* Transition probabilities can come only from longitudinal data, and full understanding of the impacts of public policy on the health status of societies can come only from such transition data. Basic knowledge of health status can come only from research of this kind.

A DIGRESSION ON THINK TANKS

In the pluralist tradition, the processes of research dissemination, advocacy, and public participation stimulated, animated, and orchestrated by think tanks play a key role in bringing research to bear on policy (as well as in probing the validity of research results and testing the limits of their application). Think tanks or policy institutes fall squarely into the chasm between researchers and policy responsibility. There are two routes to go in trying to bridge that chasm. One might follow the route of research, reason, and roundtables—what I call the "Ottawa" approach: influencing by stealth, hoping that ideas might rub off by osmosis. Or alternatively, one might pursue the avenue of profile, promotion, and press conferences—the "Toronto" approach: influencing by proximity and provocation, hoping that ideas will be adopted as pressures build.

In thinking of themselves as actors in the process of policy formation, think tanks are always asking themselves whether they should be agent, advocate, activist, or simply analyst. In the end, the point is to get the information onto the table, into the public domain, part of the debate—to worry about seeing research through to visible implementation is to enter into a frustrating and ultimately futile pursuit.

CONCLUSIONS

A forcing mechanism within the process of policy discussion may be as important as the content of analysis itself. Canada's National Task Force on Environment and Economy (Canadian Council of Resource and Environment Ministers, 1987) recommended:

1. that First Ministers demonstrate a commitment to environment-economy interaction by *inter alia* "directing that Cabinet documents and major government economic development documents demonstrate that they are economically and environmentally sound and therefore sustainable"; and
2. that all ministers must become directly responsible and accountable for the environmental and economic consequences of their policies, legislation, and program by *inter alia* mechanisms "ensuring that every major report on economic development and every related Cabinet document demonstrates that the proposal is economically and environmentally sound."

There may not soon be agreement on what is meant in concrete terms by *economically and environmentally sound* or which things qualify as such, but an inescapable requirement to acknowledge the question each time—with a mandatory section of a Cabinet document, for example—forces its own compelling logic on the discussion, and ultimately the outcome. That this is so has been demonstrated by legions of auditors general, accountants, and financial managers who have forced their values on the policy process by making a concern for the three E's (economy, efficiency, and effectiveness), the first charge on the discussion of any policy proposal.

I support a quadruple-E process (economy, efficiency, effectiveness, and environment), and would be delighted if we could find some way to add *equity in health* to the list as a fifth E. We might not know exactly what it is, but research might help to persuade us whether any particular step is moving us toward or away from that goal, and certainly the question should be continually recognized. By adding *environment* and *equity in health*, we might force reorientation of the public agenda toward programs for health rather than health care, prevention and lifestyles rather than treatment and technology, and individual responsibility rather than paternal professionalism. By discussions involving premiers and politicians directly, and by procedures requiring these questions to be addressed automatically as part of the routine paper flow, we might cement the link from these research results of the policy process.

For think tanks and researchers, academics, practitioners, and politicians, the only really practical advice to offer is, Keep the faith. Research ultimately has its impact on policy through the slow spread of new ideas. Subtle reasoning and intricate computation may rarely change specific programs or alter particular decisions, but broad policies and overall government orientations are shaped by perceptions and outlooks formed from the interplay of ideas and the contest of research findings over many years and many encounters.

In 1990 at the next conference, we can review progress toward these objectives. In the meantime, we can back measures (1) to mount nationwide health surveys, (2) to use the 1991 census as a carrier for health status review, and (3) to coordinate resources across a variety of agencies in federal and provincial governments in order to produce a more uniform, coherent patient-oriented or individual-oriented system of health statistics focused on socioeconomic status, lifestyle, and preventive measures.

After 20 years of grappling with links from research to policy, I still come back to the position expressed in lines I once wrote for the Honourable Bud Drury, quoting my old teacher Paul Samuelson, who in turn was quoting William Blake: "Truth can never be told so as to be understood and not believed." The presentation of research results in Cabinet Committees on Health Policy may be an art form in an absurd theater, but the audience is all of us, and the play really does matter.

REFERENCES

Canadian Council of Resource and Environment Ministers. (1987). *Report of the National Task Force on Environment and Economy.* (Available from Department of Environment, Safety, and Health, Province of Manitoba Legislative Assembly, Winnipeg, Manitoba)

Cohen, D., & Lindblom, C. (1979). *Usable knowledge: Social science and problem solving.* New Haven & London: Yale University Press.

Drury, C. M. (1975, Winter):. Quantitative analysis and public policy making. *Canadian Public Policy, 1*(1), 89–96.

Feeny, D., Guyatt, G., & Tugwell, P. (1986). *Health care technology: Effectiveness, efficiency, and public policy.* Halifax: Institute for Research on Public Policy.

Maslove, A. (1988). *Tax reform in Canada.* Halifax: Institute for Research on Public Policy.

Morgenstern, O. (1963). *On the accuracy of economic observations* (2nd ed.). Princeton: Princeton University Press.

Roy, D., & de Wachter, M. (1986). *The life technologies and public policy.* Halifax: Institute for Research on Public Policy.

Wildavsky, A. (1987). *Searching for safety.* Transaction Books. New Brunswick and New Jersey: Rutgers University.

Wilkins, R., & Adams, O. (1983). *Healthfulness of life.* Halifax: Institute for Research on Public Policy.

Wolfson, M. C. (1987, September). *A system of health statistics: Toward a new conceptual framework for integrating health data.* Unpublished working paper, Social and Economic Studies Division, Statistics Canada.

40. Strengthening Research-Policy Relations in the Field of Aging and Health

RONALD BAYNE

WHERE RESEARCH IS NEEDED

It is now true to say that the Canadian population is aging, that is, that the average age of the population is rising. This rise is chiefly due to a fall in the birth rate to pre-World War II levels or below, but it is also due to increasing longevity. Not only are more people reaching age 65, but even 80- and 90-year-olds have gained an increase in life expectancy in recent years (Stone & Fletcher, 1986). It is an achievement to be proud of. Years of active life potential have been added for many people.

It is generally accepted that there is a genetically determined life span for all animals, including humans. Although extension of the life span may be possible with better understanding of the aging process, further extension of life expectancy as a result of reduction of mortality is a practical reality. As life expectancy increases and approaches a relatively fixed life span, one can expect a compression of mortality into the last years (Fries, 1980). However, most people are more interested in gaining disability-free years than just years of life.

Disability is increasingly prevalent after age 60 and very common in extreme old age, and the possibility of reducing disability and dependency in old age is a relatively new consideration. Previously, disability was considered a part of aging and old age, and dependency was seen as a reward for a life of hard work. Now, people are looking forward to an interesting and rewarding retirement and seek relief from or prevention of disability.

There is some encouraging information from the U.S. Health Interview Survey (Palmore, 1986). It showed a 10–18% decline in seven measures of disability (days of restricted activities, bed disability, injuries, acute condi-

Aging and Health: Linking Research and Public Policy, © 1989 Lewis Publishers, Inc., Chelsea, Michigan 48118. Printed in U.S.A.

tions, visual impairments, severe visual impairments, and hearing impairments) in persons aged 65 or more over the period of 1961–1981. This decline is probably due to improved health of each age cohort reaching 65, as well as improved health care and improved economic status of the aged.

Origins of Disease

If the major causes of disease and disability were identified and prevented, it would greatly reduce dependency and the need for institutional care. (For example, prevention or successful treatment of senile dementias could make nursing homes as obsolete as tuberculosis sanatoria.) But to focus on the major diseases causing disability in later life, there has to be a change in perspective from immediate causes of and acute onset of disease to early origins of disease and the contributory factors that act over a lifetime. Public understanding and participation is essential because the causal factors are related to such societal issues as environmental pollution, occupational hazards, and lifestyle. Inequities in economic status and employment must also be corrected, because these are related to poor health and reduced life expectancy. Expensive high-technology research to treat the late-phase acute stages of disease should be seen as an interim measure. A major focus must be toward the origins of disease.

Treatment of Chronic Illness

The survival of large numbers of persons beyond age 65 has made them very visible. The public and scientific media repeatedly forecast a blocking up of the health care system by the aged and insupportable costs. Yet research (Roos & Shapiro, 1981) has shown that a majority of the elderly do not use the health care system more often than do younger people, and that it is a small minority of elderly patients who account for a high proportion of the use of physician's services and hospitals. The focus must be on better ways of treating the chronic illnesses of later life and on avoiding unnecessary dependency.

But piecemeal solutions do not work. For example, the provision of geriatric medical consultation in acute care hospitals has not reduced the length of stay or use of resources (Hogan et al., 1987). The provision of a coordinated geriatric assessment, rehabilitation, and follow-up for selected cases with potential for improvement is more successful. Home care programs do not reduce use of hospitals or long term institutional care. It may be better to identify a professional case-manager with defined responsibility to ensure not only that needed care is given but also that use of resources is tightly controlled. However, an important concern, sometimes not evaluated, is the objective of the patient. Reduced use of resources may not be important for the individual. Evaluation of treatment should measure relief of pain and anxiety, and improved quality of life. It is difficult to define and measure these intangibles, but research on trade-offs and quality-adjusted life expectancy is a beginning.

Health Care Expenditures

The forecasts of economic insolvency due to the health care of the aged seems more related to the current deficits of all governments and a desire to reduce expenditures than to uncontrolled rising costs. The cost of Canadian health care as a percentage of the gross national product has changed only a little since 1971 (Glaser, 1987). It is comparable to other developed countries and considerably lower than that of the United States. Clearly, the amount of money to be spent on health care is a political question. So is the allocation of the funds to the various components of care such as physicians, hospitals, long term institutional care, and community services. Research should provide the information on which decisions can be based. Such research should be independent of governments and should be used to inform and educate the public.

There are severe pressures to increase expenditures on health care. Technological innovations can be produced by research and marketed to the public before the long term effectiveness can be evaluated. Once publicized, they cannot easily be subjected to random controlled clinical trial, and they become an addition to expensive health care. Research policy should identify the areas for focused attention, likely new developments, and the place for those new technologies that can be shown to be effective.

Information for Politically Active Seniors

A factor of growing importance with the aging of the population is the political influence of seniors. When the Old Age Security Pension and the Health Insurance programs were introduced, the proportion of seniors to the total population was relatively small, and they were accepted as a dependent minority. Seniors are now increasingly visible and increasingly audible. The recent attempt of government to cease indexing the Old Age Security Pension to the cost-of-living index produced a very effective resistance from seniors.

Each cohort of seniors is better educated and economically better off. Although there continues to be a large group almost solely dependent on the Old Age Security Pension and supplements, there is another group of seniors now retiring on substantial pensions and other income. They indicate that they want to continue to be involved in ongoing societal issues, to delay retirement or seek new employment, and to be seen as middle-aged rather than as elderly.

But at present all persons at age 65 receive special consideration for tax credits, drug benefit programs, and other advantages not available to other citizens because of age. Governments may be tempted to control costs by reducing these benefits, applying some form of means testing, or postponing eligibility. Better information on possible consequences and alternatives should be acquired. Seniors need good information in order to balance their rights and their responsibilities as citizens (Hudson, 1987).

Seniors are requesting more information and greater influence in health care decisions. Some groups of seniors have accepted the responsibility of informing and helping more disabled and dependent persons in their age group. Research could help to provide them with reliable information and to evaluate the effectiveness of what they are doing.

Health service professionals sometimes seem to be suspicious that researchers use seniors inappropriately in studies, or that research is merely a way of delaying provision of needed services. The involvement of seniors and service providers in research planning and development could both inform them and give them input into research. Their experience can provide a perspective and help to identify the important questions.

The direct involvement of seniors in research would provide important information on the effectiveness of treatments in older people and the effects of aging in response to therapy. Ways should be found to involve in special research studies even patients who are unable to understand and give specific consent, to evaluate treatments that might benefit them. Proper ethical control and good scientific design would be essential.

SUPPORT FOR GERONTOLOGICAL RESEARCH

How can we promote geriatric and gerontological research? Clearly, we require a number of able scientists, trained in good research methodology, who understand these special, complex problems and are committed to a career in gerontological research. Undoubtedly, older persons benefit from research now being done in cardiovascular disease, neurological diseases, and other areas of medical diagnosis and treatment. But with such information it will still not be possible to meet the health needs of the aging population.

What is different about geriatric and gerontological research is that it must be concerned with the whole person (because usually more than one disease is present) and with the environment (if old people are to remain independent). It is characteristically interdisciplinary and collaborative. There is need for special research design, and there is often a need for longitudinal perspective.

Much of biomedical research can be done in laboratories, as can basic gerontological research. But to study the problems relevant to an aging population, the research must often involve clinical practice and care settings and service professionals with little knowledge of research methods. A research scientist needs a base from which to operate. To be effective, he or she needs the support and encouragement of a "critical mass" of researchers working in proximity on related problems.

The Social Sciences and Humanities Research Council

In 1979, the Social Sciences and Humanities Research Council (SSHRC) established a Strategic Grants program to focus on themes of national interest. A Population Aging program was established on the basis of recommendations made in 1976 by social scientists interested in gerontology and by the Canadian Association on Gerontology (C.A.G.). Five types of grants, which focused on research projects, personnel training, and institutional support, were provided. In 1984, an evaluation was done by an independent agency (SSHRC, 1984). They found that the program had made a major contribution by increasing research output, by raising the credibility of gerontology as an academic endeavor, by establishing five university gerontology centers in four provinces, and by increasing the interest of graduate students. Other universities followed this lead and developed gerontology centers on their own initiative. The Population Aging program was terminated, having met its objectives, but general research support continues.

Benefiting from the growth in interest and support, C.A.G. has greatly expanded in membership and in its educational endeavors. The membership of over 2400 persons, with the provincial affiliate gerontological associations, includes health and social scientists, researchers and educators, practicing professionals and others interested in gerontology. C.A.G. holds an annual scientific and educational conference in centers across the country. It publishes proceedings of special workshops, an educational newsletter, and the *Canadian Journal on Aging*.

Biomedical Research

Support for research in the biomedical aspects of aging and in geriatrics is less evident. The Medical Research Council of Canada and the Natural Sciences and Engineering Research Council have indicated interest in such research but have found few proposals that can meet their criteria in competition with other requests. Because aging research tends to be across disciplines, the two councils set up a committee to arrange appropriate peer review but with little success. The number of researchers continues to be very small. Proposals that involve both health and social science disciplines fall between the councils. Even if they are accepted for peer review, the reviewers often seem to lack the experience and knowledge required.

The National Health Research and Development Program

The National Health Research and Development Program (NHRDP) has provided support for research in health services, including those serving the elderly. NHRDP has indicated that problems of the aged is one of their priorities, and recently announced funding targeted to research in Alzheimer's disease and osteoporosis. This funding reflects the government's awareness of the importance of these two conditions and the effectiveness of the relevant two societies in bringing them to public attention. However, we do not know how research in these conditions relates to other gerontological research priorities. Nor do we know how the information obtained will fit with information from related studies and whether it will be in practical, usable format.

Thus, despite the dire predictions based on the aging of the population, and the need for accurate information to solve the very real challenges that face Canada, there has not been a clear statement of national policy or intent for gerontological health research. Research priorities have not been identified and funding is inconstant.

Corporations

Research requires financial support. Governments, faced with large deficits, have urged researchers—and everyone else—to turn to the public and to corporations. The greatly increased number of requests to corporations has caused them to review all requests carefully and to donate to a selected minority. Canadians have traditionally relied less on charitable donations for support of universities and research than have Americans. The level of corporate giving in Canada is, for all purposes, about one fourth that of the United States, and the level of individual giving is even lower.

A permanent Corporate-Higher Education Forum was created in 1983 to strengthen links between corporations and universities (Panabaker, 1986). A series of Task Forces were set up in 1984-85 which recommended to the forum that corporations should take an interest in how their funds are spent. The report suggested that corporations in future will want evidence of clear direction and efficiency in management of the university, and the corporation may want to be involved in projects of mutual interest. For donations to move beyond a charitable context, there must be evaluation of the value of the support to the corporation as well as to the university. The danger of skewing support toward particular faculties such as science, engineering, and business and of concentrating support in research-intensive universities was recognized. Therefore, the Task Force said, support from corporations should also go to general education and training. This stance was seen as particularly important in view of the government's program to match funding from corporations by giving equal amounts to the Research Councils. Such matching would further underscore the emphasis on technological research.

Geriatric and gerontological services tend to be low in technology and high in human services. Gerontological research is needed in order to provide services most effectively and efficiently. The research must focus on specific effects of aging in the individual and on the social effects of aging of the population. Such research is unlikely to create wealth or a product to sell on the international market. Therefore, financial support from most industrial corporations for gerontological and geriatric research is likely to continue to be on the basis of charitable donations. However, some industries may have a greater interest if the research can improve the quality and presentation of their product. There are important industrial opportunities in applying electronic technology to improving communication in service industries (Quinn, Baruch, & Paquette, 1987). Especially in community health services, we need better interprofessional communication, monitoring, and recording of confidential information. Electronic technology should be used to improve public information on specific health products and services.

The Gerontology Research Council of Ontario

In 1981, the Gerontology Research Council of Ontario (GRCO) was established by the Ministry of Health of Ontario with a substantial grant from Provincial Lottery. GRCO held a consultative conference with gerontologists and professionals providing services to the elderly to identify the focus for research support. These proceedings were published under the title *Research Issues in Aging* (Bayne & Wigdor, 1982). GRCO set up a Research Advisory Committee and peer review system. By 1987, over $1.9 million had been provided to increase participation in the field of geriatric and gerontological research through Research Scholarships, Fellowships, and Advanced Student Bursaries. It also provided small grants for exploratory studies.

In 1983, GRCO conducted a Survey of Research in Ontario and an enquiry of priorities among the research community and the professionals and administrators who use research information. Five areas of high priority for research were identified from the survey, all of them concerned with helping older persons remain in their own community:

1. Community health care to the elderly involves many disciplines. What combinations of professional and nonprofessional services are optimal? What system of monitoring and reporting is optimal for communication and control between the physician, other professionals, nonprofessionals, the family, and the client?
2. Many elderly are now placed in institutions for care. What methods are needed for early detection of breakdown in those elderly who are at greatest risk of requiring institutional care? What preventive action could be taken

both in the community and in acute care hospitals (at emergency departments and at time of discharge) to prevent readmission or institutional care?

3. The elderly are high users of medication, often with benefit, but at the risk of polypharmacy and drug toxicity. What prescribing, dispensing and monitoring systems are practical for use by physicians, pharmacists and community care services to help the elderly use drugs more effectively, and are less costly?

4. Elderly persons with impaired mental functions are at risk of injury, exploitation, or premature institutionalization. How can impaired mental function be diagnosed early yet avoid labeling? How can the family, the physician, and community care programs help the person to stay at home? What is the role of protective monitoring, protective housing, and protective residential care?

5. Not everyone has difficulty adjusting to retirement. Those who do often have not prepared for the social and economic problems to be faced. How can persons who will have difficulty with retirement be identified for help? What approaches or resources have been found to be useful and should be included in the retirement planning programs?

Research in these areas would contribute significantly to enabling older persons to maintain independence and to remain at home in their community.

GRCO has moved ahead on one of these areas: problems in the use of medication by elderly persons. It was evident that these problems are not limited by provincial boundaries but are a matter of national concern. Therefore, GRCO invited approximately 80 persons from across Canada to meet in a working conference in Hamilton in December 1987. These participants included representatives of the pharmaceutical manufacturing industries and researchers, pharmacists, pharmacologists, geriatricians, nurses, representatives of the National Advisory Council on Aging, and administrators of provincial drug benefit programs and of the national drug regulatory authority. Financial support was provided by GRCO, Health and Welfare Canada, Pharmaceutical Manufacturers Association of Canada, Medical Research Council of Canada, and the Canadian Pharmaceutical Association as well as local industries in Hamilton.

It was the task of this group of Canadians, with very different professional backgrounds, to identify the major problems in use of medications by the elderly, the obstacles to improvement, and to develop a consensus on what should be done. One and a half days were spent in intensive multidisciplinary small-group meetings, alternating with plenary reporting sessions, and consensus was achieved. A list of practical actions that should be taken was drawn up. It was recommended that action should be carried out through a national coalition of the organizations and agencies concerned, with GRCO providing the organizational support.

SUMMARY

Canada can be proud to have enabled a larger number of its citizens to achieve the age of 65 and well beyond it. Although gloomy forecasts have been made of a growing population of dependent elderly, this need not occur. Not only should life expectancy further increase, but also disability-free years. There is some evidence of improved health of seniors, but research is needed to understand aging and to help individuals to realize the benefits of old age, not just idealize them. Research must focus on the important needs and desirable goals as identified by the research community, by health professionals and caregivers, and by seniors themselves. Seniors should be encouraged to take part in research to improve its focus and to ensure its relevance and acceptance.

Researchers and persons needing research information must be regularly brought together to improve mutual understanding and to enable research to be made more available and practically useful. Funding specifically for gerontological and geriatric research is essential, because it has characteristics and requirements that are different from other research. Longitudinal research on the natural history of aging, and on illness in old age is needed.

Universities are the most appropriate location for a research team, but the research should not be limited to university premises. Research is needed in community services and programs as well, and interdisciplinary research should be encouraged and supported. More programs of gerontological research training are needed.

Although the federal government has published statements on health policy emphasizing health promotion and prevention, neither it nor the national health research agencies have identified research priorities in relation to the aging population. Research priorities could be established by a nongovernmental organization that would work with other research and professional organizations. The coordinating organization should have a board of directors—made up of researchers and private citizens—and a mission directed solely to improving knowledge and understanding of aging through education and research. Such an organization with a national mandate could work through a steering committee representing both researchers and professional service providers and seniors. It would maintain links with the gerontological research community to develop policies and priorities for gerontological and geriatric research. It could help in reviewing research requests and in obtaining funding, and it would maintain a continuous review of subsequent use of research information. Clearly, it would be closely affiliated with the Canadian Association on Gerontology, National Advisory Council on Aging, and the national research agencies.

Relying on private and corporate donations will not achieve gerontological research objectives. A strong commitment by government to gerontological and geriatric research is needed. It should support an organization that would be at arm's length from government but would work closely with government and the national research councils.

REFERENCES

Bayne, J. R. D., & Wigdor, B. T. (Eds.). (1982). *Research issues in aging*. Hamilton: Gerontology Research Council of Ontario.

Fries, J. F. (1980). Aging, natural death, and compression of morbidity. *New England Journal of Medicine, 303*, 130–135.

Glaser, W. A. (1987). International perspectives in aging with limited health resources. In *Aging with limited health resources, proceedings of a colloquium on health care, May 1986*. Ottawa: Canadian Government Publishing Centre, Supply and Services Canada.

Hogan, D. B., Fox, R. A., Badley, B. W. D., & Mann, O. E. (1987, April 1). Effect of a geriatric consultation service on management of patients in an acute care hospital. *Canadian Medical Association Journal, 136*, 713–717.

Hudson, R. B. (1987). Tomorrow's able elders: Implications for the state. *Gerontologist, 27*(4), 405–409.

Palmore, E. B. (1986). Trends in the health of the aged. *Gerontologist, 26*(3), 298–302.

Panabaker, J. H. (1986, October 1). Address to the Association of Universities and Colleges of Canada, St. John's, Newfoundland.

Quinn, J. B., Baruch, J. J., & Paquette, P. C. (1987, December). Technology in services. *Scientific American, 257*(6), 50–58.

Roos, N., & Shapiro, E. (1981). The Manitoba longitudinal study on aging—Preliminary findings on health care utilization by the elderly. *Medical Care, 19*(6), 644–657.

Social Sciences and Humanities Research Council of Canada. (1984). *Report on evaluation of the population aging program*. Ottawa: SSHRC

Stone, L., & Fletcher, S. (1986). *The seniors boom* (Statistics Canada Catalogue No. 89–515). Ottawa: Canadian Government Publishing Centre, Supply and Services Canada.

41. Research and Policy from the Federal Government Perspective

PETER GLYNN

INTRODUCTION

I spent nine years in Saskatchewan. I worked in health and in post-secondary education and, quite frankly, a lot of my biases, a lot of my approach came from my experiences in Saskatchewan, in virtually every town, village, and hamlet in this province. In this chapter, I want to clarify what is *research* and what is *public policy*. I want to talk about some themes that have emerged in this conference. I want to talk about how we—Health and Welfare and the federal government—are attempting to be of assistance, and lastly I would like to talk about where we go from here.

DEFINITIONS

My definition of research is absolutely anything that tries new approaches, examines new approaches, asks questions, does some thinking, describes, or explains. It is not nice, neat packages of academic research. It includes formal research, it includes what one might call semiformal research, and it includes informal research. One of the things I do a lot of is informal research. Larry Chambers's iterative loop approach to research and public policy (Chapter 35) is exactly what I mean. We think, we ask some questions, we involve people, we try some things, we ask some more questions, we involve some more people, and then we think again and we change some things and we just keep that rolling right along. There is no front end and there is no back end; there is a circle or a wheel. Seniors, the consumers, are all in the center of the wheel and, indeed, they are why the wheel exists.

Aging and Health: Linking Research and Public Policy, © 1989 Lewis Publishers, Inc., Chelsea, Michigan 48118. Printed in U.S.A.

Let me use an example of some informal, but very practical research. In 1983, when nursing home care was brought back into the Department of Health, Rick Roger (Chapter 33), who was responsible for hospitals; Steve Petz, who was responsible for continuing care; and I went on the road to small-town Saskatchewan and asked people a question they had never been asked before: "Which of our rules are making it impossible for you to do what is reasonable to do?" The communities did not believe we would actually ask that question, so in the initial round we did not get very good answers because they were a little skeptical. But that is just as much research as anything else that has been talked about in this symposium, and we need to remember that, and we need to do it, and we need to ask people, What are we doing that makes it impossible for you to do something that makes sense?

Now let's just throw in a few other biases: an overreliance on the scientific approach. In social policy, rigorous hypothesis testing is probably the quickest way to make sure that nothing will happen, because there are severe methodological problems. If you try to do multivariate analysis, you get so bogged down in the methodology that nothing ever happens. Another bias is against an overreliance on the role of experts. A centralization of expertise without some involvement of seniors is a mistake. (And when I say *involvement*, I mean real involvement, not just calling them in to rubber-stamp what the experts are suggesting.)

Now, public policy—what is it? Public policy is implicit or explicit policy that exists in every public setting, no matter what form it may take. It can be formulated in a home care board, a service club, a provincial government, the federal government, municipal council—you name it, it is all public policy. Public policy is not the same as government policy. As Dorothy Pringle said (Chapter 32), policy and public policy embody values and beliefs. We need to remember there is a whole set of values and beliefs dependent on the context and upon the groups you are dealing with. Research does indeed influence those values and beliefs. An illustration from one of the workshops this morning relates to the growing view that aging and incompetence do not go together.

THEMES AT THIS CONFERENCE

1. *Independence, interdependence, and the environment.* These three words are absolutely consistent with *Achieving Health For All* (1986), the health promotion framework document by Mr. Epp. That document is a good example of how research and thinking in the field of aging can influence public policy development, because thinking in the field of aging and gerontology had substantial impact on its development.

2. *The future does not need to be bleak.* It can and will be positive and progressive.

3. *We have to abandon the "us-them" approach and deal with* we *and what future* we *want—not categorizing seniors as "them."* We have been looking at this issue incorrectly as a planning problem. What we are really looking at is a natural evolution of our own society.

4. *Ethics.* I hope we will not create a number of expert opinions on the ethics of death and dying. Ethics is both a personal and a societal issue. We need to keep emphasizing the involvement of individuals in the ethics that affect them.

THE ROLE OF HEALTH AND WELFARE CANADA

The appointment of the Hon. George Hees as Minister of State for Seniors has provided at the national level and in the federal government a focal point for issues of seniors. It has created an interest—an opportunity—and as Mr. Hees would say, he is the friend at court for seniors and seniors' issues. To help Mr. Hees and to provide the operational support, we have created the Senior Secretariat. We have been putting together workshops. We had one two weeks ago on senior women's issues where we brought together 20 women. We sat the bureaucrats around the wall, told them to be quiet, and let these 20 people go at it in terms of what the real issues are for senior women. There will be a report out of that, and it will also be part of the planning for a workshop at the Canadian Association of Gerontology meeting later in 1988.

We are holding an invitational conference next week on ethnicity and aging, where we will have a representative of every ethnic association in this country we could find, plus service providers and government policy people, to identify, for the first time ever on any kind of scale in this country, the issues surrounding ethnicity and aging. At least 30% of seniors in this country have neither a French nor an English background. We need to start dealing with that explicitly.

The Laboratory Centre on Disease Control hosted a workshop on the epidemiology of Alzheimer's disease and I suspect we will see some work come out of that as well. We will assist the Canadian Medical Association in the financing of a conference on ethics and aging which grew out of their task force. Ron Bingham put together a proposal for a workshop on drugs and the elderly, which we helped finance, and we are waiting for a report.

The Seniors Independence Program announced at this conference is just as much a research program as anything else (if you take my definition of research). It is aimed at the community, however, and at helping groups experiment, learn, change, and talk about evaluation in the sense of, Is this right for us? Through the Seniors Independence Program we will be talking to the provinces about how to make sure we do not confuse or exacerbate their priorities.

The New Horizons program is just as much a research program as anything else, and the budget there has been substantially increased.

We did put some money into research on disease related to seniors' independence, but we took more of a problem-oriented approach than maybe we have in the past. We want to start dealing with, especially, the nonbiomedical part of Alzheimer's disease, which tends to be left out, and osteoporosis. And there will be a process for defining research needs and a solicitation in the next few months from the National Health Research and Development Program in terms of generating research proposals.

The National Advisory Committee on Aging has been increased both in numbers of staff and operating budget so it can do its own homework, its own research, and help the government with advice on appropriate public policy.

WHERE DO WE GO FROM HERE?

First, we must recognize the circulatory and iterative nature of what we are talking about. We recognize that consumers are at the center of this issue and that there is not a nice, neat time relationship between research and public policy. You may do something now and not see the impact of it for a number of years. You may do something now and see the impact of it tomorrow. That variability has to be allowed to occur.

Must we possibly agree with my definitions of research and public policy and take a much broader and much more holistic approach? We must make research more visible and translate it into information useful to seniors, consumers, caregivers, policymakers, health managers, you name it. We must create more opportunities for this kind of forum. This kind of discussion may be around particular issues as opposed to general issues, and that will help deal with Pringle's semipermeable membrane (Chapter 32), which is as good an analogy as any chemical engineer could have come up with.

Everyone agrees how important this work is, but we have to do more than just agree it is important—we have to continually work on it and make it work. We have to recognize there are no instant answers. We need to start where the world is—with political realities—and we need to deal with opportunities as they arise, having our homework done so that when they do arise, we can capitalize on them.

REFERENCE

Epp, J. (1986). *Achieving health for all: A framework for health promotion.* Ottawa: Health and Welfare Canada.

42. How Can Granting Agencies Respond to the Need for Research on Aging and Health?

DAVID R. J. JARRETT

INTRODUCTION

If a group of clinicians and scientists from all disciplines of medicine were asked to list what they felt were the 10 most important breakthroughs in the last decade or so, very few would include any innovation specifically related to the elderly. Yet the elderly have undoubtedly benefited from the recent explosion in knowledge in the life sciences and in clinical research. Most of the advances, such as in the treatment of Parkinson's disease and cardiac failure, or in the development of the many new imaging techniques have not evolved from research directed toward the elderly. Yet many of the acute and chronic disabling medical conditions show an exponential rise in incidence with advancing age.

So where have the many advances in medical care of the elderly come from? Much of the clinical research carried out by departments of clinical gerontology has been based on reapplying and modifying research carried out on the young and finding new and innovative ways of applying these advances to help the older adult, albeit with a varying degree of success. The most fundamental research takes place not with the elderly specifically in mind, but the practical application of this work for the benefit of the elderly has been pioneered by clinical gerontology.

Interest in the medical conditions of the elderly is relatively new. Over the last few decades, many of the fundamental principles of clinical practice have had to be critically reassessed and their relevance to the older adult tested. Demography dictates that the relative ignorance about disease and the provision of care for the elderly cannot persist. In the future, geriatric medicine must initiate major breakthroughs in medical science rather than have breakthroughs handed down from other specialties.

The romantic view of research—the Newton's apple view, whereby phenomenal and momentous ideas are generated by the collision of cranium and apple—owes much more to fantasy than reality. Serendipity may occur once in a lifetime, but cannot be relied upon as a source of inspiration. Alexander Fleming was lucky to leave his laboratory window open long enough for the *Penicillium notatum* to enter and conveniently settle on his petri dish. Most research is wrought from perspiration rather than inspiration.

THE GAP BETWEEN THEORETICAL AND CLINICAL GERONTOLOGY

The two general models of the research process are the linear model and the market-pull model. In the first, pure curiosity is the initial driving force for research. This research may suggest some practical application that can be further developed by experimentation until a true innovation emerges. In the latter model, a problem is identified and research is directed toward solving that problem or meeting some need.

Both models occur in the genesis of medical advances. The development of monoclonal antibodies gives us an example of the linear model of research. Monoclonal antibodies are revolutionizing many aspects of laboratory and clinical medicine. Their potential uses seem almost endless. Yet their development stems from parallel fields of investigation over many decades, including the major advances in the sciences of virology, immunology, and other disciplines. It is doubtful that even a decade ago nonclinical immunologists could have foreseen the immense practical implications of their research. The development of H_2 receptor antagonists show how market need can lead to innovation. A need to control gastric acidity has long been recognized. When it became known that gastric acid production was under the control of H_2 receptors, it became apparent that an H_2 receptor antagonist could have profound therapeutic implications. After much trial and error, a chemical was engineered that could block the H_2 receptors—cimetidine.

Each pure life science seems to have some natural clinical counterpart that can benefit from its research. We hope that advances in biochemistry lead to the development of a greater understanding of the course and treatment of metabolic diseases such as diabetes and renal failure. Similarly, the practical extension of microbiology involves the diagnosis, control, and treatment of infectious diseases. The practical application of pure gerontology, the study of biological aging, would seem to be the development of some elixir of youth. I am thankful such potions are only the stuff of legend. Unfortunately, gerontology has not fueled the fires of research in its clinical counterpart. The vast body of work on biological aging is poorly understood by, and mostly of no interest to, clinicians. The work on biological aging seems to have little potential application to patient care. Most texts on aging contain complex mathematical formulae relating mortality to such nebulous qualities as vitality, or they contain vast tables of the life expectancy of numerous species of bat. Such information helps neither the elderly patient nor her clinician. Nor does this help the theoretical gerontologist who dies before the date predicted by his mortality formula. Glasgow's Professor Caird, writing about research in geriatric medicine, states that the relevance of research to man is directly proportional to the nearness of the species studied to man. The rat is the most favored animal in gerontology research, but no elderly rat has to suffer the indignity of trying to put minute batteries in hearing aids with arthritic hands and poor sight. This chasm between the pure science and the practical medicine in gerontology may explain why funding for research into aging is a low priority. Recent figures from the United Kingdom show that funding for research in aging by both medical charities and the Medical Research Council is less than any other major specialty. Cancer and cardiovascular and neuropsychiatric diseases, not surprisingly, top the list in terms of research expenditure. Research that leads to some confluence of gerontology and geriatric medicine is sorely needed.

THE PROBLEM OF JUSTIFICATION

It has always been difficult for granting panels to know where to direct their limited funds. They are not helped by the obvious difficulties in predicting which fundamental science project will yield practical benefits and which market-driven technological research projects will lead to a dead end. There is a paucity of research on the nature of research itself. There is a labyrinthine pathway between the conception of an idea and its final practical outcome. It is virtually impossible to ascertain the relative importance of these steps in the evolution of an innovation. The few studies that do exist tend to reflect the biases of those investigating. Government-funded studies tend to favor business and industrial laboratories as the source of practical advances. University-based studies, not surprisingly, reach the opposite conclusion— namely, that the pure sciences are the major source of innovation. All the studies so far have been retrospective, and the results have been difficult to interpret.

There have been great advances in the provision of care for the elderly. The policies for providing services cannot be static but have to constantly change in response to the changing economic, political, and demographic structures of our society. It is not enough to put money into new policies that have not been fully researched. Jeremy Bentham's utilitarian philosophy of "the greatest good for the greatest number of people" has special poignancy for the provision of health care to the older adult. In the latter part of the 20th century, one would have to add to this adage, "for a given expenditure." Politicians tend to work from one election to the next, but lesser mortals working directly with clients, their problems, and what services are available need policies that outlast governments. Before money is put into a new scheme, a need for this scheme has to be proven. The new scheme must be critically assessed to see whether it is achieving what it was designed to achieve. All too often, new schemes are based on ideas that have been poorly tried and tested or on innovations that have worked well in one environment but are totally inappropriate in another. A Meals On Wheels service would be as unrealistic in the remote areas of northern Saskatchewan as it would be in Calcutta.

THE NEED FOR RESEARCH

In many Western societies, there is an impending crisis related to the provision of long term care beds for the elderly. Each inappropriate placement has repercussions on the rest of the system. Problems do not go away but are passed through the system, the end result often being the inappropriate hospitalization of the frail elderly. This action can have major effects on acute hospital services. A basic principle must be to have the right client in the right place at the right time. Alas, this is not happening in many societies, and research is needed to clearly define how these problems have arisen and how best to provide a reasonable solution. Medicine must meet the needs of society. Society's problems cannot be squeezed into what medicine and government have to offer as solutions.

The greatest resource that society has is the talent of its citizens, not the size of its hospitals and the technology of the equipment therein. In North America, there is a great shortage of physicians trained in the care of the elderly. Doctors and other health care workers will have to be recruited into the specialty of clinical gerontology. Granting agencies can have some influence and can encourage people to train in geriatric medicine by redirecting funds toward this underfunded discipline. More research is required to reveal why physicians are not attracted toward the care of the elderly. When the reasons are known they can be redressed.

Many areas of clinical practice of great relevance to the elderly are begging for good quality research. Most doctors know that rehabilitation works but often cannot say why it works. Until recently, there have been no trials about the effectiveness of rehabilitation. There has also been a lack of a firm theoretical foundation for many of the branches of rehabilitation medicine. The essence of research is to provide a rational basis for clinical practice. Because physical therapy has lacked this foundation, it has been unable to counter the criticism of cynics. Good quality research in these fields of practice must be encouraged.

The elderly have the largest numbers of medical problems and are the greatest consumers of medications. By implication, therefore, they are in the greatest need for good prescribing. Ironically, they are often the victims of poor prescribing and are the least studied group in many aspects of therapeutics. Only recently has it become apparent that drug absorption, distribution, and metabolism has to be studied in the elderly before a drug is marketed. It is not sufficient to extrapolate data obtained from young adults and hope that it will hold true for the elderly. The pharmacologist Professor Gaddum stated that "the ill may get better because of or in spite of drugs." In our own Unit in Saskatoon, 19% of all our admissions are due wholly or partially to poor prescribing or adverse drug reactions. Essential data on pharmacokinetics and pharmacodynamics in the elderly are absent for many drugs. Clinical gerontologists with special interest in therapeutics or clinical pharmacologists with a special interest in the elderly are few and far between. Those with their hands on the purse strings could encourage people to move into this important area of research by redirecting resources. The recent court cases in the United Kingdom over the benoxiprofen affair have highlighted the pressing need for premarketing studies involving the elderly. The delicate ethical and practical problems of investigating the older adult have all too often been used as an excuse not to perform essential research.

Pharmacists, too, should be encouraged to improve patient education. The elderly are particularly vulnerable to noncompliance and departments of pharmacy have a potentially vital role in reducing this state of affairs. The majority of disabling diseases such as strokes, osteopenia, and degenerative joint disease are essentially incurable. Vast quantities of drugs are given in the vain and unproven hope of preventing such conditions, with little hard data to support their use. As yet, there is little evidence that treating "hypertension" in people over the age of 80 has any appreciable effect on cardiovascular or cerebrovascular morbidity and mortality. Yet millions of dollars are spent annually on prescribing antihypertensives to this age group. Large multicentered, and possibly international, well-designed, long term trials are required. Such trials must emphasize particularly the relevance of treatment to the elderly, and require immense amounts of organization and funding.

All academic medical departments have three important functions—patient care, education, and research. There is no generally accepted "best" way of teaching health care professionals. Some methods of teaching are more likely to change for the better the attitude of medical students toward the care of the elderly. It is up to medical teachers, who all have their own general impressions of how best to inspire their students, to incorporate research into their educational techniques to give substance to these impressions. Armed with good data, medical teachers can constantly update and improve their educational programs. The future of clinical gerontology in North America is in the hands of those now passing or about to pass through medical schools. Good data on how best to teach these students will be a great investment for the future of clinical gerontology.

The medicine of old age is a subject still in its infancy. There are still great areas of relative ignorance, such as the most efficient ways of providing services to the elderly, all aspects of drug medication, rehabilitation, and education. Granting agencies have a duty to provide funds to research projects that are most likely to benefit society. At present, the elderly are one of the most needy groups in society. They are also a group for whom research into all aspects of their health is most sorely needed.

Index